PRACTICAL MANAGEMENT
OF PERSONALITY DISORDER

Practical Management of Personality Disorder

W. John Livesley

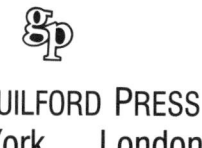

THE GUILFORD PRESS
New York   London

© 2003 The Guilford Press
A Division of Guilford Publications, Inc.
72 Spring Street, New York, NY 10012

Printed in the United States of America

This book is printed on acid-free paper.

Last digit is print number: 9 8 7 6 5 4 3 2 1

Library of Congress Cataloging-in-Publication Data

Livesley, W. John.
   Practical management of personality disorder / by W. John Livesley.
      p. cm.
Includes bibliographical references and index.
  ISBN 1-57230-889-3 (hardcover)
  1. Personality disorders. I. Title.
  RC554 .L585 2003
  616.85′8—dc21
                             2002155225

To my family—
Ann, my wife,
and my children, Adrian, Nigel, and Dawn—
while not forgetting Flint and Cole

About the Author

W. John Livesley, MD, PhD, is Professor and former Head of the Department of Psychiatry at the University of British Columbia, Vancouver, British Columbia, Canada. He is also Editor of the *Journal of Personality Disorders* and has contributed extensively to the literature on personality disorder. Dr. Livesley's research focuses on the classification, assessment, and origins of personality disorder, and his clinical interests center on an integrated approach to treatment based on current empirical knowledge about personality disorder and its treatment.

Preface

This volume deals with the treatment of severe personality disorder. The intent is to describe a practical approach based on what we know about personality disorder and interventions that work. A general framework is presented that will be useful to practitioners and trainees from all mental health disciplines working in such diverse settings as general hospital inpatient units, outpatient departments, community mental health services, managed care programs, and private offices. The approach provides guidelines for treating patients in therapies ranging from crisis intervention to long-term treatment.

In organizing my ideas about personality disorder and its treatment, I have attempted to address the questions posed by clinicians from all disciplines attending lectures and workshops that I have presented for more than two decades. Typically, two kinds of questions are raised: general and situation-specific. Questions of a general nature are usually variations on such themes as: "What is personality disorder?", "How do you treat personality disorder?", and "Can personality disorder really be treated?" More specific questions take the broad form of "What should I do when . . . ?" followed by a variety of problems including suicide threats, crises developing during long-term treatment, attempts to change the treatment plan, missing therapy sessions, attending sessions under the influence of alcohol, refusing to leave at the end of a session, demanding more time, and so on.

Both types of questions suggest that (1) the questioners would have benefited from a systematic account of personality disorder and a framework for organizing treatment, and (2) many clinicians rely on tactical interventions to deal with problems as they surface during treatment, rather than use an overall treatment strategy based on an understanding of the pathology involved. Although the clinicians were not inexperienced, uninterested, or uninformed, they probably acted in this way because personality disorder is inordinately complex, and this complexity creates a gamut of management problems. Patients typically present with multiple problems and complicated clinical pictures. Diagnosis is complicated by difficulty untangling personality pathology from the symptoms of mental state disorders. Even when the proper diagnosis is reached, it does not really help: DSM-IV and ICD-10 personality diagnoses have limited value in treatment planning. The multiple problems of a given patient are also challenging because a combination of interventions is usually needed. Furthermore, there is the challenge of managing the therapeutic relationship when patients find it difficult to trust and collaborate with the clinician.

Personality disorder has a complex etiology; multiple biological, psychological, and cultural factors contribute to its development, and the implications of these multiple causes for treatment are rarely considered. This complexity accounts for both interest in the disorder and frustration with attempts to treat it. Few clinicians are not intrigued by personality disorder, the subtle ways it presents, the involved histories of many patients, and the complex interaction between clinical course and outcome. Yet there are few clinicians who have not also been frustrated in their attempts to understand it and to treat it. For most clinicians, treatment presents a series of dilemmas, beginning with the problem of how to organize information about the multiple problems and extensive psychopathology into a coherent case formulation that facilitates treatment planning, and continuing throughout the therapy in relation to which issues to address and in what order, how to manage the inevitable relationship problems, and how to select the appropriate intervention when faced with a variety of alternatives.

Unfortunately, complexity is not only an inherent attribute of the condition; professional reactions to personality disorder are also complex. Like the old adage that psychotherapy supervision often mirrors the therapist's relationship with the patient, professional reactions to personality disorder frequently seem to reflect the complexity of the disorder and the confusion that often surrounds those who attract the diagnosis. Many clinicians have difficulty approaching patients with personality disorder in the same organized and consistent way that they approach patients with other disorders. The problem is exacerbated by the complexity of some treatments and theoretical models, which are described in language that often obscures rather than clarifies. Many clinicians do not find current theories to be of practical help in daily clinical practice. Most of these theories have minimal empirical support, and there is no evidence that one approach is better than another. There is, however, evidence showing that some interventions are effective for some problems. This finding suggests the need for an eclectic and pragmatic approach that applies interventions on the basis of what works and a rational analysis of what is needed.

This volume attempts to provide a framework that clinicians can adapt to their own style and the setting in which they work, and which can also be modified as our understanding grows. The goal is not to develop yet another treatment for the disorder but rather to define what we need to achieve in treatment and then identify the best way to accomplish these goals, based on the evidence. The approach presented here is eclectic *not* in the sense that it provides a compendium of current ideas on treatment—such is not my aim. Rather, *Practical Management of Personality Disorder* presents "reasoned eclecticism," to borrow a phrase from Gordon Allport. I have borrowed extensively from the concepts and intervention strategies of perspectives as diverse as self psychology, interpersonal therapy, psychodynamic and psychoanalytic therapies, cognitive therapy, behavior therapy, and constructivism, as well as combinations such as cognitive analytic therapy and dialectical behavior therapy. These are combined with medication, as necessary.

I had thought of giving the approach a name that could form a suitable acronym. It seems that an approach is nothing without an apt title that can be referred to as a set of letters. However, to do so seems to violate the spirit and intent of the exercise. If the study of personality disorder is to progress and treatment to become more effective, we need to break away from one-dimensional approaches and adherence to theoretical models that, despite their claims and even their elegance, are based on little more than speculation. The framework offered is clearly not the last word on the treatment of personality disorder; rather, it is a work in progress that will evolve as our knowledge about these conditions progresses from our current somewhat scanty understanding to something more systematic and profound.

As I look over the final proofs, I feel tremendous gratitude toward the patients with whom I have worked over the years. Their struggles with personality disorder were a source of stimulation. At the same time, their insightful descriptions of their problems and struggles, and the metaphors they used to communicate their distress, transformed my understanding and guided the development of an approach that could be tailored to their needs.

I am grateful to Seymour Weingarten, Editor-in-Chief of The Guilford Press, for patiently encouraging my efforts with this volume and for his support over the years, and to Rochelle Serwator, who rather amazingly managed to transform the original manuscript into something that might be understood. My assistant, Roseann Larstone, provided much valued assistance throughout.

Finally, I owe much to my family. I am deeply grateful to my wife, Ann, who has not only patiently tolerated my absorption in the task of writing in her uniquely loving and supportive way but also actively encouraged my efforts; and to my children, Adrian, Nigel, and Dawn, for their support and benign tolerance and encouragement.

Contents

CHAPTER 1

Introduction

Some years ago a patient told me that therapy was boring. Her comment was surprising, since she seemed to be making good progress. She went on to declare that before treatment, life was exciting—painful and difficult, but nonetheless exciting. Now she was not sure that she could tolerate the boredom. These comments were troubling. Not only did they indicate a problem in treatment, they also raised fundamental questions about the nature and treatment of personality disorder—questions that are not easy to answer.

The patient, an intelligent, articulate woman in her late 20s, had a long and complex psychiatric history of the kind that invariably attracts the diagnosis of borderline personality disorder. She engaged in self-harming behaviors, including frequent overdoses, and she was often rushed to the emergency room with serious self-inflicted injuries. Her mood was labile. She was impulsive. Her social life was chaotic. She sought the company of others who shared and encouraged drug and alcohol abuse. She frequently found herself in fights and arguments, and she was often the center of incidents in restaurants and bars that would culminate in arrest. The behavioral turmoil was associated with considerable affective lability and a profound disturbance in her sense of self. She was unsure of who she was; her self-image changed from one occasion to the next; and she had little sense of what she wanted out of life. Relationships with others were superficial and unrewarding. Lasting intimate relationships eluded her. Instead, she lurched from one temporary but intense relationship to another. Nevertheless, her lifestyle generated an excitement that was satisfying as well as painful. These problems had begun more than 10 years previously, and she had seen many therapists over the years. Therapy tended to mirror her life—therapeutic relationships were established only to be abandoned. At the time in question, she had been in treatment for nearly 1 year. The parasuicidal, self-harming, and impulsive acts had ceased some months previously. Her life was more stable, but she missed the excitement and activity of her previous lifestyle.

If we consider this case in a commonsense way, free from the constraints imposed by speculative theories, we see that although it has idiosyncratic features, it illustrates many key issues and dilemmas in understanding and treating personality disorder. First, the vignette reveals the diverse problems that characterize typical cases. The multiple symptoms include anxiety, cognitive disorganization, and generalized distress. Situational problems and interpersonal crises are common. There are problems with affect and impulse regulation. Traits are expressed in rigid and maladaptive ways. Interpersonal relationships involve repetitive and dysfunctional patterns of relating. Self and identity are impaired. Thus the problems of personality disorder are not circumscribed; rather, they affect all aspects of the person. Indeed, *disorder* seems to be woven into the very fabric of personality. To manage such diverse problems and pathology, we need to organize complex, multifaceted information in a systematic way that can be used to develop a treatment plan that helps clinicians to tackle problems in an effective sequence.

Second, the case provokes typically puzzling questions: Why does this patient need so much excitement and stimulation, and why is this need so strong that it threatens treatment by leading her to prefer a chaotic and painful lifestyle over a more normal existence? What is the origin of traits such as sensation seeking? What accounts for their persistence? Can they be changed?

Third, the vignette raises questions about the changes that can reasonably be expected from treatment. As the case illustrates, impulsive and self-harming behaviors can be treated effectively (Linehan, Armstrong, Suarez, Allman, & Heard, 1991). Once these problems have resolved, however, fundamental interpersonal difficulties and self and identity problems remain. The result is often what Linehan has termed "a life of quiet desperation." Follow-up studies show that even after long-term psychoanalytic therapy, core self and interpersonal problems are relatively unchanged in this population (McGlashan, 1986; Stone, 1990, 1993, 2001). The various components of personality disorder do not seem to respond similarly to treatment or to the same approach, which suggests that an array of interventions is required to treat most cases. This conclusion raises additional questions about the best way to organize treatment, manage multiple interventions, and effectively treat the self and interpersonal problems that are central to personality disorder—and so intractable. Finally, evidence of limited change prompts the question of whether there are aspects of personality that cannot be changed using currently available techniques. If so, what can be done about these untreatable aspects?

These challenging questions require answers if we are to develop a rational and comprehensive treatment that achieves something more than mitigation of impulsive and parasuicidal behavior. The answers, based on empirical findings as far as possible, will form a framework for understanding personality disorder that, in turn, will shape an approach to treatment. We begin our search by examining briefly how various common theories and treatments would view this patient's problems, and the limitations and disparities of these ideas.

CONTEMPORARY THEORIES

When we consider this case from a *psychoanalytic perspective*, we encounter the immediate problem that contemporary psychoanalysis incorporates several competing models (Wallerstein, 1988; Westen, 1990). Many therapists with an eclectic psychodynamic viewpoint would consider the need for excitement to be a defense against a profound sense of inner emptiness and a chaotic sense of self and identity: Excitement fills an otherwise painful void. This formulation is a simplified expression of the *conflict model* of classical psychoanalytic theory, which considers all personality processes to be the product of conflicts and compromises involving basic drives, especially sexual and aggressive impulses. Thus personality constellations are assumed to originate in developmental conflicts and defenses against conflicts that become translated into the trait structure of personality.

This idea was first proposed in Freud's (1908) classic paper on anal eroticism that linked a triad of traits—orderliness, miserliness, and obstinacy—to the anal stage of psychosexual development. Later, Abraham (1921, 1925) expanded the idea into a typology that related personality structure to problems encountered at specific psychosexual stages. For example, dependent traits are said to originate in oral conflicts. Reich (1949) extended this approach by suggesting that psychoanalysis should address traits that form what he referred to as "character armor." These traits were assumed to be ego-syntonic, unlike the symptoms of neuroses that were usually assumed to be ego-dystonic. Consistent with the classical model, character armor was assumed to arise from successful defenses against developmental conflicts. Contemporary extensions of the model see longstanding patterns of personality traits as "a series of compromise formations between wishes and defenses that oppose these wishes, on the one hand, and constellations of internal representations of self and others, on the other" (Gabbard, 2001, p. 360; see also Gabbard, 2000).

Treatment based on the conflict model focuses on resolving significant conflicts and developing a more coherent sense of self. The implication for the above case is that this treatment outcome should reduce the need for excitement and hence interest in an exciting but dysfunctional lifestyle. But is sensation seeking simply a defensive reaction to conflict? Is this idea consistent with knowledge about the origin of personality traits generally, and the etiology of stimulus seeking in particular? Are the self and interpersonal problems that are so central to this patient's difficulties simply the product of conflicts centered on basic drives and instincts?

Other psychoanalytic models offer alternative views on these issues. The *object relations approach* rejects the psychosexual model and conflict–compromise framework as explanations of the development of personality, in favor of the idea that personality structures, including self and identity, are shaped by interactions with significant others (Fairbairn, 1952). Problems arise from the failure to integrate different representations of the self or others, leading to fragmented images of self and others. In Kernberg's (1975, 1984) concept of borderline personality organization, which attempts to combine the classical model with object relations theory (although the formulation emphasizes the primacy of conflict), biologically determined aggressive feelings are assumed to impede integration of positive and negative object representations, resulting in splitting and other primitive defenses that lead to ego weakness. Clearly the patient in our vignette has considerable hostility and seems to hold conflicting views of the self and others. But is Kernberg's formulation a sufficient explanation of what is happening?

Self psychology (Kohut, 1971, 1977) maintains that the self is not the product of conflict and compromise but of empathic parenting. This is a *deficit model*, in which personality pathology is assumed to involve structural problems involving the failure to establish a cohesive self due to the empathic failure of caregivers (Blanck & Blanck, 1974). Following Kohut, Buie and Adler (1982) advanced a deficit model of borderline pathology that posits unsatisfactory mothering during the separation–individuation phase, leading to failed internalization of holding–soothing representations. This failing creates difficulty in self-soothing, leaving the person vulnerable to painful and panicky feelings of aloneness and abandonment. This model is radically different from that of Kernberg and leads to very different intervention strategies.

Kernberg's approach (see Clarkin, Yeomans, & Kernberg, 1999; Kernberg, 1984, 2001) with this patient would involve the clarification, confrontation, and interpretation of the primitive defenses and affective shifts associated with fragmented and split-off aspects of identity as they are manifested within the transference relationship. The expectation is that this approach would lead to a strengthening of personality and hence to a stronger sense of self or identity. The theoretical assumption of underlying problems with aggression leads to a more confrontational approach. In contrast, the Kohutian model advocates an empathic approach, with the expectation that experiencing empathic responses would facilitate the development of a more cohesive self. Two issues are important here. First, the two approaches make very different assumptions about the nature and origin of core aspects of personality disorder: *conflict* versus *deficit* models. To develop a coherent treatment, we need to consider the evidence available to resolve this apparent inconsistency. Second, the two approaches offer different explanations of change. According to the classical model and Kernberg, personality is transformed through insight achieved via the confrontation and interpretation of defenses, especially in transference. According to Kohut, in contrast, change results from an empathic therapeutic relationship. To make an informed choice about the models, we need to know how they relate to empirical knowledge about the causes of personality disorder and the factors influencing therapeutic change.

Cognitive and *cognitive-behavioral therapies* offer a different theoretical framework. Cognitive therapy would consider the patient's need for excitement to be the product of maladaptive beliefs and expectations that lead the patient to construe normality as boring. Similarly, self pathology would be understood in terms of maladaptive self schemata. The task would be to change these schemata by using the techniques of cognitive therapy—a very different method from those that characterize the different versions of the psychoanalytic model. Cognitive therapy assumes that dysfunctional cognitions are the central problem of personality disorder. But can cognitive dysfunctions account for all features of personality disorder? How does the model fit with ideas that traits such as sensation seeking have a genetic basis? With more behaviorally oriented models, social skills deficits and limited problem-solving abilities also may be invoked to explain the patient's behavioral problems. Under these circumstances, treatment might include skill training—again, a very different approach from that espoused by more psychodynamic orientations. Despite the potential utility of these techniques, it is not clear how they would change core self and interpersonal pathology.

Interpersonal theory (Benjamin, 1996; Benjamin & Pugh, 2001) postulates that the destructive, maladaptive patterns characteristic of personality disorder are directly related to behaviors learned in relationships with loved ones or attachment figures. These patterns are said to involve what Benjamin refers to as "copying processes": the person strives to be like the attachment figure (identification), acts as if the attachment figure were still present and in charge (recapitulation), or treats the self as the attachment figure did in the past (introjection). Benjamin suggests that these copying patterns repeat earlier behaviors because of a wish for reconciliation with, or validation by, the attachment figure. Treatment involves identifying these patterns and consistently addressing the underlying attachment, until the wish for reconciliation or validation is abandoned and new patterns are learned. This goal may involve interventions derived from any theoretical framework. Interpersonal theory shares, with object relations theory and self psychology, the assumption that the maladaptive patterns of personality disorder originate in early relationships with important others; it differs in that a structural model of interpersonal behavior is used to account for these patterns. The model has many attractive features, including a systematic way to describe the maladaptive interpersonal patterns that characterize personality disorder. But, like the cognitive approach, it does not seem to account for all features of personality disorder. Interpersonal difficulties are not the only problems observed in personality disorder (Widiger & Kelso, 1983). Furthermore, the model does not provide an adequate explanation of traits such as the sensation seeking observed in this patient.

Turning to *normal personality theory*, this patient's need for stimulation and excitement is characteristic of someone with a high level of sensation seeking—a trait that includes thrill and adventure seeking, experience seeking, disinhibition, and boredom susceptibility (Zuckerman, 1971, 1991). Empirical evidence suggests that sensation seeking has a genetic basis (Livesley, Jang, Jackson, & Vernon, 1993; Zuckerman, 1994a, 1994b). From this perspective, sensation seeking does not develop out of a defense against a sense of emptiness and other aspects of self pathology, or even developmental conflicts, although it may be used for defensive purposes. Rather, it is an enduring characteristic that emerges from the combined effects of genetic predisposition and experience. This perspective introduces a third model, the *vulnerability model*, that assumes that underlying dispositions, which may have a biological basis, predispose an individual to the development of personality problems. This model raises additional issues for treatment. If traits are stable entities that are partly inherited, can we expect to change maladaptive traits such as sensation seeking? What implications does the evidence of a heritable component to traits have for treatments and theories that emphasize a psychosocial etiology to personality disorder and the theoretical models underlying psychoanalytic and cognitive therapies? How do we reconcile conflict, deficit, and vulnerability models?

Finally, *biological psychiatry* would probably view the affective lability and impulsivity of this patient in terms of problems in specific neurotransmitter systems (Coccaro, 2001; Coccaro et al., 1989; Coccaro, Kavoussi, & Hauger, 1995; Siever & Davies, 1991), for which specific pharmacological interventions may be warranted (Markovitz, 2001; Soloff, 1998, 2000). This perspective raises further questions about the role of biological factors in the etiology of personality disorder and how pharmacological interventions can be integrated effectively with interventions based on other theoretical models.

This overview of common theories and therapies illustrates the many varied and often confusing ideas held about the nature and treatment of personality disorder: personality disorder as the result of conflict and compromise versus a deficit resulting from empathic failure; personality disorder as the result of psychosocial adversity versus genetic predisposition; and personality as stable versus changeable. Views on intervention also differ: confrontation and interpretation versus empathy, validation, and mirroring; and structured, skill-building approaches versus unstructured exploration. Given this range of perspectives, concepts, and strategies, it is not surprising that many clinicians are confused about how to treat personality disorder or pessimistic about the outcome. Nor is it surprising, as some authorities have commented, that many patients seem to deteriorate rather than improve through contact with the health-care system (Frances, 1992; Rockland, 1992).

As noted, personality disorder and its treatment are inherently complex. However, the plethora of theories and treatment strategies, many based on minimal evidence, makes treatment more complicated than necessary. Many therapies are presented as comprehensive or even definitive, forcing clinicians to choose among them without the evidence required to make an informed choice. With each model, an intervention strategy is offered based on an underlying theory. As a result, each approach offers a limited array of interventions, and interventions derived from other theories are ignored, even if they are known to be effective. Theory, rather than an empirical understanding of personality disorder or evidence of treatment efficacy, guides treatment decisions. The result is that personality disorder is treated as a cognitive problem, a behavioral problem, an interpersonal problem, or a motivational problem. Personality disorder, however, is all these. Few approaches, if any, offer a comprehensive set of interventions to cover the range of problems seen in most cases. Moreover, the assumptions of some approaches seem inconsistent with our contemporary knowledge about the nature and origins of normal and disordered personality.

BASIC ASSUMPTIONS OF THEORETICAL MODELS

Although the different theoretical models and associated therapies are in some ways incompatible, they share two assumptions:

1. Personality disorder is primarily a psychosocial disorder caused mainly by adverse developmental experiences.
2. Personality is malleable and can be changed with therapy.

To develop a science-based approach to treatment, we need to examine the validity of these assumptions. The advent of the *Diagnostic and Statistical Manual of Mental Disorders–III* (DSM-III) in 1980 changed the study of personality disorder from a field dominated by theories based on clinical observations of a few patients in rarefied settings to an active area of empirical research. At the same time, work in the related fields of personality psychology, cognitive science, behavior genetics, and evolutionary psychology contributed new ideas and perspectives. These developments are changing our understanding of the structure, causes, and treatment of personality disorder. Although this understanding is far from complete, a new picture of personality disorder is emerging that challenges these assumptions.

Most treatments emphasize the psychosocial origins of personality disorder, although most also acknowledge the importance of biological factors. It is as if theorists need to acknowledge constitutional factors before getting on with what is considered to be the real business of therapy— addressing the consequences of psychosocial adversity. Constitutional factors are rarely systematically incorporated into explanations of therapeutic change or taken into account when conceptualizing treatment. Thus therapy tends to focus on memories, conflicts, affects, and cognitions associated with adversity, and the cognitive structures and processes influenced by these experiences. This focus is appropriate given the well-established etiological importance of adversity.

Adversity, however, is not the only factor that influences the development of personality pathology; biological factors are also important. The evidence indicates a substantial heritable component to personality (Goldsmith, 1983; Loehlin & Nichols, 1976). Infants differ from birth in such features as emotionality, activity, and sociability (Buss & Plomin, 1975). Few approaches to treatment consider the therapeutic implications of this fact. It is not that psychosocial explanations of etiology are wrong or that the assumptions of traditional treatment models are invalid. Rather, they are inadequate as total explanations. In the case of the patient described earlier, sensation seeking may indeed be used to defend against inner emptiness, and it may be influenced by developmental conflicts—but this is not a total explanation. Sensation seeking, like other traits, is acquired and consolidated through a lengthy interaction between genetic predisposition and experience. For this reason, it seems unrealistic to assume that a resolution of self problems or developmental conflicts will inevitably lead to changes in maladaptive traits. To develop evidenced-based treatment, we need to consider how the biology of personality influences treatment, not just in the simple sense of whether biological treatments should be part of a comprehensive treatment, but in the more fundamental sense of how the biological and adaptive aspects of personality shape an overall treatment approach (Livesley, 2001c). Failure to incorporate an understanding of genetic and other biological factors into treatment models may lead to less than optimal interventions.

Most therapies implicitly assume that personality is relatively plastic and open to radical change. This idea is an obvious, although perhaps simplistic, conclusion to draw from the assumption that personality is largely environmentally determined. If psychosocial environment causes personality disorder, it is not unreasonable to assume that personality can be modified by psychosocial interventions. This is, however, a somewhat paradoxical idea, since personality disorder is defined in terms of its *stability*: According to the DSM-IV, personality disorder is "an enduring pattern of inner experience and behavior" (American Psychiatric Association, 1994, p. 630). Yet we seek to *treat* personality disorder, and treatment implies *change*.

In the early days of psychoanalysis, there was considerable optimism about the extent to which personality could be changed. Although this optimism was subsequently tempered by the recognition that personality is highly stable, the idea persists that personality—and hence personality disorder—are malleable and that they can be changed with appropriate psychological interventions. But do we really think that it is possible to help someone who has a high need for excitement and stimulation to tolerate a rather humdrum lifestyle? Or that the shy, schizoid individual can become outgoing and sociable? The idea conflicts with substantial evidence that important parts of personality, especially traits, are extremely stable and change little during the adult life span (Caspi & Bem, 1990; Heatherton & Weinberger, 1994). Although the goal of treatment is to change personality, we need to consider what this goal really means and whether it is even possible to change all components of personality disorder.

A FRAMEWORK FOR TREATING PERSONALITY DISORDER

It is argued that treatment should be based on empirical findings about the nature of personality disorder. Most treatments proposed for personality disorder, however, do not approach the problem in this way. Most are based on more speculative accounts of personality pathology that are often extensions of more general theories of psychopathology.

Conceptual Foundations

Two bodies of knowledge form the foundation for an approach to treatment: empirical knowledge about the structure and origins of personality disorder, and information on which interventions work and which do not (see Table 1.1). Ideally, treatment should be based on a comprehensive theory of personality disorder supported by appropriate evidence. Unfortunately, such a theory is not available or likely to emerge for some time. Meanwhile, a feasible alternative is to construct a framework in which to organize knowledge about personality disorder in a manner that describes *problems and pathology* using simple descriptive statements and low-level inferences, closely related to observable behavior, that avoids complex speculative formulations. The framework also should incorporate empirical

TABLE 1.1. Framework for a Treatment of Personality Disorder

Conceptual foundations

Basic features of personality disorder: Description of current knowledge about personality disorder that is relevant to the design and organization of treatment. Three kinds of information help to define the basic principles of treatment and intervention strategies:

1. Problems and psychopathology
2. Etiology and development
3. Stability and change

Evidence of treatment efficacy: Empirical evidence on treatment outcome:

1. General outcome studies that provide information on the efficacy of treatment
2. Specific outcome studies of treatments for personality disorder

Conceptual structure

Basic principles: General rules and postulates about the most effective ways to facilitate change derived from an understanding of the basic features of personality disorder and the principles of personality and behavioral change

Strategies: Clusters of interventions sharing a common objective that translate principles into therapeutic actions. Two broad sets of strategies are used to implement basic principles:

1. *General therapeutic strategies:* Strategies used with all patients at all stages of treatment to manage and treat the core or universal features of personality disorder
2. *Specific therapeutic strategies:* Strategies used to treat specific problems in individual patients. Specific strategies vary across patients, stage of therapy, and the problems that are the focus of change

Interventions: Specific therapeutic actions designed to effect change

Operational structure

Phases of treatment: The overall sequence of themes and interventions:

- *Safety:* Interventions to ensure safety of patient and others
- *Containment:* Interventions to contain affective and behavioral instability
- *Control and regulation:* Interventions to reduce symptoms, control affects and impulses, and improve self-management of affects and impulses
- *Exploration and change:* Interventions to change the cognitive, affective, and situational factors contributing to problem behavior
- *Integration and synthesis:* Interventions designed to address core pathology and forge a new sense of self and more integrated and adaptive self and interpersonal systems

(*continued*)

Stages of change: The sequence through which individual symptoms and features of personality disorder change:

- *Problem recognition:* Problem behavior or characteristics are recognized and accorded a preliminary commitment to change
- *Exploration:* Examination of the nature, causes, and consequences of the targeted behavior and the cognitive and affective mechanisms involved
- *Acquisition of alternatives:* Exploration and implementation of alternative behaviors
- *Consolidation and generalization:* Consolidation of new learning and generalization to everyday situations

---

findings about *etiology*, because in the long run, treatments that address causes are likely to be more effective than those that only address symptoms (Benjamin & Pugh, 2001). Moreover, an understanding of etiology should help to identify intervention strategies. Finally, this framework should incorporate the results of research on personality *development* and the factors that contribute to *stability and change* in personality.

The second component of a conceptual foundation for treatment is provided by evidence of treatment efficacy. Studies of therapeutic outcome provide the basis for identifying generic principles of change. These principles are used to define *general treatment strategies* that apply to most forms of disorder and therapeutic settings. Evaluations of treatment should also help to identify *specific interventions* that are likely to be effective. Unfortunately, comparatively few evaluations have been conducted on treatments for personality disorder. Although reviews of these studies indicate that substantial change can be achieved, leading to improved adjustment and enhanced quality of life (Piper & Joyce, 2001), they do not provide a systematic body of knowledge that can be used to organize a comprehensive approach. They do, however, provide valuable suggestions about the best ways to approach certain problems. For example, the evidence points to the value of cognitive-behavioral strategies in managing impulsive and self-harming behaviors.

Conceptual Structure: Basic Principles, Strategies, and Interventions

The next step in constructing an approach to treatment is to describe the overall structure of therapy and how this is related to the conceptual foundations. The system that Beutler and Harwood (2000) used to describe a systematic approach to treatment selection is adopted for this purpose. They describe treatment in terms of *basic principles, strategies,* and *techniques* or *interventions* (Table 1.1). The selection of strategies and interventions is guided by an understanding of the *basic principles* of therapeutic change. These principles specify how treatment is organized and the most appropriate therapeutic approach or stance; they also guide the selection of treatment strategies, which are based, as far as possible, on empirical knowledge of personality disorder and treatment outcome. Principles differ in range. Some are broad postulates that determine the overall therapeutic approach and help therapists to select interventions and plan the sequence with which problems will be addressed. For example, the simple idea that personality disorder involves multiple problems involving all aspects of personality suggests that treatment should incorporate a combination of interventions drawn from different schools of therapy. Similarly, the idea that pathology consists of (1) some common features that characterize all forms of personality disorder, and (2) more specific problems and features that differ across different forms of disorder and individuals suggests the basic principle that treatment should incorporate (1) general strategies used throughout treatment to treat all individuals in all settings, and (2) specific interventions that vary across individuals, treatment setting, and stage of treatment. Another broad principle derived from outcome studies is that treatment should maximize the nonspecific component of therapy. Other principles are more specific: they determine intervention strategies rather than the overall structure of therapy.

Strategies specify the ways that the basic principles are translated into therapeutic actions. Each strategy is implemented through a cluster of interventions that shares a common objective (Beutler & Harwood, 2000). For example, the basic principle of optimizing the nonspecific component of therapy is implemented through such strategies as building a collaborative relationship and maintaining a consistent and validating treatment process. *Interventions* are the specific techniques used to effect change. Interventions designed to build a collaborative relationship, for example, include providing support, recognizing progress, and reinforcing treatment goals. Other interventions include medications and specific cognitive, behavioral, or psychodynamic techniques to bring about targeted changes.

The basic principles are the most prescribed and fixed component of the framework because most are grounded in an empirically based understanding of personality disorder. For this reason, they are only likely to change with major advances in knowledge. Strategies are also relatively fixed because they represent ways in which principles are translated into therapeutic action. Interventions are the least prescribed and the most specific component. Within the limits imposed by principles and strategies, clinicians are free to select the interventions they consider appropriate.

This structure seems to fit the way most clinicians prefer to work. Most do not appear to want a prescribed set of interventions to follow slavishly. A flexible framework that clinicians can adapt to their style and that of their patients, according to the setting and duration of treatment, is far preferable. Such an approach also fits the nature of personality disorder. The problems of individual patients vary widely, so that treatment needs to be tailored to the individual. There are also extensive differences among patients in what they can tolerate and use. Hence it is not possible to define a protocol to follow with all cases. Although flexibility is dictated by the very nature of personality disorder, it is important to have a foundational conceptual framework (as opposed to merely a set of interventions), because it reduces the danger of therapists becoming too focused on the immediate problem at the expense of a wider context (i.e., not seeing the forest for the trees). A conceptual framework also provides a consistent therapeutic process that minimizes the possibility of treatment being driven by psychopathology.

Operational Structure

The implementation of treatment is guided by three ideas. First, treatment consists of general strategies to manage all forms of personality disorder, and specific interventions to treat individual differences in problems and pathology.

Second, the treatment process progresses through a series of phases, each addressing different problems through different combinations of interventions. Five phases are proposed: safety, containment, regulation and control, exploration and change, and integration and synthesis. The first phase is to *ensure safety* of patients and others. Once safety issues have been addressed, attention turns to *containment*; the goals of this phase are to contain impulses and affects. The third phase focuses on the *control and regulation* of affects and impulses. Subsequently, attention focuses increasingly on *exploration and change* of the many personality processes, maladaptive interpersonal relationships, and consequences of psychosocial adversity that influence maladaptive behavior. The final phase is one of *integration and synthesis*; at this point, therapeutic effort focuses on the formation of a more integrated and adaptive self and sense of identity and the development of more integrated representations of others.

Third, the specific thoughts, feelings, and behaviors that are the targets for change during the different phases of treatment may be managed using the stages of change model (DiClemente, 1994; Prochaska, DiClemente, & Norcross, 1992; Prochaska, Norcross, & DiClemente, 1994). A four-stage process is proposed: problem recognition, exploration, acquisition of alternative ways of behaving, and consolidation and generalization. Change begins with *problem recognition* and the development of a commitment to change. Next comes *exploration* of the problem and the events leading to it, as well as the consequences of this way of acting. Exploration eventually leads to a consideration of *alternative ways of behaving* and the development of new behaviors. Subsequently, these behaviors are *consoli-*

dated and generalized to everyday situations and until they become part of the individual's normal behavioral repertoire.

Because personality disorder involves so many complex problems, it is often difficult for therapists to decide which of the many problems and issues should be addressed at a given time. The *phases of change framework* provides guidelines about the sequence for tackling problems. The *stages of change model* is used to manage specific problems and guide the selection of interventions. The purpose of these guidelines is not to establish a prescribed sequence but rather to impose order and structure on the complexity of the change process.

OVERVIEW OF THE BOOK

We begin developing an approach to treatment by first exploring the nature of personality and personality disorder. Chapters 2 and 3 establish the conceptual foundations for an evidence-based approach to treatment, as far as this is possible within the constraints of current knowledge. Chapter 2 provides a framework for describing and understanding personality disorder. It begins by discussing what is meant by *personality* and *personality disorder*. This leads to the proposal that the overall goal of treatment is to enhance adaptation. The idea of personality as a system is introduced as a way to organize the multiple problems of personality disorder. Given this range of problems, it is unlikely that any one approach or theoretical model could serve as the foundation for a comprehensive treatment framework. It is argued that each of the different perspectives discussed earlier—psychoanalysis, cognitive-behavior therapy, interpersonal theory, normative personality theory, and biological therapy—has something to contribute. The chapter also examines the idea that personality disorder has both core components that are common to all forms of the disorder and specific/individual features. This idea leads to another fundamental element of the proposed model: namely, that a comprehensive approach must address both core and specific features, and that treatment should be organized around interventions to manage and treat core self and interpersonal pathology.

Chapter 3 examines three key areas: (1) empirical evidence on the etiology of personality disorder to determine the impact of both environmental and biological constraints on personality; (2) how these constraints influence a comprehensive treatment model; and (3) the extent to which personality can be changed and the implications of the stability of some core components of personality for the sequence with which problems are addressed within the phases of change framework.

The rest of the book examines, in detail, the different aspects of an integrated and tailored approach to treatment. Chapter 4 offers an overview of the process of change from the perspective of a generic model of treatment and discusses the stages of change model as applied to personality pathology. Chapter 5 deals with assessment, and Chapter 6, with treatment planning. Chapter 7 covers general treatment strategies, the core component of treatment. This chapter discusses ways to operationalize the nonspecific component of therapy as it pertains to the treatment of personality disorder. Four strategies are described: (1) building and maintaining a collaborative relationship, (2) maintaining a consistent treatment process, (3) validation, and (4) building and maintaining motivation for change. It is argued that interventions based on general strategies should take priority over all other interventions except those needed to ensure safety.

More individualized treatment strategies for managing specific components of personality pathology are covered in Chapters 8–13. Chapter 8 considers ways to manage crises and symptoms, thereby covering the safety and containment phases of treatment. Chapters 9 and 10 examine the control and regulation phase as applied to symptoms and impulses, including deliberate self-harm (Chapter 9), and treating the consequences of trauma and dissociative behavior (Chapter 10). Chapter 11 introduces the exploration and change phase of treatment by examining strategies and interventions for treating self and interpersonal problems. This phase continues into Chapter 12 with a discussion of the treatment of maladaptive traits. Chapter 13 introduces the final phase of treatment—integration and synthesis—wherein the goal is to promote a more adaptive understanding of the self and more integrated representations of others. Finally, Chapter 14 discusses practical ways to implement the treatment model.

COMMENT

In considering an overall approach to the treatment of personality disorder, it is useful to bear in mind what we hope to achieve. The goal is not to develop a "new treatment"—there are more than sufficient therapies described in the literature. Rather, the two-pronged goal is to (1) develop an understanding of personality disorder that allows us to select interventions that are likely to be effective, based on current knowledge of the disorder and treatment efficacy, and (2) identify an approach that is practical, credible, and capable of being modified in the light of new findings. To be *practical*, it should be relevant to treating patients with personality disorder in general clinical settings such as inpatient units, outpatient departments of general hospitals, community mental health clinics, and the offices of private-practice clinicians. Many treatments fail this requirement for practicality. Some are too labor-intensive for modern health care systems concerned with accessibility, accountability, and cost.

A treatment also should be *credible* to patients, therapists, and the profession, including the health care system. The credibility and validity of any treatment are not based upon a single line of evidence or source of support. To be accepted, any treatment should, however, possess face validity—it should appear to therapists and patients to be an appropriate way to deal with problems (Beutler & Davison, 1995). Lastly, the approach to therapy being proposed is not based upon an underlying theory of personality disorder but on a descriptive framework for organizing current knowledge that is easily modified to accommodate new findings.

CHAPTER 2

A Framework for Understanding Normal and Disordered Personality

This chapter begins to lay the conceptual foundations for treatment by developing a framework for understanding personality and personality disorder. The intent is to describe the functions of normal personality and the way these functions are disturbed in personality disorder. Ideally, a concept of personality disorder should grow out an understanding of normal personality. However, definitions of personality disorder are rarely approached in this way. The DSM-IV, for example, simply lists features thought to characterize personality disorder without a rationale for their selection. This method is not adequate for treatment purposes. If we want to put something right, we need a better understanding of what is wrong. But there is another reason for beginning with normal personality: a description of the functions and structure of personality provides a framework for (1) organizing the often overwhelming array of information that typifies most cases, and (2) understanding how personality may change. This overview of normal and disordered personality uses an array of ideas and concepts drawn from personality theory, personality assessment, cognitive theory, evolutionary psychology, clinical accounts of personality, and psychoanalytic theory.

WHAT IS PERSONALITY?

Students of personality agree that the term *personality* refers to regularities and consistencies in behavior and forms of experience (Bromley, 1977).

These enduring features are usually described in terms of traits that vary across individuals, such as dependency, suspiciousness, and impulsivity. They also agree that personality is not just a collection of traits; instead, most approaches emphasize the integrated and organized nature of personality (Hall & Lindzey, 1957) and the "consistency and coherence of normal personality and view the individual organism as an organized and complexly structured whole" (McAdams, 1997, p. 12). Hence a central task for personality research is to explain this coherence and organization of personality (Cervone & Shoda, 1999) and describe the means by which people forge a coherent sense of self that gives direction and meaning to their lives from the diversity of their experiences.

The themes of *enduring characteristics* and *coherence* are both pertinent to personality disorder. Psychiatric classification seeks to describe stable individual differences in maladaptive behavior patterns, as reflected in the DSM-IV definition of personality disorder as "an enduring pattern of inner experience and behavior" (American Psychiatric Association, 1994, p. 633). The organization and coherence of personality has received scant attention from psychiatric nosologists. However, clinicians have noted the significance of the problem, as illustrated by Kohut's (1971) descriptions of impaired cohesiveness of the self in narcissistic conditions and Kernberg's concept of identity diffusion, involving poorly integrated images of self and others, in individuals with borderline personality organization. To treat personality disorder, we need to know more about these integrative processes and how they fail so that we can help patients to construct a more coherent and authentic sense of self that gives them greater stability in their behavior and more control over their lives.

Another way of viewing personality that contributes to understanding personality disorder is by considering its functional aspects. As Allport (1937) noted, "personality is something and personality does something" (p. 48). The study of personality (and personality disorder) has been more concerned with what personality *is* rather than what personality *does* (Cantor, 1990). Research has concentrated on identifying the characteristics that describe personality and the diagnostic features of different disorders. Less attention has been paid to the functions of personality and the dysfunction associated with personality disorder (Livesley, 1995). Yet the structures and processes that constitute personality serve an adaptive purpose. To understand personality disorder, we need to understand the functional aspects of personality.

Starting with Allport's statement, Cantor (1990) suggested that a major function of personality is to solve major *life tasks*—the problems that confront individuals in everyday life—such as developing the capacity for satisfying relationships and establishing meaningful goals. Although many life tasks differ from person to person, some are universal tasks that everyone shares due to a common biology and culture (Cantor, 1990). Life tasks that have evolutionary significance are especially important; these are the tasks that faced our remote ancestors when they lived as hunters and gath-erers, and adaptive mechanisms probably evolved to help them solve these problems. Knowledge of these tasks may help us to identify the basic func-tions of personality and develop a definition of personality disorder that can be applied across different cultures (Livesley, 1998; Livesley & Jang, 2000; Livesley, Schroeder, Jackson, & Jang, 1994).

Plutchik (1980) described four universal tasks:

1. The development of a sense of identity.
2. Solving problems of dominance and submissiveness that arise with the social hierarchies that are critical elements of primate social behavior.
3. The development of a sense of territoriality or belongingness.
4. Resolving problems of temporality that occur when dealing with loss and separation.

Essentially, these tasks could be summarized as developing a *coherent sense of self or identity* and *the capacity for effective relationships with others within kinship and social groups*. Adaptive solutions to these tasks were critical to function and survive in the ancestral environment. They are equally nec-essary to function effectively in contemporary society.

DEFINING PERSONALITY DISORDER

These ideas about the functions of personality suggest that personality dis-order may be defined as the *failure to achieve adaptive solutions to life tasks* (Livesley et al., 1994). These adaptive failures involve one or more of the following:

1. Failure to establish stable and integrated representations of self and others.
2. Interpersonal dysfunction, as indicated by the failure to develop the capacity for intimacy, to function adaptively as an attachment figure, and/or to establish the capacity for affiliative relationships.
3. Failure to function adaptively in the social group, as indicated by the failure to develop the capacity for prosocial behavior and/or cooperative relationships.

To complete this definition it is necessary to add that these failures or def-icits are only indicative of personality disorder when they are enduring and can be traced to adolescence or early adulthood, and when they are not due to a pervasive mental state disorder, such as a cognitive or schizo-phrenic disorder.

This definition, derived from evolutionary psychology and normal personality theory, is remarkably compatible with clinical concepts. The clinical literature suggests that personality disorder involves two related problems: *severe and chronic difficulties with interpersonal relationships*, and *problems with a sense of self or identity*. Rutter (1987), for example, argued that personality disorder primarily involves chronic interpersonal dysfunction. Similarly, Vaillant and Perry (1980) noted that personality disorder is inevitably manifested in social situations, and Pincus and Wiggins (1990) noted that impaired interpersonal functions are a defining feature of personality disorder (see also Benjamin, 1993; Keisler, 1986; McLemore & Brokaw, 1987). The significance of self pathology is recognized by other contributors. As noted, identity diffusion is central to Kernberg's (1975, 1984) concept of borderline personality organization, and Kohut (1971) emphasized the importance of self pathology in narcissism. Constructivist approaches to psychotherapy (Neimeyer & Mahoney, 1995) also assume that the consolidation of a self is a pivotal organizing principle that brings meaning to experience.

Cloninger incorporates both interpersonal and self problems in his definition of personality disorder as low cooperativeness and low self-directedness (Cloninger, 2000; Cloninger, Svrakic, & Przybeck, 1993). Similarly, Blatt and colleagues (1994) suggested that personality development involves two fundamental tasks: the achievement of a stable, differential, realistic, and positive identity, and the establishment of enduring, mutually gratifying relationships with others. Both tasks are also represented, in their problematic forms, in the four general criteria that the DSM-IV proposed for diagnosing personality disorder. Criterion 1 refers to deviations from the norm in "ways of perceiving and interpreting the self, other people, and events," and criterion 3 refers to deviations in "interpersonal functioning" (p. 633). (The other two criteria refer to "the range, intensity, lability, and appropriateness of emotional response" and "impulse control" [p. 633]). Putting aside differences in theory and terminology, there is consensus that (1) *chronic interpersonal dysfunction* and (2) *problems with the structure of the self* lie at the heart of personality disorder.

Defining personality disorder as an adaptive failure is consistent with the *deficit model* discussed in the previous chapter. This does not mean, however, that the conflict and vulnerability models are unimportant. Adaptive failures inevitably lead to conflicted relationships, and they develop in the context of genetic predispositions to develop certain traits. Nor does the definition imply that everyone with personality disorder shows the same maladaptive responses to life tasks. Personality traits influence the way adaptive failures are expressed. The failure to develop a coherent self may take the form of fragmented and unstable self-images in individuals with borderline traits, or an impoverished concept of self and lack of authenticity in individuals with schizoid traits. Similarly, problems establishing lasting intimate relationships may lead to brief, intense, and chaotic relationships in individuals with borderline traits, whereas individuals with schizoid traits may simply avoid relationships. Despite these differences, the failure to establish adaptive solutions to life tasks is common to all disorders. As will be seen later, this idea has major implications for treatment. For now we should note that it suggests the following basic principle concerning the broad goals of treatment:

> Basic Principle: The overall goal in treating personality disorder is to improve adaptation.

This goal orientates the therapist to the way treatment should be approached and acts as a reminder of what is to be accomplished and what is not. As applied to the defining features of personality disorder, the goal is to help patients to find more adaptive solutions to universal life tasks.

THE PERSONALITY SYSTEM

It is useful to think of personality as a system of interrelated structures and processes (Costa & McCrae, 1994; Mischel, 1999; Vernon, 1964). The basic framework is formed by *traits* such as affective lability, introversion, impulsivity, and compulsivity. Traits are enduring qualities that differ across individuals. They have a substantial genetic component and influence the development and functioning of other parts of the system. Also important are the constructs used to process information, impose meaning on experience, and predict events. Constructs that are important for understanding personality are those used to organize information about the self and those used to organize information about the interpersonal environment. These construct systems are referred to as the *self* and *interpersonal* or *person systems*, respectively. The latter consists of beliefs, expectations, and associated behavioral strategies that influence how we think about and relate to other people and the affects aroused by these processes. An important part of the construct system is an understanding of the rules governing behavior that are used to understand self and others and predict other people's actions.

Constructs are shaped by experiences, especially with significant others, and the individual's salient traits. For example, introverted people are likely to see themselves as more socially inept than others, and anxious individuals are likely to think of themselves as more dependent and ineffectual than those who are calmer or more phlegmatic. Constructs, in turn, shape perceptions of the environment and influence the way traits are expressed. Because constructs are so important in shaping behavior, personality can be conceptualized as an information-processing system that receives, selects, and transforms information about the self and the world, thereby structuring experience and influencing action (Neimeyer & Mahoney, 1995).

The output of the personality system is *behavior*, which includes emotional responses and cognitions. These *characteristic responses or expressions* represent the way personality is expressed as consistent behavior patterns and forms of experience. The overall system is controlled by *integrative and regulatory processes* that manage feelings, impulses, and behavior, and combine information to form the self and interpersonal systems.

Finally, any account of personality would be incomplete without reference to the *environmental context* in which behavior occurs. Unfortunately, environmental issues are often neglected due to the emphasis traditional clinical explanation places on internal personality dynamics. Context is important, however, and close attention needs to be given to how the social situation shapes behavior and maintains the repetitive maladaptive patterns that characterize personality disorder. People seek out environments, including social relationships, that are conducive to their personality. Consequently, the environment helps to consolidate and maintain maladaptive patterns, and patients may need to acquire the skills that would enable them to change their environments and manage them more effectively.

The components of personality are not distinct entities but rather interacting structures and processes that form an organized system. Figure 2.1 is a simplified representation of this system and the links between the subsystems. The division of personality into subsystems is not a substitute for a theory of personality and personality disorder. It is merely a heuristic that helps us to (1) organize the information that facilitates treatment planning and (2) generate ideas for effecting change. Because the self and interpersonal systems are crucial in understanding personality disorder, and trait structure is important in describing individual differences in personality pathology, both are discussed in more detail later. But first we need to consider the treatment implications of viewing personality as a system.

IMPLICATIONS FOR TREATMENT

The personality system provides a simple scheme by which to describe the multiple problems of typical cases. The idea also has implications for organizing treatments and the selection of interventions to treat the different components. Using this framework, six overlapping problem domains can be identified, plus a domain of symptoms:

1. Symptomatic: self-harming behavior, cognitive and affective symptoms, and symptoms associated with a concurrent Axis I disorder

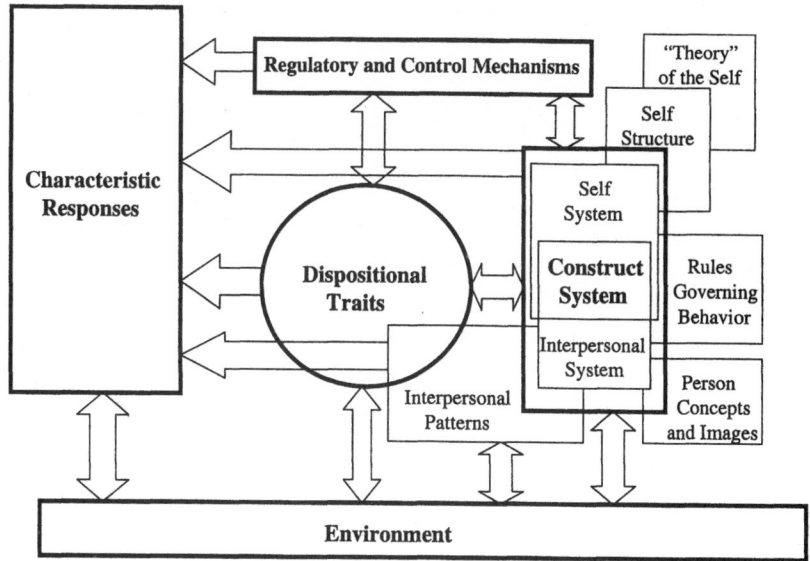

FIGURE 2.1. The personality system.

2. Situational or environmental: past and present situational problems, including dysfunctional relationships
3. Regulation and control: problems managing emotions and impulses
4. Dispositional traits: maladaptive expressions of traits
5. Interpersonal: maladaptive interpersonal schemata and relationship patterns, and problems forming integrated representations of others
6. Self system: maladaptive schemata, and problems forming an integrated sense of self

The six domains of psychopathology encompass most of the problems typically addressed in treatment. Although DSM-IV diagnostic criteria were not selected systematically to represent these problem areas, they cover the psychopathology defined by the personality system, as illustrated in the following examples:

Domain	Diagnostic criteria	Personality disorder
Symptomatic	Suicidal behavior	Borderline
	Ideas of reference	Schizotypal
Situational	Lacks close friends	Schizoid
Regulatory	Difficulty controlling anger	Borderline
	Impulsivity	Antisocial
	Constricted affect	Schizotypal

Dispositional traits	Rigidity and stubbornness	Obsessive–compulsive
	Overly conscientious	Obsessive–compulsive
	Lacks empathy	Narcissistic
Interpersonal system	Unstable relationships	Borderline
	Interpersonally exploitive	Narcissistic
Self system	Identity disturbance	Borderline
	Chronic feeling of emptiness	Borderline
	Views self as socially inept	Avoidant

This range of problems has implications for conceptualizing treatment because each domain may respond to different interventions, and domains may change at different rates. The evidence suggests that treatment outcome and the effectiveness of a given intervention vary across domains and that various approaches, including behavioral interventions, cognitive therapy, and dynamic psychotherapy, are effective (Piper & Joyce, 2001). Symptoms such as parasuicidal behavior and impulsivity respond to behavioral and cognitive-behavioral interventions (Davidson & Tyrer, 1996; Lieberman & Eckman, 1981; Linehan, 1993; Linehan et al., 1991; Perris, 1994). Symptoms of social anxiety respond to social skills training (Argyle, Tower, & Bryant, 1974; Marzillier, Lambert, & Kellett, 1976). Symptoms of impulsivity and cognitive dysregulation involving transient or quasipsychotic features often respond to medication with selective serotonergic reuptake inhibitors (SSRIs) and neuroleptics, respectively (Markovitz, 2001; Soloff, 1994, 2000); Gabbard (1998) also observed that the optimal treatment of borderline personality disorder may be a combination of medication and psychotherapy. Dysfunctional cognitions, on the other hand, are likely to respond to cognitive therapy (Beck, Freeman, & Associates, 1990; Young & Lindemann, 1992). These differential effects suggest the following principle for conceptualizing treatment:

> *Basic Principle: Comprehensive treatment requires a combination of interventions to treat the range of psychopathology typically associated with personality disorder.*

The general relationship between domains of psychopathology and therapeutic modality may be summarized as follows:

Psychopathology	Most appropriate therapeutic model
Symptomatic	Cognitive-behavioral therapy
	Chemotherapy
Situational	Cognitive-behavioral therapy
	Skill training
Regulatory	Cognitive-behavioral therapy
	Chemotherapy
Dispositional traits	Cognitive-behavioral therapy

Interpersonal system   Psychoanalytical psychotherapy
                            Interpersonal psychotherapy
                            Cognitive therapy
Self system   Psychoanalytical psychotherapy (especially self psychology)
                            Interpersonal psychotherapy
                            Cognitive therapy

This list suggests that structured interventions are most likely to be effective in managing psychopathology at the top of the list and that both biological and psychological interventions are useful. The list is, of course, an oversimplification. Some therapies have broader effects than shown, and interventions not included may be effective. Moreover, the six domains form an integrated system, so that change in one domain may spread to others. Nevertheless, the list makes the general point that different domains are likely to respond differentially to a given intervention. This differentiation suggests that (1) general questions such as "Are treatments of personality disorder effective?" need to be refined to specify the type of intervention and the kind of problem addressed, and (2) outcome criteria need to be domain-specific (Piper & Joyce, 2001).

Although the treatment of personality disorder is dominated by therapies based on specific theoretical models, the value of using a combination of interventions is widely recognized. Vaillant (1992), for example, argued that therapists "can use help from every competent theorist that they can find. Drives, people, reality, and culture are all significant. Psychoanalysis, family systems theory, and behavior modification can all play valuable roles" (p. 119). Similarly, Aronson (1989) suggested that a comprehensive set of strategies is required to treat the multiple problems associated with borderline personality disorder; Andrews (1984) maintained that the effective treatment of histrionic personality disorder required psychoanalytic and behavioral interventions. Empirical support for these ideas is indirectly provided by a randomized control trial of a psychodynamic day treatment program conducted by Piper, Rosie, Joyce, and Azim (1996). Treatment consisted of participation in a large daily group and several small groups that included (1) unstructured and insight-oriented groups and (2) structured skill-oriented groups. Treated patients showed greater improvement than controls on multiple variables, and improvement was maintained at follow-up. The authors attribute the program's success to the use of a comprehensive set of interventions delivered in a group format.

The evidence indicates that no single approach or school of therapy has a monopoly in treating personality disorder. Comprehensive treatment requires an array of interventions drawn from diverse schools of thought. This perspective is consistent with evidence on the effectiveness of psychotherapy. As Luborsky (1995) noted, most therapies lead to therapeutic change in significant numbers of patients, but no single form of therapy appears be effective for all problems and all persons. This perspective implies another general principle:

> Basic Principle: Interventions should be tailored to the problems presented by a given case, the problems that are the focus of immediate therapeutic effort, and the personality style of the patient.

Although the value of tailoring treatment to specific patient needs has been emphasized (Beutler & Clarkin, 1990; Frances, Clarkin, & Perry, 1984), the treatment of personality disorder is rarely approached in this way. Different schools are often presented as if they were the most effective, and evidence of effectiveness in treating one problem, such as self-harm, is taken to imply effectiveness for all problems. Comparisons are made between therapies, as if the task were to select the best therapy, rather than recognizing that each may have components that merit attention.

Tailored treatment is usually associated with integrated or generic models of therapy (Norcross & Goldfried, 1992). However, the need to tailor treatment to patient variables is also recognized within specific schools of therapy. For example, Horwitz and colleagues (1996), discussing psychoanalytic treatment of borderline personality disorder, noted:

> The majority of writers have used a "lumping" strategy in which they proposed one general approach to the average, modal patient, while mentioning some exceptions for those persons who deviate from the majority. We believe that clearer diagnostic differentiations based on ego functions, relationship patterns, and developmental considerations will lead to the appropriate treatment approaches for a particular type of patient. (p. 29)

Although Horwitz and colleagues were discussing a combination of psychoanalytic approaches, not a combination of interventions from different schools, their comment indicates growing recognition that the complexity and range of psychopathology associated with personality disorder demand a combination of approaches. Piper and Joyce (2001), reviewing the literature on treatment outcome, concluded that the best results occurred when treatment was individually tailored and the patient and therapist agreed on a specific contract.

The task of a tailored approach is to select interventions to treat targeted problems based, when possible, on proven efficacy or, if this is not available, on a rational consideration of what is likely to be effective, given current knowledge of the disorder and the nature of therapeutic change. Selected interventions may be used in combination or sequentially, as different problems become the focus of attention. When used in combination, the different interventions may target different problems, or an array of interventions may be used to focus on a single problem, as illustrated by the use of medication and cognitive and behavioral interventions to treat impulsivity and self-harm.

SELF AND INTERPERSONAL SYSTEMS

Having considered the implications of viewing personality as a system, we can now return to a more detailed examination of the way the construct system and traits contribute to an understanding of personality disorder, beginning with the self and interpersonal systems. Many approaches to personality and psychopathology, including psychoanalysis, cognitive therapy, interpersonal models, and constructivism, share the idea that the cognitive structures used to interpret the world, especially interpersonal relationships, are core components of personality (Barnett, 1980; Holt, 1989) and that reorganization of the construct system is the goal of treatment. This concurrence suggests that self and interpersonal constructs have the potential to serve as integrating concepts (Eells, 1997; Gold, 1996). These constructs are variously labeled object relationships, working models (Bowlby, 1980), self and object representations (Gold, 1990a, 1990b; Ryle, 1990, 1997; Wachtel, 1985), cognitive schemata (Beck et al., 1990), and self or interpersonal schemata (Guidano, 1987, 1991a; Horowitz, 1988, 1998). Here the term *schema* is used because is it is a relatively neutral term with a long history in psychology, being first used by Piaget (1926) and Bartlett (1932).

Schemata are categories used to organize information and interpret experience. In Segal's (1988) words, they are "organized elements of past reactions and experience that form a relatively cohesive and persistent body of knowledge capable of guiding substantial perception and appraisal" (p. 147). The term *schema*, as used here, however, differs from its meaning in cognitive therapy, where generally the term is applied only to core beliefs such as "I am bad," "I am unlovable," or "The world is hostile and everyone is against me" (Layden, Newman, Freeman, & Morse, 1993; Young, 1990). Here the concept is used more generally to describe any category or cluster of information. Core beliefs are merely one form of self-schema. Because they have a pervasive influence on self and interpersonal functioning, they are referred to as *core schemata*.

Theories based on the schema concept propose that knowledge is organized in units consisting of attributes (items of knowledge) and an explanation of how these attributes are connected (Komatsu, 1992; Rumelhart, 1980). For example, the schema of bicycle is more than just a list of parts (set of attributes), such as wheels, pedals, seat, and handlebars. It also includes an understanding of how these attributes are related to each other and how they work together. A schema may also include specific examples of the concept. The schema of bicycle, for example, may include memories of the first bicycle received as a birthday present, or the bicycle from which one fell and suffered injury. These examples are memorable because they are unusual or associated with strong feelings. Schemata are not separate and unrelated "islands" but organized into a hierarchy. The schema of bicycle, for example, may be part of a higher-order schema of nonmotorized vehicles along with scooter and tricycle. This higher-order schema is in turn part of a more general schema of vehicles.

Application of Schema Construct to Self and Interpersonal Systems

The idea that (1) a schema consists of attributes, a theory explaining the relationships among these attributes, and memories of specific instances and (2) that schemata are organized into a hierarchy is useful in understanding how the self and interpersonal systems are organized. Images of the self or another person include information about personality characteristics and behaviors that is integrated to form a coherent impression. A schema representing the self as "kind" consists of behaviors such as "being helpful," "acting in a generous way," and "being solicitous of others' well-being" that are assumed to characterize this quality. The schema of kindness may itself be part of a more general schema representing a global image of the self. People usually form multiple self-images, viewing themselves differently in their various roles of parent, partner, friend, and so on. The schemata defining different self-images are linked to form more general representations that culminate in an overall conception of the self. For example, a person may form a schema of the self as therapist, defined by such attributes (more specific schemata) as competent, helpful, kind, intermittently puzzled, and having occasional feelings of inadequacy (Fig-

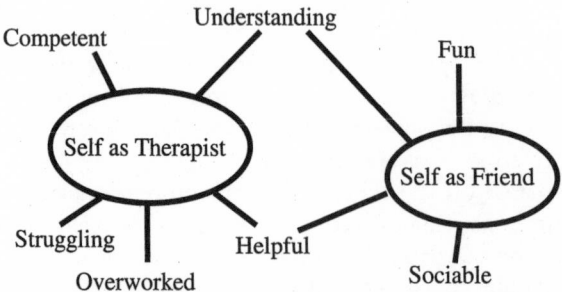

FIGURE 2.2. Self schemata.

ure 2.2). The same person may have a schema of the self as friend that includes being sociable, outgoing, fun, concerned, helpful, and kind. These schemata are linked by the attributes *kind* and *helpful*. These links help to integrate the self by connecting different self-images. The schemata of *therapist* and *friend* could be considered part of a higher-order schema of the self as a kind and helpful person. This schema, in turn, will be related to other higher-order schemata, and so on, to form a global schema of the self (Figure 2.3).

The interpersonal system may also be understood in the same way (Horowitz, 1998). For example, the schema of another person may include characteristics such as kind, loving, cheerful, and yet irritable at times, and ideas about the way that these behaviors are related, although this explanation may not be very elaborate. For example, we may notice that a person is normally cheerful and kind but irritable when stressed. Schemata also incorporate memories of things the person did, important experiences shared with him or her, and so on. These memories are usually salient because they evoke strong feelings. In this way, feelings are incorporated into schemata.

The network of schemata forming the interpersonal system consists of (1) person schemata representing specific individuals; (2) generalized person schemata that describe designated groups of individuals (e.g., men, authority figures, sexual partners, and so on); and (3) generalized ideas and beliefs that constitute the individual's understanding of the principles and rules governing human behavior (Figure 2.4). *Person schemata* form the basic level of the interpersonal schema hierarchy; these are the impressions formed of different individuals. When the other person is significant and well known, the person schema is likely to include several facet schemata that represent different impressions of the person. For example, the child's experience of mother responding sensitively to his or her needs may lead to a schema of mother as caring and loving. Other experiences of mother as less responsive are likely to produce a schema of her as uncaring or withholding. As the child's cognitive skills and memory mature, the realization dawns that the different images apply to the same person. Under normal conditions, these disparate images will be integrated to form a global image of mother.

A second achievement of the interpersonal system is the establishment of *generalized person schemata* that consist of general impressions of specific groups of individuals. For example, experiences with men may give rise to a generalized schema of how men typically behave, think, and react, which is used to understand, anticipate, and predict the behavior of any new male who is encountered. Generalized schemata enable us to draw upon experience to predict the likely behavior of a member of a designated group. To be adaptive, generalized person schemata should be sufficiently flexible to accommodate the behavior of specific individuals. If applied rig-

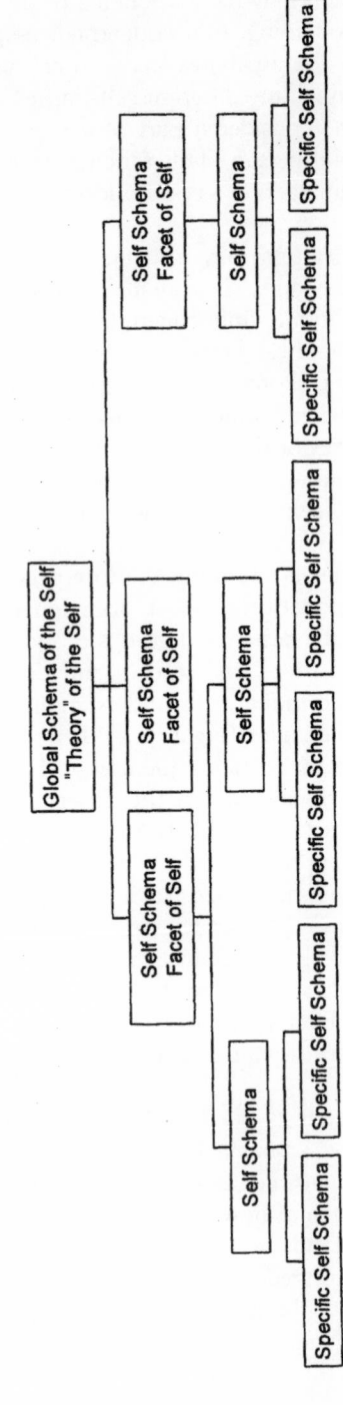

FIGURE 2.3. Hierarchical structure of the self system.

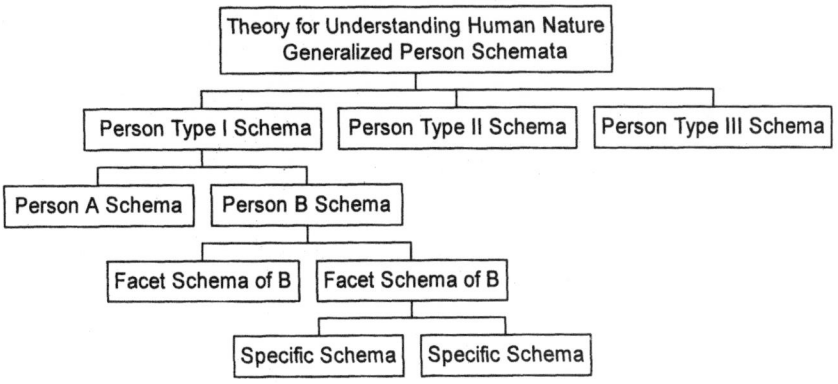

FIGURE 2.4. Structure of the interpersonal system.

idly, such schemata lead to stereotyped reactions that are based more on the group to which the person is considered to belong than on his or her actual behavior.

Over time, experiences with other people also are likely to lead to a *generalized understanding of people and the principles and rules governing human behavior* (Figure 2.5). The ability to relate effectively to a wide range of people requires a sophisticated understanding of human behavior. Under most circumstances, interpersonal encounters proceed smoothly without much conscious thought about how we should behave or what the other person is likely to do. This automaticity suggests that interpersonal actions are guided by an intuitive understanding of how people are likely to act and what they expect of us, which was probably acquired by generalizing and integrating diverse experiences with different people across a wide variety of situations. The emergence of what Mead (1934) referred to as a concept of the "generalized other" is facilitated by the realization that other people have minds and hence experience things similarly (relatively speaking) to oneself. This generalizability enables the child to understand that human behavior is predictable and follows rules (Livesley & Bromley, 1973). However, these rules are difficult to articulate because they are part of procedural or implicit memory and hence applied intuitively and automatically. It is only when understanding or prediction fails in some way that one becomes aware of the process. Failure creates a sense of puzzlement about the other person. This intuitive understanding is poorly developed in many personality disordered individuals, leading them to feel uncertain and puzzled about how to behave toward other people, what is expected of them, or how others are likely to respond.

Although the self and interpersonal systems have been discussed separately for clarity, obviously they are closely interrelated. Both emerge from the same interpersonal matrix that is influenced by genetic dispositions and adaptive mechanisms. Self and interpersonal schemata are also functionally intertwined: The activation of self-schemata invariably leads to arousal of interpersonal schemata, and vice versa, and the rules developed to understand behavior apply to self and others. The development of both systems involves a balance between assimilation and accommodation (Piaget, 1952). *Assimilation* involves the categorization and integration of experiences into existing schemata; through this process, a stable view of the self and interpersonal reality is maintained. *Accommodation* involves changing cognitive structure to incorporate new experiences that are discrepant with already existing schemata. The ongoing interplay between assimilation and accommodation ensures a degree of stability in the construct system that allows prediction of interpersonal events, while also allowing the system to change in response to new experiences. In personality disorder, assimilation and accommodation processes are often disturbed: Core schemata that determine the person's construction of reality are remarkably stable, and discrepant information is readily discounted; at other times, the comments and actions of others are too readily assimilated, so that experience of the self is excessively dependent on the reactions of others.

The construct system develops through simultaneous processes of *differentiation* and *integration*. Self-experience becomes increasingly refined over time to create a more detailed understanding of the self. This progression is illustrated most clearly with emotions: early global feelings differentiate into more subtle feelings. Similar processes occurring with other aspects of the self give rise to an increasing variety of self schemata. As differentiation proceeds, boundaries develop that differentiate self from others. Differentiation is paralleled by integrative processes that organize more general conceptions of the self. Viewed in this way, the self may be considered a network of self schemata (self-images) that form a hierarchical structure (Horowitz, 1998). The interpersonal system evolves similarly. For example, the child's initial concepts of another person are usually broad evaluations of whether the person is good or bad (Livesley & Bromley, 1973). Over time, diverse experiences with the person cause global impressions to differentiate into more precise images. Gradually these schemata are integrated to form a coherent representation of the person.

Integration and Coherence

Adaptive self and interpersonal systems incorporate integrated representations of self and others to produce a sense of unity in the experience of self. Since integrated conceptions of self and others are impaired in personality disorder, we need to understand the mechanisms that contribute to integration in order to develop treatment strategies. Integration arises from (1) cognitive processes that organize information about the self or another person into a hierarchy of schemata, and (2) the consequences of goal-directed behavior.

Cognitive or Structural Component of Integration

The subjective experience of self-cohesiveness and unity is the product of extensive connections within self-knowledge (Toulmin, 1978). This *cognitive* contribution to integration has several components. At the most elemental level, *a sense of cohesion arises from the naturalness and cohesiveness of any schema.* The qualities we attribute to ourselves, such as friendly, reliable, and cheerful, seem to us to be real qualities—like the schemata for bird, tree, or cat seem real. The perceived naturalness of a schema arises from the fact that organizing information into categories is an inherent feature of the way in which we handle information about the world (Komatsu, 1992). Hence a sense of clarity and certainty about one's personal characteristics is a prerequisite for, and actually promotes, integration by providing a stable understanding of one's enduring qualities.

Integration also arises from *the links among self schemata and self-states.* The more equipped the person is to organize "multiple self schemas into a coherent whole, the more likely the individual is to experience a sense of identity cohesiveness and continuity over extended periods of time" (Horowitz, 1998, p. 87). The integrative links within self-knowledge often depend on images and feelings that connect different aspects of self. Experiences of being accepted and cared for and being recognized as competent get linked by feelings of satisfaction and pleasure. Over time, these linkages crystallize into a sense of self as loved and lovable and competent. As cognitive functions develop, these links become cognitively mediated (Livesley & Bromley, 1973).

At the highest level, integration comes from the formation of a *higher-order understanding of the self* or *"theory" of the self* (Epstein, 1973, 1990). Integration and the subjective experience of wholeness are enhanced by the sense of continuity that occurs when we integrate self-experiences to construct a coherent and stable life story that imposes structure and meaning on our experience of ourselves and our lives and that is updated periodically to incorporate past experiences as well as future hopes and aspirations (Greenwald, 1980; McAdams, 1994; Ross, 1989). To paraphrase Murphy (1947), the self is the person as known to the person. Although these statements are in a sense tautological and have limited value as definitions, they are useful metaphors that capture the sense of cohesion that is central to an adaptive self structure.

This model assumes that the self emerges from the way self-information is processed and organized. The subjective experience of continuity and unity results from connections within self-knowledge and the integration of experiences across time. The value of this conception is that it expresses vague but important clinical ideas about the cohesiveness of the self and identity diffusion in a way that leads to ideas for change. For example, it suggests that interventions may be required to promote interpersonal boundaries, help patients identify self schemata and develop clarity about their knowledge of themselves, build connections within self-knowledge, and facilitate the synthesis of a more adaptive understanding of the self. The emphasis on cognitive processes in the emergence of the self and interpersonal systems may be seen as "too cognitive" and as neglecting emotional processes. However, this framework recognizes that schemata have an emotional element and that meaning can be laden with affects and defined by emotions.

Self-Directed or Conative Component of Integration

As used in contemporary psychology and by many clinical thinkers, the term *self* does not refer only to the organization of self-referential knowledge but also "to the more-or-less integrated center of agentic activity" (Sheldon & Elliot, 1999, p. 483). The establishment of direction and purpose to action and a sense of agency and autonomy are crucial components of adaptive self-functioning (Carver & Scheier, 1998; Shapiro, 1981). This self-directed or *conative* component involves setting and working toward goals, which are important because they energize and give meaning, purpose, and direction to lives (Baumeister, 1989; Carver & Scheier, 1998; Pervin, 1992).

Meaningful goals help to promote integration by drawing together different aspects of personality; they link needs and wishes with the abilities and skills needed to attain them. As Allport (1961) noted, it is striving toward a goal that confers integration, not its attainment. "To reach a goal we have to overcome distractions, discords, and obstacles. The effort involved welds unity" (p. 380). Major goals imply subordinate goals. For example, the decision to pursue a career as a mental health professional has a powerful organizing effect on a person's life, because it implies a variety of subgoals such as studying to get into university, working to support educational objectives, and so on. It also affects day-to-day goals, such as whether to study on a particular evening or socialize. This hierarchical arrangement facilitates integration by organizing and directing large segments of behavior.

The cognitive and conative aspects of integration are related. A clear understanding of the self is needed to define enduring personal goals, because the selection of goals is influenced by personal assessments of ability and mastery (Bandura, 1999). Established goals contribute to integration by connecting different aspects of self-knowledge and linking personal goals with expectations and beliefs about the self (Dweck, 1996).

Self-States

Although the self may be experienced as integrated, the process of integration is never complete. Self-experience usually varies across occasions because some self schemata persist when aroused, creating enduring states of mind or *self-states* (Horowitz, 1979, 1998; Ryle, 1997). Most people experience several self-states, some conflicting, such as confident and buoyant, confused, incompetent, discontented, and so on. Individuals with adaptive self systems recognize these states as different facets of the self, such that their sense of integration and unity is not impaired. However, the self-states associated with personality disorder are more extreme and contribute to a sense of fragmentation.

Horowitz (1998) defined self-states or states of mind as "a combination of conscious and unconscious experiences with patterns of behavior that can last for a short or long period of time" (pp. 13–14). Each state involves a specific pattern of emotions, ways of thinking about the self and others, interpersonal relationships, and coping strategies. Self-states are important in understanding the structure of self-experience and the flow of interpersonal behavior. They define characteristic ways of experiencing the world and relating to other people. For example, in an exuberant and confident self-state, the person may feel self-confident and energetic and be seen by others as cheerful and fun to be around. In an angry and disgusted state, the same person may feel disillusioned and act in an angry, withdrawn way, leading to different reactions from others.

The basic schema that defines and establishes a self-state is triggered by specific events (usually interpersonal) or mood changes. Once activated, the schema arouses strong emotions and possibly other schemata that help to maintain the state (Figure 2.5). Self-states also include char-

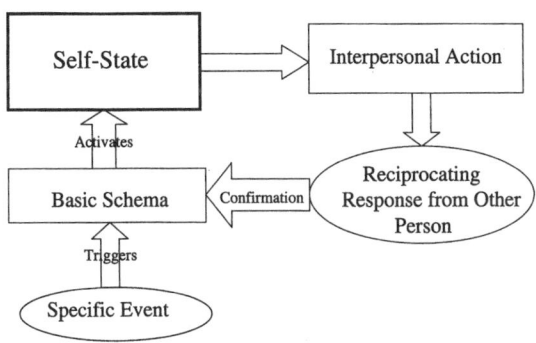

FIGURE 2.5. Self-state arousal and maintenance.

acteristic interpersonal behaviors that tend to evoke reactions from others that confirm the triggering schema (Ryle, 1997). For example, a dependent individual in a submissive self-state may act in ways that elicit abusive or controlling responses from others, thereby confirming the basic schemata and maintaining the state. The sequence of (1) a triggering situation evoking (2) basic schema that, in turn, evoke (3) an experiential state, (4) behavioral response, (5) reciprocating responses from others, and (6) evaluation of outcome leading to confirmation of the basic belief creates a cyclical interpersonal dynamic that is self-maintaining and difficult to disrupt. Recognition that the social environment contributes to maladaptive patterns suggests that, in addition to addressing basic schema, patients may also need to learn social skills for managing the social environment more effectively if these cycles are to be disrupted.

This formulation of self-states resembles traditional object relations concepts. The important difference is that object relations theory emphasizes the significance of the "inner world" of object relations in shaping perceptions of the external world and interpersonal behavior, whereas the current conceptualization also recognizes the role of external events, especially other people's behavior, in maintaining self-states and repetitive maladaptive patterns (Ryle, 1997).

Major self-states are assumed to originate in early dyadic relationships (Siegel, 1999). Repeated experiences with caregivers are "summated" to form schemata of the caregiver. Infants with a secure attachment to their caregiver experience consistent nurturance, sensitivity, and predictability that contribute to the formation of schemata of a responsive and available attachment figure. When activated, such schemata evoke feelings of safety and security that help infants to regulate their own emotional states and form the basis for self-soothing throughout life. In contrast, infants with less responsive and predictable caregivers are likely to form schemata of insecurity, unresponsiveness, and even fear. The activation of these schemata arouses unpleasant or frightening affects that make it difficult to learn ways to regulate emotions and self-soothe. Different experiences with caregivers give rise to multiple schemata that form the basis for different self-states. Each state typically involves (1) a specific self-image, (2) an image of the other person, and (3) a representation of the relationship between the two. The cognitions, affects, and behaviors that characterize a given state are likely to be supplemented with specific memories when these are emotionally charged. Under normal circumstances, early self-states are likely to be modified in the light of new experiences. As cognitive mechanisms mature, the various self-states originating from different experiences with significant others are likely to be integrated into a more global self-structure. Nevertheless, for most individuals different self-states are common, and each tends to be recurrent.

SELF AND INTERPERSONAL PATHOLOGY

The previous description of the self and interpersonal systems provides the basis for understanding the self and interpersonal pathology that form critical elements of personality disorder. Pathology encompasses (1) the *contents* (maladaptive schemata and maladaptive patterns of interpersonal relationships), (2) the *organizational or structural* aspects of the self and interpersonal systems, and (3) the *self-directed or conative* aspects of the self (see Table 2.1).

Maladaptive Schemata and Interpersonal Behavior

Maladaptive ideas about self and others and maladaptive interpersonal patterns are extensive in personality disorder (Beck et al., 1990; Young, 1990, 1994; Young & Lindermann, 1992). Although some maladaptive schemata are specific to the individual, many are organized around adverse developmental experiences related to issues of trust, cooperation, attachment, intimacy, and control (discussed in the next chapter). Maladaptive schemata

TABLE 2.1. Pathology of the Self and Interpersonal Systems

	Self system	Interpersonal system
Cognitive problems		
Maladaptive content	Maladaptive schemata	Maladaptive schemata Repetitive maladaptive interpersonal patterns

Maladaptive differentiation	Poorly defined boundaries
	Impoverished self-concepts
	Global, poorly differentiated
	  self schemata
		Poorly defined boundaries
		Impoverished and stereotyped
		  representations of others
		Poor discrimination among
		  others
		Global interpersonal schemata

Maladaptive integration	Fragmentary self-
	  representations
	Unstable self-images
	
	Poorly integrated self-states
	Lack of a coherent theory
	  of the self
		Separate or poorly integrated
		  images of another person
		Unstable representations of
		  another person
		Poorly developed concepts of
		  human nature and behavior

Conative problems	Low self-directedness Low motivation	

give rise to repetitive and cyclical patterns of maladaptive interpersonal behavior. These patterns, acquired in past relationships, underlie many of the difficulties for which patients seek help. Typically, maladaptive interpersonal patterns are based on a cycle of events involving (1) a state within the person that may be described in terms of fears, wants, wishes, goals, or expectations; (2) actions arising from this state; (3) the other person's perception of these actions and responses to them; and (4) the self's perceptions of, and reactions to, the other person's perceptions and actions (see Leary, 1957; Luborsky, 1977, 1997a, 1997b; Schacht, Binder, & Strupp, 1984). The repetitive nature of these cycles is readily explained by the schema concept. Schemata tend to be self-perpetuating because they influence what is noticed and the way events are interpreted (Guidano & Liotti, 1983). They also influence responses to events. As with self-states, these responses often evoke reactions from others that confirm the schema and perpetuate the cycle (i.e., a self-fulfilling prophecy).

Structural Problems

Problems with the organization and structure of the self and interpersonal systems (core features of personality disorder) are readily understood in terms of the concepts of differentiation and integration discussed earlier (see Table 2.1).

Problems of Differentiation

Inadequate differentiation leads to poor interpersonal boundaries and consequent difficulty in differentiating the self from others (Akhtar, 1992; Kernberg, 1984) and to self-experiences that are confused with those of others. This confusion creates the fear of losing oneself by merging with the other person. As one patient expressed it, "I lose myself in another person and forget about myself." Another realized, "I am afraid that one day there will be no real 'me' left." Differentiation problems also create global and nonspecific schemata, uncertainty about personal qualities, impoverished self and person concepts, and a sense of inner emptiness. The simple question, "What sort of person are you?" often elicits a puzzled and vague response. One patient responded to this question: "There are only a few things that I am sure of about myself. I would not kill anyone. I like dogs—in fact, all animals. I like music. I like the color green. This is how I felt when I was 4. It's as if I have not changed. I got stuck." It is instructive to compare this adult's self-description with that of a 7-year-old girl: "I am 7 years old. I have one sister. Next year I will be eight. I like coloring. The game I like is hide-the-thimble. I go riding every Wednesday. I have lots of toys. My flower is a rose, and a buttercup, and a daisy. I like milk to drink and lemon. I like to eat potatoes as well as meat. Sometimes I like jelly and syrup as well" (Livesley & Bromley, 1973). Both descriptions are simply lists of preferences with little awareness of personal characteristics or organized understanding of the self.

Lack of clarity about personal qualities leads to reliance on context and input from others to define the self, leaving the individual open to exploitation and control. One patient noted: "I am like a chameleon; I change my color according to what other people expect. I simply play the role that others expect of me." Another patient said, "I am not sure what I want or who I am. I just do what people expect of me." This is the quality that Deutsch (1942) referred to as the "as-if" personality. Lack of clarity also affects self-directedness; it is difficult to set goals when one is unsure about oneself and has difficulty identifying salient qualities, abilities, and wants.

Problems of Integration

Integration problems produce fragmented self and person representations. For one patient, this fragmentation created a sense of being divided: "I am divided into two—the rational me and the irrational and crazy me. My job is to put them together." Others express this feeling with such phrases as, "I feel as if I am many different people," and "I feel fragmented." These statements reveal major fractures in the individual's experience of the self—labeled *self-state disjunctions*—in which different self-states are experienced as separate and unrelated, with abrupt transitions from one state to another. This quality is captured in the DSM-IV criterion for borderline personality disorder: "Identity disturbance: markedly and persistently unstable self-image or sense of self" (American Psychiatric Association, 1994, p. 654). However, this characteristic is not specific to borderline personality disorder, although it is most obvious when intense feelings make it difficult to connect disparate states or even recall experiences in other states.

Integration problems may also involve another form of fracture in self experience: a *real self–false self disjunction*, in which a disconnection is experienced between the experience of the self that is presented to the world and the real self that is keep hidden and protected. Such individuals present a facade or false self (Winnicott, 1960) that masks what they believe is their true self. They often comment that even when talking about themselves, nothing seems real, and that their "real self" is rarely revealed because it is precious and vulnerable. Although it is difficult to conceptualize the idea that the "me" who is experiencing and interacting is in some way different from the "real me," particularly when the person does not feel in touch with the "real me," the idea captures a significant aspect of the self-experience of many patients. The underlying problem usually involves a separation of the feelings and related thoughts, leading to self experiences that lack richness and authenticity.

Similar integration problems occur with person schemata (see Table 2.5). Rather than combining different images (facet schemata) of a person into an overall understanding of that person (person schema), distinct images are retained, as described by object relations theory. Kernberg (1984), for example, suggested that a defining feature of borderline personality organization is the mechanism of splitting, in which good and bad representations of significant others are maintained as separate images. Splitting is assumed to serve the defensive function of preventing "good" objects from being destroyed by "bad" objects or the person's inherent aggressiveness. Here it is assumed that the emergence of separate and unrelated facet schemata for a given person represents a failure of integration rather than the consequence of motivated, defensive behavior. The formation of a cohesive representation of a person depends on the capacity to integrate information and the degree of inconsistency in information about the other person. Mild neuropsychological deficits observed in some cases of personality disorder (van Reekum, Links, & Boiago, 1993) may limit the capacity to integrate information, leading to disconnected person schemata (and self system). Highly inconsistent information may exceed the integrative capacity of even intact cognitive processes, as occurs when someone behaves inconsistently (e.g., a parent who is both loving and abusive).

Despite the differing assumptions, both conceptions agree that the failure to form integrated representations of others is a core feature of personality disorder that leads to unstable relationships. Instability occurs because behavior toward another person varies according to the facet schema that is active at the time. This variability is illustrated by a patient who began a regular treatment session by saying that she had nothing to say because she did not trust the therapist and thought that he did not care about her. Later it emerged that she had been looking forward to the session. Even on the journey to the office, she was looking forward to talking about an important event that had occurred a few days earlier, anticipating the therapist's understanding and helpfulness. As she walked into the office, however, her self-state suddenly changed. She "realized" the therapist could not be trusted and that she should not confide in him. When the therapist noted that the patient seemed to have two very different images of him, the patient agreed but added that it was difficult to recall how she had felt on the way to the office. She also noted that she thought in this way about everyone who played a major role in her life.

Consequences of Structural Problems

Structural problems in the self system compromise the sense of personal continuity and historicity that is fundamental to adaptive functioning. A sense of continuity comes from (1) the perception of the self extending through time, and (2) the integration of events across time. When experience of the self and the world changes constantly, individuals experience a "temporal discontinuity in the self" (Akhtar, 1992, p. 30). The self is defined by the moment and there is little sense of the self extending into the past and future. Patients sometimes note that it feels as if they do not have a past and that they have difficulty recalling how they felt even a short time earlier. Such individuals feel that their lives are "lived in pieces" (Pfeiffer, 1974). Or, as one patient expressed it, "My life is a series of snapshots, not a movie." This discontinuity heightens despair when circumstances are difficult, because such individuals lack the temporal perspective that would allow them to recall that things were once better and thereby feel hopeful that things will change—after all, they have felt this way before and survived. In treatment, this quality of temporal discontinuity makes it difficult for the patient to link events across time and conceive that change is possible.

One of the more fundamental consequences of structural pathology is the failure to acquire an intuitive understanding of the rules guiding behavior. Many individuals with personality disorder are often puzzled about themselves and others. One apparently socially skilled patient expressed the problem this way: "I don't know how to describe the problem. I just don't understand relationships. I'm different from other people, even people as mixed up as I am. They know how to make friends. I can't make friends. I can't relate to people; I just don't know how." These were not the words of a socially isolated person with schizoid traits and obviously defective social skills but of someone with more labile affects. The statement captures the conviction that something important but difficult to define is wrong. At a deep intuitive level, the patient simply did not understand how to relate to others. Another patient expressed it differently: "I am like an electrical receptacle without the right connections. People just can't connect to me. I don't know how to let them; I don't understand what I should do." Both patients are struggling to find words for something that they intuitively believe about themselves; they do not understand how relationships work or how to make them work. Resolving this problem is not simply a matter of learning appropriate social skills but requires something deeper. As noted, these individuals lack an intuitive understanding of the basic principles governing interpersonal behavior; they also lack empathy, not in the sense of being unable to feel or care for others, but in the more primary sense of not understanding people and relationships.

A further consequence of severe self-pathology is a pervasive sense that there is something seriously wrong with oneself—that one is fundamentally flawed. Sometimes such individuals describe themselves as "frauds," "fakes," or "shams," terms that reflect the lack of authenticity that occurs with serious self-pathology. The fluid nature of self-experience, permeable self-boundaries, and lack of authenticity combine to create deep-seated anxieties about whether one really exists and doubts about who one really is. For many, life is an ongoing existential struggle to define oneself: a continuous battle against feelings that one does not exist. For some, this leads to a fear of thinking too deeply about themselves lest they discover that "there is really nothing there." These fears are often experienced as a sense of emptiness and hollowness that they desperately seek to fill by clinging to other people, as if a relationship would fill the void; using medications, drugs, and alcohol; overeating; or even hurting and harming themselves. Feeling pain is often better than feeling nothing, especially when the nothingness evokes fears of annihilation. Although originally proposed as a feature of borderline personality disorder, patients with other forms of personality disorder also experience these distressing feelings about themselves.

Conative Problems

Self-directedness, conative striving, and feelings of autonomy are crucial features of an adaptive self system that are poorly developed in individuals with personality disorder (Cloninger, 2000). The establishment of anything other than short-term goals requires the ability to envision future possibilities in the form of goals to be attained and lifestyles to be achieved (Markus & Norius, 1986). Personality disorder limits the capacity to envision an optimal life or even possibilities other than what the present moment holds, or else leads to such unrealistic and inflated goals that disappointment is inevitable. To identify meaningful goals and imagine future possibilities, one needs a measure of clarity about one's interests and abilities. Without clarity, enduring goals are rarely maintained because wants and aspirations change with mood and circumstance.

It is not that people with personality disorder do not have goals; most are crippled by negative goals. Their lives are often defined more by what they want to avoid than by what they want to achieve. Where more positive aspirations exist, they tend to be influenced by perceptions of what other people expect rather than want they want to do. Many patients have a strong sense of what they *ought* to be—a sense that incorporates feelings of obligation and responsibility that often originated in perceptions of parental expectations (Higgins, 1987, 1989, 1996). People who are dominated by thoughts of who they ought to be are very attuned to avoiding negative outcomes (Higgins & Tykocinski, 1992). Goals defined in this way are rarely attained, and even more rarely, a source of meaning and satisfaction; instead the goals generate conflict and compulsion and do not feel authentic or provide a sense of identity or coherence because they do not arise from a sense of who one is or what one genuinely wants to accomplish.

This aspect of self pathology includes passivity and the conviction that one is unable to influence the direction of one's life. However, these

features may not be apparent in the personality disordered individual because they frequently coexist with powerful tendencies to control and
dominate others. Feelings of autonomy grow out of basic trust (Erikson,
1950) that is consolidated during development into beliefs that one has
some control over one's experience and a degree of mastery over one's life
and environment. Psychosocial adversity hinders the emergence of agency
and autonomy. At the same time, impoverished self-knowledge enhances
feelings that things are outside one's control. Patients often dread losing
what little sense of autonomy they possess. This precariousness makes close
relationships especially threatening: They engender primitive fears of being
overwhelmed, taken over, and engulfed—feelings that are further intensified by boundary problems. A passive–aggressive variant is fear of losing
autonomy and independence. Therapeutic relationships therefore constitute a serious threat. Patients with borderline features react to this fear by
alternating between overinvolvement and withdrawal, those with more
schizoid traits by withdrawal and noninvolvement.

IMPLICATIONS FOR TREATMENT

The idea that personality disorder involves core failures common to all
cases suggests a simple model in which individual differences are organized
around core self and interpersonal pathology (Figure 2.6). This model suggests another principle for organizing treatment:

> *Basic Principle: Treatment involves (1) general strategies for managing
> and treating core self and interpersonal pathology, and (2) specific
> strategies for managing and treating individual differences in problems
> and psychopathology.*

With this approach, treatment is organized around general strategies designed to manage the consequences of adaptive failures and promote integration. Specific interventions, which are more concerned with directly
changing pathology, are inserted into this framework, as required, to treat
individual differences in symptoms, maladaptive personality characteristics,
and other problems specific to the individual. Thus the treatment model is
isomorphic with the model of personality disorder.

Conceptualizing treatment in terms of general and specific strategies
suggests that the same general strategies may be used to treat all forms of
personality disorder in all settings (with the possible exception of extreme
psychopathy). The emphasis on general features contrasts with that of
most treatments, which tend to highlight individual differences and recommend different approaches for different DSM-IV personality disorders.
Effective treatment, however, requires careful attention to managing core

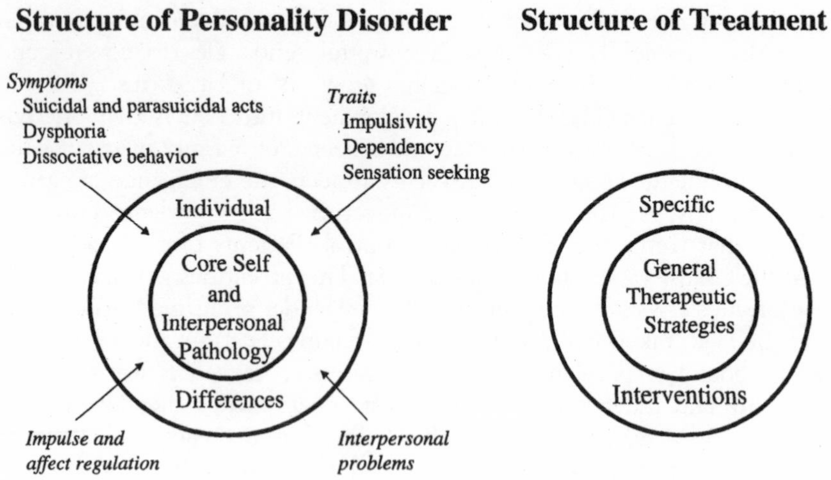

Structure of Personality Disorder   **Structure of Treatment**

Symptoms
Suicidal and parasuicidal acts   *Traits*
Dysphoria   Impulsivity
Dissociative behavior   Dependency
                                         Sensation seeking

Individual   Specific

Core Self   General
and   Therapeutic
Interpersonal   Strategies
Pathology

Differences   Interventions

Impulse and   *Interpersonal*
affect regulation   *problems*

FIGURE 2.6. The structure of personality disorder and the structure of treatment.

pathology and promoting more adaptive self and interpersonal systems, which, in turn, requires an approach that fosters integration (Ryle, 1997). A combination of interventions delivered separately from each other is unlikely to be effective. Attention has to given to delivering multiple interventions in an organized way that facilitates integration. Later in this chapter and in subsequent chapters, several broad organizing principles and guidelines are suggested to circumvent these problems.

Problems with cooperation and collaboration lead to difficulty in establishing an effective working relationship, and the tendency for maladaptive patterns to disrupt treatment makes it difficult to maintain a consistent therapeutic process. For these reasons, we need to consider the optimal way to manage and treat core pathology. Unfortunately, evaluations of the treatment of personality disorder do not provide much guidance. The general literature on psychotherapy outcome, however, contains useful suggestions. Meta-analyses show similar outcomes across different therapies (Beutler, 1991; Luborsky, Singer, & Luborsky, 1975). This similarity implies that different therapies share common elements associated with successful outcome (Norcross & Newman, 1992). About 40% of outcome effects is due to common factors and about 10% is due to specific factors involving intervention or type of therapy. Patient characteristics account for the remaining effect. This breakdown of efficacy factors suggests the following principle:

> *Basic Principle: Treatment should seek to maximize the effects of common factors.*

The common factors share a relational and supportive component, based on the therapeutic relationship, and a technical component that provides new learning experiences and opportunities to apply new skills (Lambert, 1992; Lambert & Bergen, 1994). As Beutler and Harwood (2000) noted, "therapeutic change is greatest when the therapist is skillful and provides trust, acceptance, acknowledgement, collaboration, and respect for the patient and does so in an environment that both supports risk and provides maximal safety" (p. 56). Research on treatment outcome consistently reveals that the treatment alliance is a major predictor of outcome. Unfortunately, the disclosure of personal information required for therapeutic work demands levels of trust, closeness, and cooperation that are the antithesis of the characteristic relating styles shown by personality disordered individuals. This clinical reality suggests a second reason for emphasizing a common factors approach when treating personality disorder: Because core pathology creates problems in establishing a collaborative working relationship, even more attention needs to be paid to the relationship component of treatment. This formulation leads to the following principle:

Basic Principle: Core pathology is most effectively managed and treated using interventions based on a common factors approach.

An emphasis on the therapeutic relationship is the most effective strategy for building the collaboration required for positive outcomes and to minimize treatment disruptions arising from maladaptive patterns. Clinical observation suggests that supportive and validating interventions—key ingredients of generic treatment—place less pressure on the therapeutic relationship (Winston, Pinsker, & McCullough, 1986), whereas the more confrontational strategies used in some forms of expressive therapy strain the relationship and tend to evoke reactions that adversely affect the alliance (Horowitz & Marmar, 1985).

Given the evidence that supportive interventions are effective in achieving change (Horowitz, 1974; Wallerstein, 1986), it seems that both core pathology and outcome studies point to the importance of this nonspecific component of treatment. Both lines of evidence place the following factors at the center of the treatment process: building a supportive and collaborative relationship, the treatment alliance, validating interventions, building and maintaining a consistent therapeutic process, and fostering motivation. Clearly, systematic attention needs to be given to ways to incorporate the common factors into a set of general therapeutic strategies (Goldfried, 1980, 1982, 1983, 1995).

Core pathology also involves boundary problems that make patients feel vulnerable and exposed in treatment and lead to difficulty in maintaining a consistent therapeutic process and prompt attempts to alter the therapeutic frame. The magnitude of these boundary problems has implications for the frame of therapy, the working relationship, and the way therapy is approached. The ubiquity of boundary problems means that treatment needs to be organized and delivered in ways that reduce the impact of these problems and provide opportunities for patients to learn appropriate boundary functions. These objectives are achieved by giving careful attention to establishing and maintaining an explicit therapeutic frame that establishes the practical and functional boundaries of treatment and provides the structure required to support and contain the treatment process. Another principle emerges from these considerations:

> *Basic Principle: Change results from general and specific interventions and from the way treatment is organized and delivered.*

Often the structure and process of therapy are as important, or even more important, than specific interventions in effecting change, and patients learn much more than what is imparted by the therapist's explicit methods of working (Chessick, 1977). This is especially the case with patients who have core pathology: The structure of treatment and the treatment relationship provide an opportunity for the patient to experience a more adaptive relationship. This gradually draws the patient into ways of relating that counter their maladaptive patterns.

PERSONALITY TRAITS

Traits form the cornerstone of a framework for understanding individual differences in personality and personality disorder. Maladaptive traits define the personality disorders listed in the DSM-IV and the International Statistical Classification of Diseases—10 (ICD-10), and the management of maladaptive traits is central to treatment. Traits also affect the way other problems, including core pathology, are expressed. For these reasons, we need a system to describe clinically important traits. Several models are available, derived from studies of people with normal and disordered personalities. These studies describe personality using anything from two to seven dimensions. Although this variability suggests substantial disagreement regarding the number of traits needed to represent personality adequately, the evidence suggests that only a handful of broad dimensions underlie individual differences in personality (Maddi, 1968) and personality disorder (Mulder & Joyce, 1997). There is also substantial agreement on the more important dimensions.

Normal Personality Traits

Eysenck (1987) suggested that three traits—extroversion, neuroticism, and psychoticism—are sufficient to account for individual variation. Recently, however, attention has focused upon the five-factor model as a unifying conception of normal personality (Goldberg, 1990, 1993; John & Srivastava, 1999; Wiggins, 1996) as well as a framework for classifying personality disorder (Costa & McCrae, 1990; Costa & Widiger, 1994, 2002). Costa and McCrae (1992) labeled these factors Neuroticism, Extroversion, Openness to Experience, Agreeableness, and Conscientiousness. Each higher-order trait is subdivided into six lower-order traits or facets, as follows:

- *Neuroticism:* Anxiety, hostility, depression, self-consciousness, impulsivity, and vulnerability
- *Extroversion:* Warmth, gregariousness, assertiveness, activity, excitement seeking, and positive emotions
- *Openness to Experience:* Fantasy, aesthetics, feelings, actions, ideas, and values
- *Agreeableness:* Trust, straightforwardness, altruism, compliance, modesty, and tender-mindedness
- *Conscientiousness:* Competence, order, dutifulness, achievement striving, self-discipline, and deliberation

Although other trait models have been proposed (Cloninger, 1987, 2000; Cloninger et al., 1993; Zuckerman, 1990), the three- and five-factor approaches are the most influential and have the most empirical support. Substantial overlap exists between the two models: factors of neuroticism and extroversion are common to both, and there is some agreement on psychoticism. According to Eysenck, *psychoticism* does not refer to psychotic features but to a constellation of traits resembling antisocial or psychopathic personality disorder. This factor is represented by the negative pole of agreeableness in the five-factor model.

Personality Disorder Traits

In contrast to these approaches, the DSM-IV uses 10 categories to represent individual differences in personality disorder, each category described by a cluster of traits. Substantial overlap exists among diagnoses, suggesting that personality disorder is best represented by a dimensional system. Eysenck (1987), for example, argued that individual differences in personality disorder could be described adequately using his three-factor model. Similar suggestions also have been made regarding the five-factor framework (Costa & Widiger, 1994, 2002).

The evidence supports a modified version of the five-factor approach. Statistical analyses of personality disorder criteria and traits consistently identify four factors that are similar to the five-factor domains of neuroticism, extroversion (introverted pole), agreeableness (negative pole), and conscientiousness (Austin & Deary, 2000; Clark, Livesley, Schroeder, & Irish, 1996; Livesley, Jang, & Vernon, 1998). The robustness of the four-factor solution across studies led Mulder and Joyce (1997) to describe dimensions of personality disorder in terms of the four A's: asthenic (personal distress), antisocial, asocial, and anankastic (compulsivity). It seems that analyses of people with normal and disordered personality converge on the same broad dimensions. Only openness to experience is not represented, and doubts have been expressed about its value for clinical purposes (Clark et al., 1996; Schroeder, Wormsworth, & Livesley, 1992).

Here the four patterns are labeled and defined as follows:

1. *Emotional dysregulation:* A general tendency toward behavioral disorganization and lability that is manifested by unstable and reactive affects, unstable cognitions, and unstable relationships. Component traits, in approximate order of factor loadings, are: anxiousness, affective lability, cognitive dysregulation, submissiveness, anxious attachment, social avoidance, oppositionality, narcissism, and suspiciousness.

2. *Inhibitedness:* Difficulties expressing emotions and sharing personal information, and avoidance of intimate and social relationships. Component traits are: intimacy problems, restricted expression, and social avoidance.

3. *Dissocial behavior:* Callous disregard for the feelings and concerns of other people and tendencies toward cruelty, sadism, cynicism, and contempt. Component traits are: callousness, rejection (hostile, dominating, and judgmental interpersonal behavior), conduct problems, stimulus seeking (which includes impulsivity), and narcissism.

4. *Compulsivity:* A general need for order and structure. The only component is compulsivity (orderliness, preciseness, and conscientiousness).

In this structure 16 traits define the four patterns, and unlike the five-factor model, the number of traits defining each pattern differs. This difference reflects empirical findings, as does the association between narcissism and emotional dysregulation and dissocial behavior.

Since the four factors have strong empirical support and describe clinically recognizable constellations of psychopathology, they are used throughout this volume to describe individual differences in personality disorder. Readers who are more comfortable with DSM-IV diagnoses should note that the 16 traits cover all criteria defining DSM-IV personality disorders. For example, dependent personality disorder is represented by submissiveness and insecure attachment, and narcissistic and obsessive–compulsive personality disorders are represented by a single dimension. Moreover, the four patterns resemble the more prevalent personality disorder diagnoses and may, for clinical purposes, be considered interchangeable. Emotional dysregulation resembles Cluster B diagnoses, especially borderline personality disorder, and hence will also be referred to as the *borderline pattern*. Inhibition will also be called the *schizoid–avoidant pattern* because it includes the social withdrawal, restricted emotions, and intimacy problems that are important elements of Cluster A diagnoses, especially schizoid personality disorder and avoidant personality disorder. Although the dissocial pattern resembles antisocial personality disorder, it is also referred to as the *psychopathic pattern* because the closest resemblance is with psychopathy as described by Cleckley (1976) and Hare (1991). Finally, compulsivity is also described as the *obsessive–compulsive pattern* because it clearly resembles compulsive personality disorder. Despite the resemblance to DSM-IV diagnoses, these patterns are not discrete categories, in the DSM-IV sense, but rather broad dimensions that are continuous with normal personality variation. Patients with personality disorder may show features of several or even all patterns.

The four patterns are a parsimonious way to discuss the treatment of different forms of personality disorder. The borderline or emotional dysregulation pattern will be considered in detail because it is the most prevalent and encompasses an extensive array of features. Strategies for treating this pattern cover a wide range of pathology and most forms of disorder. Empirical studies show that the traits defining emotional dysregulation are associated with all DSM-IV personality disorders (Bagge & Trull, 2003; Pukrop, Steinbring, Gentil, Schulte, & Klosterkötter, 2002), as is neuroticism (Clarkin, Hull, Cantor, & Sanderson, 1993). The schizoid–avoidant or inhibited pattern offers an important contrast to emotional dysregulation. Together these patterns provide an opportunity to discuss the management of most aspects of personality psychopathology. The dissocial or psychopathic pattern is discussed in less detail because a moderate level of this pattern may be treated similarly to emotional dysregulation. However, the management of extreme levels of this pattern, which occurs in prototypically psychopathic individuals, is not discussed because they may not respond to current therapeutic interventions. Finally, compulsivity is discussed only briefly because it does not appear to be as pervasive or dysfunctional as the other patterns (Livesley, 1998).

PATTERNS OF PERSONALITY DISORDER

Emotional Dysregulation: The Borderline Pattern

The hallmark of emotional dysregulation is instability in emotions, interpersonal relationships, cognitive functioning, and sense of self. The pattern is organized around two core emotional traits: *affective lability*, which involves unstable and reactive moods, including labile anger, and *anxiousness*, manifested by a lifelong tendency to worry and ruminate and to feel guilt for little reason. Often the emotional core includes hypersensitivity—a tendency to experience everything intensely, so that emotions and other forms of stimulation feel intrusive and overwhelming. This emotional core is associated with *cognitive dysregulation*, a tendency toward confused and disorganized thinking, especially in times of stress. In more severe cases, cognitive disorganization may include experiences of depersonalization, derealization, and schizotypal cognitions, as well as the tendency to experience brief psychotic episodes. The pattern also includes the interpersonal traits of *submissiveness, insecure attachment, social avoidance,* and, to a lesser degree, *oppositionality.*

Several additional traits, most notably *narcissism* and occasionally *suspiciousness*, are associated with emotional dysregulation and the dissocial or psychopathic pattern, although the association with emotional dysregulation is not strong. Narcissism, when present, leads to the dramatic expression of feelings, whereas suspiciousness tends to encourage more reactive, distrustful behaviors.

Core Pathology

Ever-changing emotions contribute to unstable self and person representations and uncertainty about personal characteristics, leading to a fragmented self structure characterized by major self-state disjunctions and poorly integrated representations of others. Intense, reactive emotions along with strong dependency needs also encourage enmeshed and unstable relationships and problems with interpersonal boundaries.

The traits comprising emotional dysregulation and associated core pathology intermesh to form a structure that is "stably unstable" (Schmideberg, 1947). Much of the stability of the self derives from a perceived continuity of experience that depends on a consistent affective experience. Labile and reactive affects, driven by constitutional factors, create a continually changing affective experience that is not conducive to the development of a coherent self or stable relationships. At the same time, instability in the self increases affective lability: people with more differentiated and complex self schemata generally show less variability in mood (Singer, Sincott, & Kollinen, 1989), and complex self schemata are less susceptible to fluctuations due to shifts in affect (Linville, 1982). A stable sense of self seems to provide a broad perspective on events that allows the individual to view affect changes as short-term phenomena against a background of stable life experiences. Without this perspective, the individual tends to focus solely on immediate experience. This tunnel vision exacerbates emotional responses and creates a positive feedback system.

Other components of emotional dysregulation contribute to this instability. Ever-changing wants, driven by affective lability and an unstable self, lead to unstable relationships. These, in turn, increase affective lability and contribute to an unstable self. A stable self comes, in part, from the reflected appraisals of others not only during development but also throughout life (Sullivan, 1947). Without consistent feedback from a stable social matrix, self-appraisals fluctuate. Tendencies toward cognitive dysregulation exacerbate these problems. When the world looks different or the ability to process information is impaired, self-perceptions change dramatically. At the same time, a reduction in coping due to cognitive disorganization reduces control over affects and impulses, thereby intensifying interpersonal problems and creating the conditions for the crises that are common with these patients and contributes to self problems. The result of this pattern is a structure that is remarkably stable yet prone to behavioral instability.

Relationship to Other Constructs

The broad array of features delineating emotional dysregulation that emerges from empirical research is consistent with clinical observations that most patients with borderline personality disorder meet the criteria for other personality disorders. This convergence suggests that the DSM-IV borderline personality disorder diagnosis is artificially circumscribed to distinguish it from other diagnoses. As Berkelowitz and Tarnopolsky (1993) concluded, the disorder is probably more an indication of severe personality dysfunction than a distinct diagnostic entity. The factor of emotional dysregulation is similar in breadth to Kernberg's (1984) concept of borderline personality organization, which encompasses schizoid, paranoid, borderline, antisocial, and some narcissistic and dependent personality disorders. The factor also resembles Linehan's (1993) description of borderline personality disorder in terms of emotional, interpersonal, behavioral, cognitive, and self dysregulation. The conceptualization of emotional dysregulation concurs with Linehan's argument that emotional dysregulation is the core feature of borderline pathology. Others have suggested, however, that the core feature is impulsivity (Links, Heslegrave, & van Reekum, 1999). Within the current framework, many impulsive acts, such as deliberate self-harm, are considered secondary to emotional dysregulation: They often represent attempts to regulate dysphoria. Moreover, many so-called impulsive acts are planned; some patients anticipate when and how they are next going to harm themselves. Impulsivity seems to be more complex than is usually recognized (Parker & Bagby, 1997).

Inhibitedness: The Schizoid–Avoidant Pattern

Inhibitedness is characterized by fearful and socially inhibited behavior that affects all aspects of personal and interpersonal life. The core features are *intimacy problems* and *restricted expression of inner experience, including feelings.* Underlying these traits is a fear of closeness. Other people are perceived as intrusive; these individuals feel overwhelmed, drained, or engulfed by others—feelings that are increased when the other person appears needy or demanding.

The behaviors defining *restricted expression* are difficult to label succinctly. They include difficultly showing feelings, a reluctance to discuss or disclose personal information, and a preference for self-reliance or self-sufficiency. Such individuals may appear unemotional and even cold. However, as Kretschmer (1925) noted, many schizoid individuals are also exquisitely hypersensitive (a trait that is also associated with emotional dysregulation), although this response is usually hidden beneath a mask of restricted affective expression. The lack of social and emotional responsiveness often irritates others, who respond by being even more intrusive and demanding a response. This reaction is something therapists need to avoid because it merely leads to further the patient's withdrawal.

Restricted expression is consistent with *intimacy problems.* Emotions establish bonds; it is difficult to be close to someone who does not show feelings. Many inhibited or schizoid individuals are also secretive (Fairbairn, 1952) because they feel exposed and vulnerable if they reveal information about the self. One inhibited man tried to reveal as little about himself as possible because he felt that any action could reveal information that might be used to judge him. He was even reluctant to introduce a girlfriend to other people because the impression she created would reflect on him, and his choice of girlfriend could reveal information about himself to them. Similarly, he worried about selecting clothes lest his choice reveal too much personal information. Excessive *self-reliance* is consistent with these concerns. Such individuals seek to be self-sufficient because they are afraid of revealing themselves through their needs. Care- or help-seeking behavior is also avoided because it requires contact with other people.

Like emotional dysregulation, the inhibited or schizoid–avoidant pattern strongly influences the expression of core pathology. Two major problems are *difficulties with interpersonal boundaries* and a *lack of authenticity.* Many also experience *real self–false self disjunctions.* Boundary problems are illustrated by feelings of vulnerability that occur with any interpersonal encounter. Such patients comment that they feel engulfed by others and are unable to protect themselves from others' needs and demands; hence they withdraw either physically or into a "shell" of their own making. As one patient expressed it, "It feels as if I don't have a skin. People get right through to me." Another patient found group therapy intolerable. Although he said very little and group members thought that he was cold and unresponsive, he found it extremely painful to listen to their problems. Between meetings, he worried constantly about others in the group. Eventually he left the group because he was unable to tolerate the worry. As is typical of these patients, he did not give a reason for his decision, and most group members thought that he left because he was uninterested and uninvolved. With some individuals, there is also the reciprocal fear that their needs will overwhelm others. In the language of object relations theory, they fear that their love will be damaging (Fairbairn, 1952; Guntrip, 1968).

A further feature of self pathology that has important implications in treatment is *lack of authenticity*: the experience that one's feelings and thoughts are not genuine and that the self presented to the world is not genuine but rather a facade. This experience of inauthenticity seems to be related to the cleavage between cognition and emotion that characterizes all aspects of mental life, leading to a concomitant uncertainty about all aspects of experience and to an impoverished self-concept. Many inhibited individuals find it difficult to describe themselves in any depth, as if there were an inner blankness and uncertainty in place of a sense of selfhood. This problem with self-definition is seen most clearly in additional problems with self-directedness: Many of these individuals fail to establish a coherent sense of direction and purpose in life.

Dissocial Behavior: The Psychopathic Pattern

The essential feature of this pattern is disregard for other people, often combined with conduct problems and antisocial behavior. Moderate levels of dissocial behavior are observed in many cases of personality disorder. Antagonism, callousness, and disregard for others are common traits that have major consequences for treatment planning and choice of treatment modality. For example, such individuals are often difficult to treat in heterogeneous groups because their callousness makes them insensitive to others.

The core features of this pattern are *callousness* and *rejection*. *Callousness* consists of lack of empathy, little concern for other people, lack of remorse for the way one's actions may adversely affect other people, exploitativeness, a tendency to view relationships in an egocentric way, and sadistic pleasure in the suffering and humiliation of others. *Rejection* includes hostile, dominating behavior and a judgmental attitude. These characteristics are also associated with a rigid cognitive style. The core traits are associated *conduct problems*—disregard for society's rules, tendencies toward violence, and drug and alcohol misuse. The idea that a dissocial pattern involves interpersonal traits and antisocial behavior is consistent with the finding that two factors underlie the Psychopathy Checklist (Hare, 1991)—an interpersonal component defined by traits such as callousness and entitlement, and a behavioral component defined by antisocial acts (Harpur, Hakstian, & Hare, 1988). Although the two components are correlated, they can occur separately. Not all individuals who are at the extremes of callousness and rejection show high levels of conduct problems.

Statistical analyses show that three additional traits are often associated with the dissocial pattern: *narcissism*, *suspiciousness*, and *stimulus seek-*

ing. Narcissism and suspiciousness were discussed in the section on the emotional dysregulation pattern. The association between antisocial personality disorder and narcissism has been extensively described in the literature (Hare & Hart, 1995). It seems that the grandiose component of narcissism is more closely linked with dissocial behavior, whereas the attention-seeking component tends to be more closely associated with emotional dysregulation. Not surprisingly, the tendency to treat others in a contemptuous and hostile way is sometimes associated with suspiciousness about the intent and actions of others. Stimulus seeking includes sensation seeking, recklessness, and impulsivity. These traits increase maladaptive responses to affect arousal because impulsive and self-harming behaviors often provide relief from acute distress and satisfy the need for stimulation and excitement. For these reasons, stimulus-seeking behavior is also observed in some patients who have the emotionally dysregulated pattern. The trait tends to amplify maladaptive expressions of other traits and leads to more reckless and impulsive forms of conduct problems.

The dissocial pattern is less clearly related to specific features of core self and interpersonal pathology than the other patterns. In terms of the defining features of personality disorder, it is probable that the dissocial pattern largely affects the interpersonal and societal components of core pathology: There are major difficulties in establishing attachment relationships, in functioning effectively as an attachment figure, and with prosocial behavior.

Compulsivity: The Obsessive–Compulsive Pattern

This pattern, which is less pervasive than the other higher-order patterns, consists of a tightly delineated cluster of traits: *orderliness*, *preciseness*, and *conscientiousness*. From a clinical perspective, compulsivity probably predisposes the person to a variety of Axis I disorders, including major depression and anxiety disorders. When it occurs in the absence of extreme scores on other trait dimensions, it is rarely associated with severe personality pathology. Its significance for treating personality disorder arises when it occurs in association with other higher-order patterns or extreme scores on other basic traits. Moderate levels of compulsivity may be beneficial. Kernberg (1984), for example, noted that borderline (emotionally dysregulated) patients with compulsive tendencies tend to respond better to treatment than those who are less compulsive.

COMMENT

This overview suggests that a simple descriptive analysis of normal and disordered personality, without major theoretical assumptions or postulates, is sufficient to determine the broad outlines of treatment. The wide range of structures and processes that comprise the personality system draws attention to the need for a combination of interventions, which, in turn, sets the structure of treatment and creates the need for a framework to manage multiple interventions. A model of personality disorder that describes (1) core features characterizing all cases, and (2) individual differences in symptoms, problems, and traits that are organized around this core leads directly to a treatment model involving (1) general therapeutic strategies based on generic change mechanisms, and (2) specific interventions to manage and treat discrete problems and individual differences in personality pathology. This model also has significant implications for diagnosis: It suggests that diagnosis has two components: (1) the diagnosis of personality disorder, and (2) the assessment of individual differences in personality and psychopathology.

CHAPTER 3

The Origins of Personality Disorder

This chapter continues to lay the foundations for an evidence-based approach by examining the way current knowledge about the origins of personality disorder helps to identify appropriate intervention strategies and define the changes we seek to achieve in treatment. Although knowledge about the origins of personality pathology has increased in recent years, it remains fragmented and rudimentary. Nevertheless, an understanding of the known factors involved helps to shape an approach to treatment. Evidence that personality disorder arises from a complex array of psychosocial and biological factors implies that psychosocial and biological inventions may contribute to change. However, no single psychosocial or biological factor is either necessary or sufficient to cause personality disorder. Instead, disorder arises from the cumulative effects of multiple factors, each having only a small effect. Under these circumstances, it is somewhat misleading to speak of the *causes* of personality disorder (Livesley, 1999; Paris, 2001). Instead it is more helpful to think about *the factors that increase the risk of developing personality disorder*. When considering these factors, our concern is not to review them in detail but rather to identify general etiological and developmental principles that are relevant to treatment.

PSYCHOSOCIAL FACTORS

The common assumption that adverse life experiences are important etiological factors is supported by numerous studies documenting the effects of multiple factors, including familial dysfunction, traumatic experiences, and social stressors (Paris, 2001). It does not appear, however, that adversity invariably leads to personality disorder, nor is there a relationship between the kind of adversity experienced and the form of personality disorder that ensues. Instead adversity appears to have a relatively nonspecific effect on psychopathology. Moreover, the effects of psychosocial factors are more complex than originally thought. Earlier studies of clinical samples without comparison information overestimated the effects of adversity. Community studies show that adversity does not invariably lead to psychopathology. The effects of adversity appear to be modulated by factors that influence vulnerability and resilience. This finding suggests that the treatment of the consequences of adversity should seek to modulate the traits, such as anxiousness and inhibitedness, that are known to contribute to adverse outcomes.

Familial Dysfunction

Family breakdown, parental psychopathology, and various forms of parenting behavior are associated with personality disorder (Paris, 2001). Borderline and antisocial personality disorders and antisocial characteristics such as aggression and criminality have been studied the most. The results indicate that *family breakdown* is a risk factor for borderline personality disorder (Paris, Zweig-Frank, & Guzder, 1994a, 1994b), although the effects of specific forms of breakdown (e.g., parental loss) are inconsistent with some studies reporting an increased incidence (Bradley, 1979; Links, Steiner, Offord, & Eppel, 1988; Paris, Nowlis, & Brown, 1988; Soloff & Milward, 1983) and others not finding a significant relationship (Ogata et al., 1990; Paris et al., 1994a; Zanarini, Gunderson, & Marino, 1989).

Evidence that *parental psychopathology* increases the risk of developing personality problems is most extensive for dissocial and antisocial traits. Aggressive and antisocial behavior runs in families (Jary & Stewart, 1985; Mednick, Moffit, Gabrielli, & Hutchings, 1986; Miles & Carey, 1997; Rowe, Rodgers, & Meseck-Bushey, 1992): Antisocial and psychopathic features in a parent strongly predict antisocial traits in the child (Cadoret, 1978; Robins, 1966). Similarly, the relatives of patients with borderline personality disorder show more features of impulsivity, such as characterizes borderline or antisocial personality, as well as substance abuse (Links, Steiner, & Huxley, 1988; Zanarini, 1993) and an increased prevalence of mood disorders (Nigg & Goldsmith, 1994). These familial patterns seem to be the product of both genetic and environmental influences. For example, in one study, adopted children who have a biological parent with antisocial personality disorder were more likely to show antisocial behavior when there was significant adversity in the adoptive family (Cloninger, Sigvardsson, Bohman, & van Knorring, 1982). Similarly, a meta-analysis of 24 genetic studies (Miles & Carey, 1997) showed that both family environment and genetic factors influence the prevalence of aggressive behavior in youths.

Two types of *parenting behavior* are also associated with borderline personality disorder: neglectful (as opposed to loving and supportive) and overprotective (as opposed to encouraging independence and autonomy) (Frank & Paris, 1981; Paris & Frank, 1992; Torgersen & Alnaes, 1992; Zweig-Frank & Paris, 1991). These studies relied on retrospective recall of childhood events; such recall may be biased by the effect of psychopathology. However, similar findings were reported in a community study using more objective information about neglect and abuse, such as court records (Johnson, Cohen, Brown, Smailes, & Bernstein, 1999).

Emotional maltreatment by parents may involve emotional abuse (verbal assaults and demeaning comments) or emotional neglect (the failure of caregivers to meet the child's needs for love, nurturance, and support). Both form separate factors that are moderately correlated with other forms of maltreatment (Bernstein & Fink, 1998). Emotional neglect in childhood was related to self-harming behavior in hospitalized adolescents (Lipschitz, Bernstein, Winegar, & Southwick, 1999) and to schizoid personality disorder in male drug-dependent patients (Bernstein, Stein, & Handelsman, 1999). Emotional abuse had greater and more widespread effects than sexual abuse: it was related to all three clusters of DSM-III–R personality disorders (Bernstein et al., 1998).

Physical and Sexual Abuse

Patients with personality disorder generally report having experienced high levels of all forms of abuse. Physical abuse increases the risk of various personality problems (Johnson et al., 1999), including antisocial personality disorder (Pollock et al., 1990); 25–73% of patients with borderline personality disorder report severe physical abuse (Zanarini, 2000) and verbal abuse (Zanarini et al., 1989).

Most attention has been paid to the relationship between sexual abuse and borderline personality disorder. Upwards of 70% of patients with borderline personality give a history of abuse (Byrne, Cernovsky, Velamoor, Coretese, & Losztyn, 1990; Herman, Perry, & van der Kolk, 1989; Links et al., 1988; Ludolph, Westen, & Misle, 1990; Ogata et al., 1990; Paris et al., 1994a, 1994b; Paris & Zweig-Frank, 1992; Perry & Herman, 1993; Westen, Ludolph, Misle, Ruffins, & Block, 1990; Zanarini, 2000; Zanarini et al., 1989; for reviews, see Gunderson & Sabo, 1993; Paris, 1994; Sabo, 1997). These findings prompted the conclusion that trauma is a major etiological factor for borderline personality disorder (Herman & van der Kolk, 1987). Such a conclusion, however, does not appear to be supported by the evidence (Paris, 2001; Rutter & Maughan, 1997). A meta-analysis of 21 studies involving 2,479 subjects found only a moderate association between childhood sexual abuse and borderline personality disorder (Fossati, Madeddu, & Maffei, 1999). Sexual abuse appears to be only one of many risk factors, and it is not specific to borderline personality disorder. A strong association also occurs with narcissistic, histrionic, sadistic, and schizotypal traits (Norden, Klein, Donaldson, & Pepper, 1995) and antisocial behavior (Pollock et al., 1990). In one study, 73% of patients with borderline personality disorder reported sexual abuse compared with 53% of patients with other personality disorders (Paris et al., 1994a, 1994b). Nor is abuse necessary for the development of borderline personality disorder. After reviewing the literature, Paris (1994, 2001) concluded that about one-third of patients with borderline personality disorder report severe abuse involving an incestuous perpetrator, severe sexual acts, and high frequency or duration; about one-third report milder forms of abuse that do not necessarily lead to psychopathology in community samples; and about one-third do not report abuse.

Studies of the prevalence and effects of sexual trauma in general population samples are a further reason for caution in assuming that abuse causes personality disorder. Many individuals who report abusive experiences do not develop personality disorder or other forms of psychopathology (Paris, 1994). Moreover, community studies suggest that the effect of sexual abuse depends on the identity of the perpetrator, the nature of the abusive act, and the duration of abusive experiences (Browne & Finkelhor, 1986; Finkelhor, Hotaling, Lewis, & Smith, 1990).

Invalidating Environments

Theorists from different perspectives note that the experience of *invalidation* is an important consequence of adversity. Kohut (1971), for example, noted the significance of empathic failure and inadequate mirroring for the development of the self; Linehan (1993) described the role of invalidating environments in the development of borderline personality disorder. Although empirical evidence of the significance of invalidating experiences is minimal, clinical evidence supports these ideas.

Invalidating experiences may be active or passive in nature. *Active invalidation* occurs when others behave in an invalidating way, such that the child's feelings, thoughts, or actions are not accepted, not taken seriously, dismissed, trivialized, or rejected as socially undesirable, and when the child is told he or she is wrong or bad for having such thoughts or feelings. It also occurs when the child's experience is denied and the child is told what he or she should be thinking or feeling (Linehan & Kehrer, 1993). Abusive acts invalidate the recipient by ignoring personal boundaries, needs, and wishes, and by violating expectations of autonomy, respect, and freedom of choice. The impact of active abusive acts is increased when they are portrayed as acts of love or caring that should not be revealed to anyone.

Passive invalidation involves the failure to show the positive regard and mirroring needed to develop a sense of worth or basic trust. Its effects may be as pervasive as that of active invalidation.

The individual's traits may increase the risk of experiencing invalidation. For example, individuals with the emotional dysregulation (borderline) pattern are likely to feel invalidated because others do not understand the intensity of their feelings (Robins, Ivanoff, & Linehan, 2001); similarly, the emotional unresponsiveness of inhibited (schizoid–avoidant) individuals is likely to elicit invalidating behavior from others, such as irritation and frustration because people do not recognize that the individual is not deliberately unresponsive and withholding but lacks the ability to relate emotionally.

Consequences of Adversity

Although the evidence suggests that adversity contributes to the development of personality disorder, there is limited evidence as to how this development occurs (Rutter & Maughan, 1997). Nevertheless, an understanding of the mechanisms through which adversity exerts a lasting influence on adaptive functioning is crucial for effective treatment. The presence of three factors seems to be important (Figure 3.1): traumatic memories, the symptomatic consequences of trauma, and effects on personality structures and processes. First, adverse experiences lay down *traumatic memories* that color feelings about the self and lead to conflicted relationships. Given the extent to which dysfunctional relationships are reported in the histories of most personality disordered patients, a considerable amount of treatment time is likely to be spent working through these experiences and resolving conflicts with specific individuals. Second, severe trauma gives rise to enduring symptoms, including *reexperiencing or intrusive symptoms* such as flashbacks, unwanted thoughts, images of trauma and associated events, recurring, ruminative thoughts, and nightmares; *symptoms of hyperarousal* such as hypervigilance, anger, irritability, increased startle response, sleep disturbance, and impaired concentration; and *avoidant behaviors* consisting of decreased interest, emotional numbness, restricted affect, feeling detached from others, and avoidance of thoughts, feelings, and experiences associated with event. The prevalence of these symptoms in patients with personality disorder prompted the suggestion that some disorders, most notably borderline personality disorder, are forms of chronic posttraumatic stress disorder (Herman, 1992). However, posttraumatic stress disorder is not identical to personality disorder generally or borderline personality disorder, in particular (Kroll, 1993). Personality pathology involves more

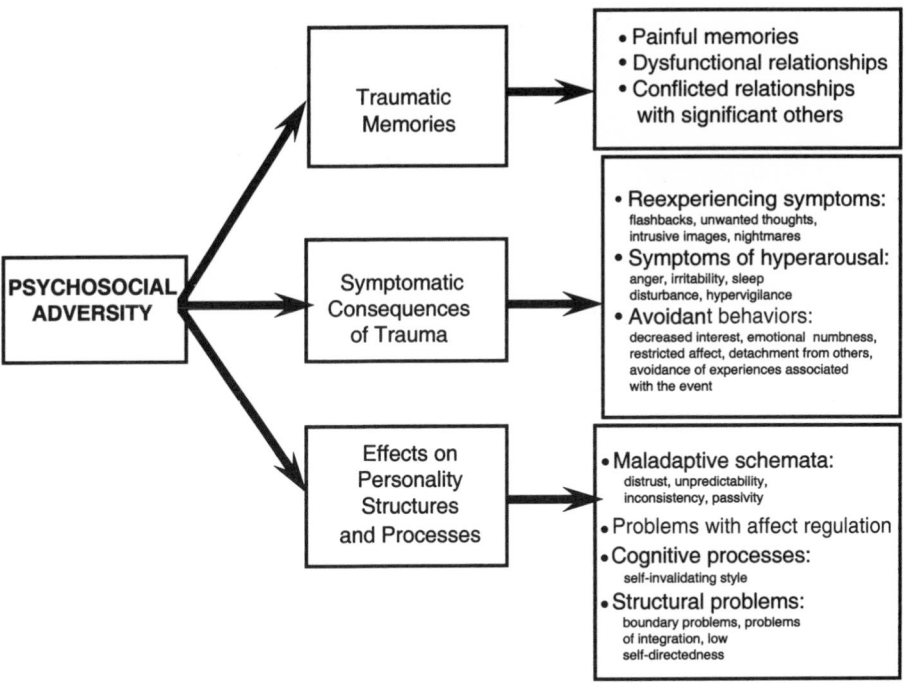

FIGURE 3.1. The effects of psychosocial adversity.

than the symptoms of trauma. Although the direct consequences of abuse are important, they are not the whole story.

Third, repeated exposure to adversity affects all aspects of the personality system. Adversity influences the *schemata* developed to understand the self, others, and the world and associated interpersonal patterns and the capacity for affect regulation. It also affects *cognitive processes* and leads to *structural* problems in the personality system through its influence on interpersonal boundaries and the organization of self-knowledge.

Schemata

Trauma and adversity lead to negative interpersonal expectancies (Meyer & Carver, 2000) and maladaptive schemata that shape responses to others and create self-fulfilling prophecies that are part of the repetitive patterns of maladaptive interpersonal behavior that characterize personality disorder. Because maladaptive schemata develop in the context of adversity, they incorporate intense affects and traumatic memories.

Although adverse experiences affect individuals differently, according to the individual personality, similarities in these experiences are likely to lead to schemata organized around such issues as trust–distrust, abandonment, lovability, unpredictability, powerlessness, and incompetence. Young and colleagues (Bricker, Young, & Flanagan, 1993; Young, 1990, 1994) described 15 maladaptive schemata that are organized into four domains:

I.   *Autonomy:* Dependence, subjugation/lack of individuation, vulnerability to harm and illness, and fear of losing control
II. *Connectedness:* Emotional deprivation, abandonment/loss, mistrust, and social isolation/alienation
III. *Worthiness:* Defectiveness/unlovability, social undesirability, incompetence/failure, guilt/punishment, and shame/embarrassment
IV. *Expectations and Limits:* Unrelenting standards, and entitlement/insufficient limits.

Subsequent analysis of a version of the Schema Questionnaire (Young, 1994) developed to assess these schemata identified three factors: *loss of interpersonal relations*, defined by schemata of abandonment, abuse, emotional deprivation, mistrust, personal defectiveness, emotional inhibition, and fear of losing control; *social dependence*, defined by functional dependence, enmeshment, vulnerability, and incompetence/inferiority; and *perfectionism*, defined by unrelenting standards and self-sacrifice (Schmidt, Joiner, Young, & Telch, 1995).

Schemata are influenced by the kind of adversity experienced. Severe physical, sexual, and emotional abuse, for example, are likely to result in schemata related to defectiveness, shame, emotional dyscontrol, mistrust, victimization, humiliation, and vulnerability, whereas physical and emotional neglect and deprivation tend to evoke schemata related to deprivation, abandonment, isolation, and basic distrust that one's needs will be met. Maladaptive schemata do not, however, show specific relationships with given personality diagnoses (Petrocelli, Glaser, Calhoun, & Campbell, 2001). Schemata defining the first two factors, loss of interpersonal relations and social dependence, occur in most forms of personality disorder. Especially important for treatment and the therapeutic relationship are schemata related to core pathology. These include schemata related to attachment and intimacy (trust, abandonment, rejection, closeness), validation, predictability of human behavior, competence or worth (incompetence or failure, defectiveness or fundamental flaws in the self, and social desirability), and cooperation and prosocial behavior.

Distrust. Some of the more pervasive consequences of adversity are due to the development of distrust. Negative expectations about the responsiveness and availability of attachment figures to meet one's needs develop into the "working models" of attachment relationships that adversely affect social relationships throughout life (Bowlby, 1973). Distrust also leads to difficulty in being cooperative, a quality basic to prosocial behavior. Individuals engaged in cooperation assist each other to obtain the same end (Hinde & Groebel, 1991). Cooperation depends upon mutual expectations that the other in the relationship can be trusted to meet his or her obligations and commitments. Adversity hinders the development of this degree of confidence in others, leading to characteristic unwillingness to engage in cooperative behavior and the need to control others.

The effect of adversity on attachment and intimacy is likely to be influenced by the person's traits. Individuals with the inhibited (schizoid–avoidant) pattern are likely to form schemata involving the avoidance of attachment and intimacy. Those with emotional dysregulation (borderline) traits are more likely to form fearful attachments, and feelings of security are likely to depend on the physical presence of the attachment figures. These individuals fail to establish a "working model" of others as available and dependable (Bowlby, 1971), leaving them fearful, needy, and dependent. Patients with dissocial (psychopathic) traits are likely to have difficulty acquiring the behaviors and attitudes required to function as responsible caregivers; egocentric traits lead to their own needs taking priority over those of others and to difficulty delaying personal gratification in order to provide for those dependent upon them. Despite these differences, each pattern is characterized by the failure to acquire adaptive attachment behavior and the capacity for intimacy. It is this failure, as much as the form that the failure takes, that leads to relationship problems.

Problems with trust arise from both deprivation and abuse, although the ways distrust is expressed may differ according to whether deprivation or abuse predominated. Clinical opinion suggests that trauma is activating, whereas deprivation tends to evoke apathy and resignation. Giovacchini (1979) distinguishes between deprivation and "privation." He suggests that borderline (emotionally dysregulated) patients are unable to form expectations of helpful relationships because they were not gratified early in life. He refers to this as *privation*, as distinct from deprivation, because such individuals do not know what it is like to be gratified and hence have not formed images (schemata) of gratification. This absence of appropriate schemata leads to difficulty with self-soothing and self-regulating affects.

Unpredictability. An important feature of adversity is that it is inconsistent. Many abusive individuals are unpredictable; they are abusive on one occasion and caring on another. Abusive acts by caregivers are often associated with changes in mental state that are difficult for the child to predict. Anyone who has treated the children of alcoholic and abusive parents is familiar with the fearfulness, bordering on terror, of the child who waits for a parent to come home from a drinking episode, not knowing whether he or she will be in a loving or abusive frame of mind. Since abusers are often people with whom the child has an affectional bond, their actions create the sense that other people, and life generally, are unpredictable. Given the lack of adequate models for understanding stable relationships, combined with dispositional tendencies toward instability, it is not surprising that many patients with personality disorder are themselves extremely unpredictable, form unstable relationships, and live chaotic lives.

Powerlessness. The unpredictability of abusive parents invariably leads children to feel powerless and to form beliefs that nothing can be done to control or change events that influence one's well-being. Over time, these feelings and beliefs crystallize into a loosely structured set of schemata that incorporate a sense of powerlessness, doubts about competence or self-efficacy (Bandura 1977, 1982), and beliefs that the locus of control is external to the self (Rotter, 1966). These schemata contribute to the feeling that one's life is fated to be a certain way. Passivity and problems with self-directedness often emerge, further affecting the perceived cohesiveness of the self and forming major obstacles to change. Beliefs about powerlessness and a perceived lack of control over one's life also increase dysphoria and distress; people deal with stress better when they feel a sense of agency (Heckhausen & Schulz, 1995; Skinner, 1996; Taylor, 1983; Thompson & Spacaman, 1991).

Some patients compensate for their feeling of powerlessness by developing the belief that everything is their fault; they harbor a painful sense of responsibility for all the terrible things that have happened to them or those they love. These feelings, although painful, are often less overwhelming than feeling that there is nothing they can do to alter a terrible situation; indeed, the feelings offer the comfort of believing that if only one had done something differently, another outcome may have occurred. This perspective replaces the pain of helplessness and vulnerability and offers the illusion of being in control.

Cognitive and Regulating Processes

Repeated adversity and dysfunctional relationships not only affect the contents of thought but also influence (1) the development of cognitive processes that shape the way information is processed, and (2) self-regulatory mechanisms that control emotions and impulses. General *cognitive processes* influence information management by increasing sensitivity to specific events and biasing the way information is interpreted. For example, parental physical abuse leads the child to be hypervigilant to hostile behavior, attribute hostile intent to others more readily, and evaluate the consequences of aggression more favorably (Dodge, Pettit, Bates, & Valente,

1995). One of the most pervasive ways adversity influences development is through the formation of a *self-invalidating cognitive style* that causes individuals to question the authenticity of their feelings, ideas, and experiences. This insidious doubt hinders the development of an adaptive self system and makes it difficult to establish goals and develop a sense of agency. Invalidation of achievements or attempts to attain personal goals undermines self-esteem and beliefs about self-efficacy, thereby promoting self-doubt and dependency. Similarly, invalidation of wants and preferences—for example, by telling children that they are inappropriate or wrong—hinders the formation of a stable conception of the self because early stable preferences help to define who one is.

It is also evident from clinical observation that abuse and associated attachment problems impair the development of *self-regulatory mechanisms* that control affects and impulses. Early relationships, especially those with attachment figures, are central to the development of emotional regulation (Bradley, 2000; Schore, 1994). The important factor is the caregiver's sensitivity to the child's emotional states. Sensitive caregiving modulates the level of emotion experienced by the child and helps the child to avoid the extremes of emotional states (Emde, 1989). In the earliest stages of development, the child's emotions are regulated by the caregiver's sensitive responses to the child's distress. In the process, the infant learns that actions can be taken to reduce distress. Gradually, infants learn how to regulate their own distress and take an increasing role in managing their feelings (Sroufe, 1991). This initial learning is an early precursor to beliefs of self-efficacy and positive expectations (hope) that distress will dissipate. Furthermore, it forms the template for developing self-regulatory mechanisms and contributes to expectations that the environment is predictable (Gable & Isabella, 1992; Sroufe, 1989a, 1989b). Inadequate caregiving, in contrast, leads to the schemata of unpredictability, noted earlier, which are increased in the child who is also exposed to abuse. At the same time, sensitive caregiving also lays down precursors for feelings of self-worth and self-esteem, which are especially reinforced when complemented by positive mirroring, as described by Kohut. The quality of these early relationship experiences has widespread effects. The occurrence of adversity not only produces negative schemata that influence self and interpersonal functioning but also hinder the development of positive schemata and control mechanisms.

Support for the importance of caregiver behavior for the development of affect regulation is provided by evidence that sensitive caregiving correlates with higher levels of positive affect, lower levels of negative affect, greater self-esteem, and greater social competence (Suess, Grossman, & Sroufe, 1992) in the child, and with more emotional openness and the capacity to label and share feelings (Greenberg, Kusche, & Speltz, 1992). Similarly insensitive caregiving is associated with more negative affect (anger and anxiety) and lower social competence and self-esteem (Suess et al., 1992).

The effects of adversity appear greatest when they occur in the context of predispositions for affective lability and impulsivity. Psychosocial factors appear to increase emotional dysregulation by amplifying the effects of genetic predispositions and hindering the acquisition of emotion-regulating mechanisms and skills. The interaction of genetic predisposition and adversity lead to serious deficits in the self-regulation of emotions that need to be addressed in treatment.

Personality Structure and Coherence

Adversity also affects the structure of the personality, especially the development of a coherent self system and integrated representations of others. At the most basic level, abuse impedes the formation of interpersonal boundaries, and repeated invalidating experiences hamper the emergence of a differentiated self structure. Strategies used to cope with repeated adversity contribute to the problem. Attempts to suppress painful experiences and dissociative reactions compartmentalize experience and undermine integration. Abuse and trauma also negate personal integrity and autonomy. Deprivation similarly evokes self-definitions of nonexistence, of not being a person: to be neglected or ignored is to be negated and invalidated as a person.

The emergence of a coherent self depends upon consistent experiences of the self in relationship with significant others and consistent interpersonal feedback. The inconsistency and unpredictability of abusive individuals lead to relationships that fail to provide the constancy needed for self-development. Moreover, in abusive relationships the child often learns the role behaviors of both victim and abuser, which are difficult to integrate and set the stage for discontinuities in self-experience. Similar fragmentation occurs in the representations formed of others when the range of experiences with that abusive parent exceeds the child's capacity to integrate.

The contribution of abuse and invalidation to the emergence of core self and interpersonal pathology is especially pernicious when automatic emotional reactions are questioned, rejected, or scorned. Invalidating adults are often intolerant of negative feelings and tell their children that they should not have such feelings as anxiety, anger, and sadness. It is criticism of the child for *having* the feeling, rather than criticism for expressing the feeling, that is important. The invalidation creates conflict between what is felt (the child's reality) and what the child is told to feel (the parent's reality). In the struggle to conform to the demands of the significant other, the child suppresses his or her feelings, wishes, and natural reactions; this act of suppression, instigated by the parent's invalidation, undermines the authenticity of the experience and creates confusion about what the child actually feels. Telling the child consistently that his or her feelings are wrong, or that his or her impressions of others are wrong, undermines confidence in the intuitive processes that guide social interaction and gives a rise to a sense of puzzlement that the patient may later express as, "I don't know what to do"; "I don't now what to think"; "I just don't understand people."

Treatment Implications

This overview of psychosocial influences leads to several proposals for *intervention strategies* that extend ideas about the structure of treatment and the therapeutic stance developed in the last chapter. The widespread effects of psychosocial adversity on the personality system indicate that it is not sufficient to deal with resulting symptoms and conflicted relationships. Attention also has to be given to (1) changing the maladaptive schemata and cognitive processes that maintain symptoms and contribute to maladaptive patterns of relating to self and others, and (2) managing and treating the impact of adversity on the core self and interpersonal systems. This formulation suggests the following principle:

> *Basic Principle: Intervention strategies should address both the symptomatic consequences of adversity and its enduring effects on personality contents, processes, and structure.*

Adversity contributes to both *deficit* and *conflict pathology*. Although intervention strategies are needed to cover both sets of problems, deficit pathology takes priority because of its impact on the therapeutic relationship. Recognition of the effects of adversity on the core personality confirms the importance of an explicit frame of therapy and a validating stance. In addition to these implications, an understanding of the way adversity exerts an enduring influence on personality functioning also helps to identify specific intervention strategies (see Table 3.1). Especially important, as noted, are the effects on maladaptive schemata and associated cognitive styles. A variety of interventions are required to manage the effects of maladaptive cognitions on the treatment process and to effect schema change. Schemata organized around *distrust* hinder the development of a collaborative treatment relationship. These problems are probably best approached through empathic and supportive interventions that focus on *building and maintaining a collaborative treatment alliance*, and a treatment process that emphasizes *collaboration in describing, understanding, and changing problem behavior*. Invalidation and self-invalidating styles require active *validation strategies* to maintain the relationship and counteract these ways of thinking and their effects on the self. Beliefs and expectations

TABLE 3.1. The Implications of Adversity Effects on Personality
for Treatment Strategies

Effects on personality	Treatment strategies
Structures	
Differentiation and boundary problems	Establish an explicit therapeutic frame and maintain a consistent treatment process Promote differentiation of self schemata
Integration problems	Integrating and synthesizing interventions
Cognitive processes	
Self-invalidation	Validation
Regulatory processes	
Affect and impulse control	Develop affect and impulse regulation and self-management skills
Schema	
Distrust/cooperation/attachment	Establish a collaborative treatment process Build and maintain an effective treatment relationship Validation
Unpredictability	Establish and maintain a consistent treatment process
Powerlessness and low motivation	Build competence and autonomy Build motivation

about the *unpredictability and unreliability* of other people and relationships
are countered by establishing and maintaining *a consistent therapeutic process*, which also addresses problems with interpersonal boundaries and feelings of distrust. Finally, feelings of *powerlessness* and beliefs that there is little that can be done to change one's life and circumstances, leading to
poor motivation and passivity, may be countered by an active focus on
building motivation, promoting autonomy and competency, and on *acquiring the
skills* required to regulate feelings and impulses more adaptively. Adversity
also leads to deficits in the regulation and control of affects and impulses,
so that it is important to adapt an affect-regulating approach, especially in
the early stages of treatment, and to provide opportunities for the patient
to learn how to self-regulate emotions and impulses.

It appears, therefore, that a commonsense analysis of the effects of adversity allows us to identify important interventions. It also provides further support for (1) using a combination of interventions from different therapeutic models, delivered in a way that promotes integration; and (2) an approach that emphasizes generic mechanisms.

GENETIC FACTORS

Psychosocial adversity is not the only factor contributing to personality disorder that is relevant to treatment. Genetic factors also have important implications, albeit of a very different kind: they raise questions about the extent to which personality can change and the kinds of changes that are likely to result from treatment. Evidence for genetic contributions to personality disorder come from studies of the (1) genetics of specific DSM-IV personality disorders, and (2) genetic and environmental contributions to personality traits.

Genetics of Specific Diagnoses

The evidence suggests that DSM-IV personality disorders have a substantial genetic component (see reviews by Dahl, 1994; McGuffin & Thapar, 1992; Nigg & Goldsmith, 1994; Thapar & McGuffin, 1993). Most of the early studies evaluated the frequency of the disorder in the relatives of individuals diagnosed with Cluster A disorders and borderline and antisocial personality disorders. Schizotypal and paranoid personality disorder are more prevalent in the relatives of schizophrenic probands, although the increase in paranoid personality disorder is relatively small (McGuffin & Thapar, 1992; Nigg & Goldsmith, 1994; Thapar & McGuffin, 1993). Since schizophrenia is understood to have a genetic basis, these findings suggest that schizotypal personality disorder, in particular, shares the same genetic etiology. An increased prevalence of disorders is also found in the families of patients with borderline and antisocial personality disorders (Nigg & Goldsmith, 1994).

Although these findings are consistent with the assumption that personality disorder has a genetic basis, they are not conclusive because family studies cannot disentangle genetic and environmental factors, either of which (or a combination of both) could account for the increased incidence of personality disorder in the relatives of affected individuals. This limitation is particularly pertinent to personality disorder because psychosocial theories of causation also predict an increased incidence in family members. Adoption or twin studies are required to separate genetic and environmental contributions; hence, more convincing evidence for a genetic basis to personality disorder comes from twin studies. These studies have tended to focus on personality traits rather than personality disorder diagnoses. However, one twin study found a strong genetic component for all DSM-IV personality disorders (Torgerson et al., 2000).

Heritability of Traits

The twin-research method involves assessing a given trait in sets of identical and fraternal twins and comparing the correlation for identical twins with that of fraternal twins. A genetic influence is suggested when the correlation for identical twins is higher than the correlation for fraternal twins. The difference between identical and fraternal twin correlations is used to estimate *heritability*, that is, the proportion of variability in a trait due to genetic factors. The twin-research method also provides estimates of the magnitude of common and nonshared environmental effects. *Common or shared environmental effects* are influences shared by both members of a twin pair—for example, being the same age, having the same socioeconomic class, occupying the same position in the family, and being treated in the same way. These effects increase the similarity of a pair of twins. *Unique or specific environmental effects* involve differences in the way each twin is treated—for example, parental favoritism toward one twin, different life experiences, or different peer relationships. These effects tend to make a pair of twins more dissimilar.

Studies of normal personality reveal a consistent picture of genetic and environmental effects (Loehlin & Nichols, 1976; Plomin, Chipeur, & Loehlin, 1990). The heritability of personality traits (assessed by self-report measures) is typically 40–60%. Unique environmental effects usually account for approximately 50%, and common effects account for less than 10% of the variability in the trait (Loehlin & Nichols, 1976). The finding that common environmental factors contribute relatively little to the variance of personality traits may seem surprising because it runs counter to beliefs that the family has a substantial impact on personality. Although familial effects influence some aspects of personality, nonspecific factors seem to have a greater impact on trait variability. For example, it appears that we are extremely sensitive to being treated differently from others (Loehlin & Nichols, 1976; Plomin et al., 1990). The implication for the clinician is that experiences of differential treatment, especially during the formative years, are likely to figure prominently in the histories of many patients.

A similar picture of genetic and environmental effects emerges for personality disorder traits. The heritability of the four patterns of personality disorder is:

emotional dysregulation, 47%
dissocial behavior, 50%
inhibitedness, 48%
compulsivity, 38%

Unique environmental effects accounted for the remaining effect (Jang, Livesley, Vernon, & Jackson, 1996; Livesley et al., 1993, 1998).

The finding that genetic and environmental factors have approximately equal effects led to the suggestion that it is possible to distinguish between *temperament*, the genetic component of personality, and *character*, the aspect of personality influenced by experience. The idea is appealing and it introduces clarity into treatment formulations: The implication is that biological interventions should target temperament, and psychotherapeutic strategies should focus on character. Unfortunately, the idea is based upon the false assumption that because traits are 50% heritable, it is possible to distinguish traits with low heritability from others that are largely environmental. Twin studies consistently demonstrate, however, that all traits assessed by self-report measures have a heritable component, including those considered to be characterological (Jang, Livesley, & Vernon, 1996b). For example, cooperativeness and openness are said to be characterological traits. Nevertheless, they are as heritable as so-called temperament traits. It appears that all aspects of personality are shaped by the interaction of genes and environment and that all individual differences in human behavior are heritable (Turkheimer, 1998).

The heritability of personality does, however, have implications for treatment. The most obvious is that it provides a rationale for using medication. The evidence suggests that medication is effective in treating impulsivity and cognitive dysregulation and that pharmaceutical agents may modify trait expression in normal individuals (Knutson et al., 1998). Nevertheless, pharmacology, at least in the immediate future, is likely to play a modest, although important, role in treating traits. Of more immediate relevance are the implications of the heritability of traits in relation to the stability of personality and our ideas about the extent to which personality can change. It is a fallacy to assume that genetically based traits cannot be changed. Phenylketonuria, for example, is a genetic disorder that results in mental retardation; this outcome is prevented with an appropriate diet. Genes require specific environmental conditions to exert their influence. In the absence of these conditions, they may not be expressed. With personality, however, the genetic underpinning to traits raises fundamental questions about the stability of personality and the extent to which traits can change.

STABILITY AND CHANGE

Surprisingly, research on stability and change in personality has received little attention in the literature on treatment. As noted in Chapter 1, most treatments seem to imply that major changes in personality structure are possible. The evidence, however, reveals that many aspects of personality are remarkably stable and resist change (Caspi & Bem, 1990; Heatherton

& Weinberger, 1994; Tickle, Heatherton, & Wittenberg, 2001). Although many details are lacking, a general picture about the stability of personality is emerging, which provides an empirical basis for understanding the changes that can be expected from treatment.

Traits

Intellectual traits are the most stable, followed by broad personality traits such as neuroticism and extroversion, although personality traits are nearly as stable as intelligence (Brody, 1994). From the late 20s onward, little change occurs in basic traits (Caspi & Herbener, 1990; Costa & McCrae, 1980): Approximately 60% of the variance in trait scores is stable over the full adult life span (Costa & McCrae, 1992), and the rank order of a group of individuals remains stable when followed for as long as 30 years (Costa & McCrae, 1994). Modest changes, however, do occur: neuroticism, extroversion, and openness to experience decrease slightly over the life span, and agreeableness and conscientiousness increase a little (Costa & Mc-Crae, 1994). Between the mid-20s and middle adulthood, psychological adjustment improves, sociability decreases, and social concern and responsibility increase (Haan, Millsap, & Hartka, 1986; Helson & Moane, 1987; Jessor, 1983; Mortimer, Finch, & Kumka, 1982). In short, it appears that people mellow a little with age and become more reliable.

Personality traits are a little less stable during childhood. Nevertheless, even during childhood there is remarkable consistency. Temperament styles in childhood, for example, have predictive utility throughout the life span (Caspi, Bem, & Elder, 1989). Similarly, aggression is stable and predicts later antisocial traits (Huesmann, Eron, Lefkowitz, & Walder, 1984; Olweus, 1979). Any greater plasticity of traits in early childhood probably occurs because the cognitive structures associated with these dispositions are not fully developed. Once these cognitions are formed, they contribute to stability. Personality may also be a little less stable between late adolescence to early adulthood. For example, Helson and Moane (1987), using the California Psychological Inventory, reported that personality was more stable between 27 and 43 years of age than during the shorter period of 21 to 27 years. Personality appears to crystallize in the late 20s and changes little thereafter (Costa & McCrae, 1994; Helson & Moan, 1987). As William James noted, "by the age of thirty the character has set like plaster, and will never soften again" (1890/1981, p. 126).

The remarkable stability of personality throughout adulthood indicates that change does not occur under normal circumstances. This does not mean that change *cannot* occur. Likewise, the modest variation that occurs in traits until the late 20s does not mean that therapeutic interventions will also lead to change—it merely indicates that, under normal circumstances, change occurs, probably due to maturation. Given the genetic basis to personality traits and evidence of stability, it seems unlikely that major changes in traits can be achieved, using the interventions currently available. This conclusion has major implications for conceptualizing personality change and for treating a major component of personality pathology. The following principle is suggested:

> Basic Principle: The goal of treatment is to help individuals to adapt to their basic personality traits and express them more constructively, rather than to change the trait structure of personality.

This principle is a more specific version of the overall treatment goal of enhancing adaptation (see Chapter 2). Therapists who are used to thinking about changing personality through exploration of conflicts, modification of defenses, recalling and working through traumatic experiences, and so on, may be uncomfortable with the idea of working with traits not with the intent of changing them but of helping patients to adapt to their traits and express them more constructively. As MacKenzie (1994) noted, both psychoanalytically oriented and cognitive therapists may find it "somewhat a culture shock to consider personality as something that one simply has and must live with, like being excessively tall" (p. 238).

Self and Interpersonal Systems

The stability of other components of the personality system has been studied less systematically than traits. In the case of the self, a reasonable hypothesis is that its contents (schemata) are less stable than its organization or structure. This hypothesis is consistent with evidence that (1) self-attitudes and self-esteem are less stable than basic dispositions (Conley, 1984a, 1984b, 1984c; 1985), and (2) clinical observations that identity problems and object relationships change relatively little, even with long-term therapy.

Self schemata vary in stability (Kelly, 1955). Some are continuously revised in the light of experience, whereas others are remarkably persistent. Everyday impressions suggest that our ideas about ourselves change across the major epochs of our lives. As circumstances change, interpersonal relationships grow, and social roles are modified due to new responsibilities, we come to think of ourselves differently. We do not attribute the same qualities to ourselves in adult life as we did in adolescence and early adulthood. The carefree young adult becomes the responsible partner and parent, and these attributes become incorporated into the self. At the same time, there is also considerable evidence for continuity. Although we think about ourselves differently at different ages, we also feel that we are the same person; we recognize continuities in our experiences and in our major qualities.

Cognitive therapists have noted that core schemata that are central to the self and identity are difficult to change, although change is possible. Similarly, the proponents of dialectical behavior therapy note that negative core self-images resist change long after more overt impulsive and parasuicidal behaviors have improved (Robins et al., 2001). Core schemata are usually associated with strong affects. Information that challenges these schemata, even if the schemata are negative, is likely to be experienced as threatening and anxiety provoking, leading to the mobilization of self-protective and self-maintenance mechanisms that reduce threats to the stability of self-image. Self schemata that are more peripheral to the self may be more amenable to change, because challenges to these schemata are less likely to arouse defenses. In summary, *changes in self, person, and relationship schemata are related to the centrality of these schemata and the intensity of associated affects.*

The interpersonal system is likely to show a similar pattern of stability and plasticity. Views of other people, and schemata used to understand and guide interpersonal behavior, will change in the light of new information according to the extent to which it mobilizes associated affects or challenges highly valued beliefs. For example, person schemata that evoke important, affect-laden memories are likely to resist change because the affect involved is liable to evoke coping reactions that minimize the effects of change mechanisms. The network of links with other schemata, feelings, and behaviors promotes stability and persistence, even for schemata that lead to undesirable consequences.

Nevertheless, the evidence suggests some plasticity in important interpersonal behavior. For example, the attachment system, especially insecure attachment patterns (Bartholomew, Kwong, & Hart, 2001), seem to change during development, and appears to be more stable in adulthood, although there is some evidence that the preoccupied attachment may decrease over time and security increase (Klohnen & Bera, 1998).

Symptoms and Diagnoses

When the stability of personality disorder diagnoses is examined, a more variable picture emerges. Although the concept of personality disorder implies stability, the evidence suggests that many clinical features fluctuate over time and that diagnoses of specific personality disorders are unstable (Grilo & McGlashan, 1999). Although diagnostic agreement among clinicians is satisfactory (Zimmerman, 1994), when diagnoses are reassessed over time, there is considerable diagnostic instability. A review by David and Pilkonis (1996) showed that the number of patients retaining a diagnosis ranged from 25% to 78% across studies, with a mean of 56%. The general diagnosis of personality disorder, however, was more stable. The low stability of specific diagnoses led David and Pilkonis to question the validity of the very concept of specific categories of personality disorder. In general, stability decreases with time interval and fluctuates with level of psychological distress (Johnson et al., 1997).

One factor that contributes to poor diagnostic stability is that the DSM-IV criteria include both state and trait components. The state or symptomatic component is less stable than trait components (Clarke, Vittengl, Kraft, & Jerrett, in press). For example, in a longitudinal study of HIV-positive individuals, the features of personality disorder fluctuated with level of psychological distress (Johnson et al., 1997). A follow-up study of adolescents with borderline personality disorder, reassessed after 3 years, showed that symptoms such as self-harm and self-mutilation, para-suicidal behavior or threats, derealization and depersonalization, and brief paranoid ideation were unstable and decreased more over the 3-year period than conflict about giving and receiving care and dependent and masoch-istic behaviors (Meijer, Goedhart, & Treffers, 1998). Changes in state lead to diagnostic instability because variations in symptoms can lead to (1) in-dividuals failing to meet the cut-offs for a categorical diagnosis, even if the other components of the disorder are unchanged; and (2) changes in responses to items that measure other features of personality disorder. This conflation probably explains why dimensional assessments of DSM-IV diagnoses made by counting the number of criteria present are more than categorical diagnoses (Crawford, Cohen, & Brook, 2001; Lenzen-weger, 1999).

Despite evidence of diagnostic instability, there is also evidence of stability. Nonaffective traits are more stable than affective traits (Hirshfeld et al., 1983; Mann, Jenkins, Cutting, & Cowen, 1981). Coping strategies are also highly stable (Drake & Vaillant, 1985; Pope, Jonas, & Hudson, 1983). Diagnoses based on nonaffective traits, such as those for schizoid personality disorder, show remarkable stability from childhood to adult-hood (Wolff & Chick, 1980).

These findings suggest that symptoms and general distress are likely to change more readily than established behavior patterns and trait-based behavior, and that affective traits are less stable than nonaffective traits. This is useful information for treatment planning: It suggests that *an early focus on symptom relief and the affective components of a disorder is likely to yield the most benefits in the shortest time.* Furthermore, successful interven-tions early in treatment are likely to enhance the therapeutic alliance and the patient's commitment to treatment.

Sources of Stability

An understanding of the factors contributing to stability should (1) sensi-tize therapists to the obstacles patients face when trying to change, and (2) encourage therapists to make optimal use of interventions that take into account the mechanisms that promote stability. Stability arises from multiple factors, both internal and external to the person (Caspi & Bem, 1990). Internal factors include genetic predispositions that probably place constraints on the range of options that are available during development and the extent to which traits can be modified. Genetic factors continue to exert an influence throughout life, and this influence appears to increase with age (Jang et al., 1996a). Internal factors also include psychological structures and processes that promote stability. Externally, environmental factors promote stability by constraining the person to react in certain ways, by limiting the behavioral options available, and by reinforcing some actions but not others. Because individuals seek out environments that are conducive to their characteristic ways of thinking and behaving, stability also arises from interaction between personal dispositions and environmental factors.

This view of stability provides an additional perspective on "resistance" to change. Psychodynamic therapists traditionally focus on motivational factors that obstruct change. However, *many obstacles to change are not motivational: They arise from the structure of personality and the interconnections within the personality system.* This does not mean that motivational obstacles to change do not occur. It does, however, mean that therapists need to be sensitive to structural obstacles to change, and they need to communicate this understanding to patients. This new knowledge helps to reduce patients' frustrations about the lack of change and their tendencies to blame themselves for not changing faster. Awareness of this issue also helps to reduce problems that can arise when traditional views of resistance lead to a more confrontational stance.

Structural Factors

The connections among the components of the personality system—traits, self system, person system, and environment—create a structure in which change to one component tends to be dampened by its effects on other parts of the system. This dynamic operates at the level of the overall system and within subsystems. Within the overall system, traits influence self-experience and self and interpersonal schemata. At the same time, these schemas reinforce trait-based behavior. Together they form a stable structure. Similarly, self and person schemata are interconnected: Changing one set of beliefs is difficult because of the effect on other beliefs.

A similar situation occurs within subsystems. Traits are complex structures of subsystems, consisting of cognitions, emotions, and behaviors based on an underlying genetic architecture. The trait of anxiousness, for example, consists of emotions such as anxiety, tension, and panic; behaviors such as expressions of worry and concern, restlessness, and signs of stress and tension; and cognitions such as beliefs that the world is threatening and that it is difficult to cope with feelings. Linked to these components are cognitive styles, such as brooding and rumination, that amplify and maintain trait expression. The different components of traits and associated thinking patterns interlock to create a highly stable way of perceiving and relating to the world.

Although structural stability may obstruct change, the extensive connections within the personality system may also be useful because if *change is achieved in one part of the personality system, it may have a ripple effect that extends change to other parts of the system.* This possibility suggests that change in one area may be consolidated and extended by exploring the way the change has affected other aspects of personality. For example, improved control over parasuicidal behavior may be extended by exploring the way it effects self-esteem and beliefs about self-efficacy. Similarly, an increase in assertive behavior may be used to improve self-esteem and decrease anxiousness.

Environmental Factors

Although clinical explanation emphasizes the role of internal personality dynamics in maintaining maladaptive and symptomatic behavior, the empirical reality is that much of the stability of behavior is due to regularities and consistencies in the environment, and much of the stability in personality occurs because the environment remains the same (Caspi & Bem, 1990). Regular events, frequently occurring situations, stable social networks, and enduring relationships tend to evoke similar responses and consistent behaviors, giving rise to the impression of internal stability and continuity. As individuals, we tend to attribute stability in behavior and personality to internal factors. As clinicians, we do the same. Longitudinal studies, however, reveal considerable stability throughout childhood in environmental factors, such as the encouragement of verbal expression and parental teaching of language behavior (which is associated with intelligence) (Hanson, 1975). More directly related to personality is the often remarkable stability of parenting behavior (Pianta, Sroufe, & Egeland, 1989; Roberts, Block, & Block, 1984); this stability consolidates established behavior patterns. Similar processes occur in adulthood.

Many behaviors are difficult to alter because the environment remains the same even though the patient begins to change. For example, interventions to help a submissive individual become more assertive are likely to have little impact if the person returns from treatment to an abusive relationship that provides little opportunity to apply what was learned, a relationship in which attempts to be assertive are scorned or rejected. Similarly, attempts to validate self-experience are unlikely to enhance self-esteem and self-cohesiveness if patients return to families that continually invalidate their experiences. In short, how can patients develop a new self-image if they remain in the situation that instilled and maintained the old one? Even if changes do occur, a return to an environment that promoted maladaptive behaviors may result in the reestablishment of old patterns, once treatment had ended. This recidivism is typical, for example, when delinquent children are treated in residential settings. Gains in prosocial behaviors are lost if the child returns to a home environment that fosters delinquent acts (Rutter, 1987). This finding suggests that treatment may need to incorporate interventions to (1) change situational factors that foster maladaptive behavior through conjoint or family therapy (MacFarlane, in press), and (2) "inoculate" against environmental influences by teaching patients the skills required to manage relationships more effectively and to recognize and anticipate potential problem situations.

Environmental contributions to stability suggest that *personality change will be most extensive and more enduring when accompanied by changes in relevant environmental circumstances.* This formulation gives rise to the following principle:

> Basic Principle: *Treatment should incorporate strategies and interventions to change, modulate, or manage the environmental factors that contribute to the initiation and maintenance of maladaptive patterns.*

Person–Environment Interactions

Although the environment plays an active role in maintaining behavior, individuals are not merely passive participants or observers of environmental events. Instead they often provoke or catalyze the events to which they respond, thereby constructing the world in which they live by actively selecting environments that are conducive to them (Caspi & Bem, 1990). These person–situation relationships make a substantial contribution to the stability of adaptive and maladaptive behavior.

The simplest form of person–environment relationship occurs when individuals *react* differently to the same event. For example, highly suspicious individuals are more likely to interpret minor events as personally significant and threatening than less suspicious people. In this way, the schemata used to interpret the world in which the person lives also create that world by determining what is noticed and what is ignored.

People do not just react differently to situations—they also *evoke* different reactions from others. Inhibited (schizoid–avoidant) individuals, for example, who are cautious and distant tend to evoke cool responses that reinforce their fears. Similarly, hostile and coercive behavior by aggressive boys provokes parental anger, to which the boys respond aggressively until the parents withdraw, thus reinforcing the boys' behavior. Through evocative interactions, maladaptive patterns are continually reinforced by events that the person believes are unrelated to his or her own actions. This dynamic helps to explain the stability of fears and expectations that originate in early maladaptive relationships (Wachtel, 1977). Evocative interactions also are important in maintaining a stable self system: People selectively attend to, and elicit, information that is consistent with their self-concept (Swann, 1983, 1987, 1990). Clinically, this dynamic is important. Patients with personality disorder are especially attentive to events that support their preconceptions, including their views of the self. These processes are powerful obstacles to change. However, they are also fundamental to the stability of personality and hence serve an adaptive function that should be acknowledged rather than simply interpreted as resistances to be overcome.

The term *proactive interaction* refers to the process of selecting and creating environments that are compatible with one's personality. At birth, parents largely determine the child's environment, but this monopoly quickly diminishes as innate dispositions begin to shape the child's responses. Gradually, this emergence of dispositionally related likes and dislikes promotes a more active search for situations that facilitate expression of basic traits, and even the creation of such situations. The person with strong tendencies toward sensation seeking searches for opportunities for thrill seeking. The inhibited individual seeks situations that minimize social contact and provide opportunities for solitary interests. This active search for congenial environments means that traits become self-perpetuating (Caspi & Bem, 1990).

Proactive interaction is especially powerful when social and interpersonal relationships are involved. People seek friendships and relationships with people who have personalities, values, and attitudes that are similar to themselves (Newcomb, 1961). The other person's actions then reinforce the personality characteristics that led to the decision to interact with him or her in the first place. This dynamic even applies when negative feelings about the self are involved. Studies show that people prefer to interact with others who share their views of themselves; those with negative self-images prefer people who also think poorly of them (Swann & Pelham, 2002; Swann, Wenzlaff, Krull, & Pelham, 1992). These intimate relationships help to maintain dysfunctional behaviors (Clarkin, Marziali, & Munroe-Blum, 1991).

The cumulative effect of person–environment interactions is that people live in worlds that are, to some extent, their own creation—in self-designed personal niches that allow expression of their personality (Willi, 1999). Once created, these worlds help to maintain the personality characteristics that created them. Life events help to perpetuate old patterns and reduce the impact of attempts to change. For this reason, it may not be sufficient to focus only on changing the way patients perceive and think about their worlds. They may also need help in understanding the way the environment influences their behavior and developing strategies to deal with these pressures.

Additional Clinical Implications of Stability

Research on the stability of normal and disordered personality indicates that *components of the personality system differ in stability and potential for change.* The features of personality disorder form an approximate hierarchy of changeability, ranging from most amenable to change to most stable (hence, less amenable to change) (Figure 3.2). The features of personality disorder that are most amenable to change are symptoms and some situational problems; many symptoms associated with personality disorder vary naturally. At the next level of stability are interpersonal patterns, maladaptive modes of thinking, characteristic expressions of traits (although not the underlying disposition), and some self-attitudes (especially self-esteem); regulatory processes also vary in stability, and many respond to appropriate interventions. Finally, dispositional traits (general tendencies as opposed to their behavioral manifestations), maladaptive core schemata (schemata that are central to self-esteem and identity), and core self and interpersonal pathology (unstable or fragmented representations of self and others) are highly stable and difficult to change.

This hierarchy of changeability is useful in treatment planning (see Chapter 6) and suggests the following principle:

> *Basic Principle: Treatment goals and intervention strategies should take into account the stability of personality and the anticipated duration of treatment. The early stages of treatment and briefer treatments should focus on the more changeable components of personality disorder.*

COMMENT

The evidence briefly reviewed in this chapter indicates that personality disorder is a biopsychological entity with a complex etiology involving

- Symptoms and some situational factors
- Affect and impulse control; interpersonal problems and patterns; maladaptive modes of thinking; more peripheral self-attitudes, including self-esteem; characteristic expressions of basic traits
- Dispositional traits (general tendencies, as opposed to their behavioral manifestations); core self and interpersonal pathology

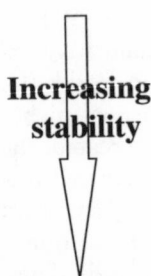

Increasing stability

FIGURE 3.2. Stability and change across domains of personality pathology.

multiple genetic and psychosocial factors. The resulting pathology extends to all facets of the personality system, combining deficits in the structure of the self and interpersonal systems and in emotional regulation with conflicted patterns of relating. All emerge under the influence of underlying genetic predispositions. These ideas about etiology and development have extensive implications for the way treatment is approached and the selection of interventions. Etiological and developmental factors support the view that treatment is primarily concerned with enhancing adaptation, as proposed in the previous chapter. These factors also raise questions about the limits of change and the feasibility of changing personality traits. Recognizing a potential ceiling to change is not a reason for pessimism but rather a way to optimize treatment of personality pathology by focusing interventions for maximum effect.

Understanding the effects of psychosocial adversity helps to define strategies and interventions that complement and extend the basic principles for organizing therapy proposed in the previous chapter on the basis of an explication of the structure of personality disorder. The enduring effects of psychosocial adversity on the contents of thought, the way information is processed, and the structure of the self and interpersonal systems points to the need to create a comprehensive set of strategies to deal with the pervasive effects of adversity.

Knowledge about the origin and stability of personality and personality disorder suggest the need for a new understanding of the role and significance of the environment. Rather than something independent of the individual, the environment to which the individual reacts is created, at least in part, during development to facilitate the expression of basic personality features. Once established, the individual's environment makes a substantial contribution to the stability of both adaptive and maladaptive functioning. This suggests that therapeutic effort should be directed not only toward helping the individual to adapt to the environment, as psychotherapy has always sought to do, but also toward helping the individual to manage the environment more effectively and to select or create an environment that fits his or her personality and needs.

CHAPTER 4

The Process of Change

A key component of any treatment is a conception of therapeutic change: what changes, the mechanisms and interventions that bring about change, and how change occurs. This chapter examines the mechanisms and interventions through which change is achieved, using a generic approach, and the therapeutic processes and stages through which they are applied. Generic sources of change include the therapeutic relationship, increased self-knowledge, the provision of new experiences, and the acquisition of new behaviors. It is suggested that the basic work of treatment is the collaborative description of problems and pathology. Changes in specific problems are described using a four-stage process that begins with problem recognition, progresses to exploration, then the acquisition of alternatives, and, finally, the consolidation of new behaviors and skills.

MECHANISMS OF CHANGE

Evidence that different therapies yield similar outcomes has prompted attempts to classify generic change mechanisms (see for example, Karasu, 1986; Lambert, 1986; Orlinsky & Howard, 1987; Prochaska, 1984; Prochaska & DiClemente, 1992; Winston & Muran, 1996. Although these formulations differ, they agree on two sets of general factors: those relating to the relationship between the patient and therapist, and instrumental interventions that increase self-knowledge, offer new experiences, and promote new behaviors.

The Therapeutic Relationship

Most therapies, including the more structured cognitive and behavioral therapies, recognize the significance of relationship factors (Beck, 1995; Fishman & Lubetkin, 1983; Goldfried & Davison, 1976). Even in behavior therapy there is general acknowledgment that technical aspects take up only a fraction of most sessions; the remainder is spent providing empathy, understanding, encouragement, support, and finding alternative behavioral solutions (Fishman & Lubetkin, 1983; O'Leary & Wilson, 1987). There is also agreement that particular attention needs to be paid to the relationship when treating personality disordered patients (Pretzler & Beck, 1996). For descriptive purposes it is convenient to divide relationship factors into the therapeutic alliance, the frame of therapy including the treatment setting, the therapeutic contract, and the therapeutic stance. Most of these factors are discussed in later chapters. Here the therapeutic stance is examined to identify therapist variables associated with positive outcomes.

Therapeutic Stance

The *therapeutic stance* refers to "the interpersonal positions, responsibilities, and activities that define and frame the interaction between patient and therapist" (Gold, 1996, p. 72). Since the stance sets the tone of therapy and shapes intervention strategies, it needs to be defined before treatment begins. In Chapter 2 it was suggested that the systematic application of generic mechanisms offers the best approach to managing and treating core pathology. This idea suggests the following:

> Basic Principle: The most appropriate stance for treating personality disorder is to provide support, empathy, and validation.

This proposal is consistent with ideas about an effective treatment relationship, such as the importance of empathic responding (Ryle, 1997), creating a holding and facilitating environment (Winnicott, 1965), providing mirroring (Kohut, 1971) and optimal responsiveness (Lichtenberg, Lachmann, & Fosshage, 1992), and a general emphasis on a supportive approach (Adler & Buie, 1979a, 1979b; Buie & Adler, 1982; Zetzel, 1971). Given the evidence, this stance represents a reasonable "default" position for treating personality disorder. The Rogerian dimensions of accurate empathy, nonpossessive warmth and regard, and genuineness capture the key elements of the stance, although other components, such as the level of therapist activity and the balance between didactic and consultancy roles, are also important.

Empathy. Outcome studies suggest that therapy is ineffective, regardless of the therapist's technical competence, when the therapist does not relate to the patient in a warm and empathic manner, and that patients with successful outcomes tend to describe their therapists as warm, attentive, interested, understanding, respectful, experienced, and active (Strupp, Fox, & Lessler, 1969). It appears that a stance that combines support, respect, and empathy with an active therapeutic style is the most effective. As noted in previous chapters, the deficits arising from psychosocial adversity also point to the importance of an empathic stance. Thus, multiple lines of evidence point to the significance of this dimension of the therapeutic relationship for the treatment of personality disorder. In this context, empathy includes skillful listening and attempts to clarify and amplify patients' experiences and understand their meaning. Empathy here does not imply identification with patients' problems. Indeed, therapists who identify closely with their patients' problems often have poorer outcomes, probably because they collude with the patient's psychopathology, rather than attempt to change it (Miller & Rollnick, 1991), and inadvertently exacerbate boundary problems.

Differences in therapist empathy probably help to explain why some therapist characteristics are associated with a favorable outcome and influence premature termination regardless of the kind of therapy being practiced (Luborsky, McLellan, Woody, O'Brien, & Auerbach, 1985; Miller, Taylor, & West, 1980). Although therapist empathy has not been studied directly in the treatment of personality disorder, studies of therapy for substance abuse (which is strongly associated with personality disorder) showed that therapist empathy accounted for two-thirds of the variance in outcome at 6 months, 50% at 12 months (Miller et al., 1980), and 25% at 2 years (Miller & Baca, 1983).

Therapist Activity. The proposed stance implies a high level of therapist activity, especially early in treatment when the alliance is being established. The need for higher therapist activity when treating personality disordered patients is widely recognized. Waldinger and Gunderson (1989), discussing patients with borderline pathology, noted that increased therapist activity was a feature of most intensive psychodynamic treatments. High activity emphasizes the therapist's presence and promotes engagement. It also anchors the patient in reality and prevents the transference distortions that tend to occur with limited structure (Ryle, 1997; Waldinger & Gunderson, 1989). Furthermore, activity promotes a holding or containing relationship, and by structuring the situation, reduces the tendency for severely disturbed patients to regress (Zetzel, 1971).

The need for structure is most apparent with emotionally dysregulated and dissocial patients, with whom therapist activity helps to contain dysphoric affects and potentially disruptive behavior. Ryle (1997) also noted that therapist talk is especially helpful when patients become overwhelmed and disorganized, and when they begin to dissociate. Those with an inhibited pattern also benefit from an active therapist who is careful not to be intrusive.

Collaboration and Consultation. The current approach assumes that the therapist's main task is to engage patients in the collaborative pursuit of treatment goals by making his or her expertise available to them. This formulation of the therapeutic relationship is similar to that of existential therapy, which has been described as the patient's hiring of the therapist as a consultant (Bugenthal & Kleiner, 1993). Support, acceptance, advice, exploration, and confrontation are all part of the relationship. This role prescription also incorporates cognitive therapy's characterization of the relationship as "collaborative empiricism," although the process envisioned here is less didactic.

The value of this component is clarified by Benjamin's (1993) concept of complementarity. The therapist's focus on the patient is matched by the patient's focus on the self; when the therapist listens, the patient is placed in the complementary position of revealing; conversely, when the therapist is nondirective, the patient is encouraged to be more active. A collaborative and consultative stance structures the relationship in a way that automatically draws the patient into a more therapeutic interaction.

Self-Knowledge

The instrumental component of a generic framework involves increasing self-knowledge, offering new experiences, and promoting new behaviors. The development of self-knowledge is an almost universally recognized therapeutic factor: Most therapies seek to extend and reframe patients' views of their problems and to enlarge self-knowledge by drawing attention to unrecognized aspects of the self. In keeping with a generic approach, a combination of interventions may be used to increase self-knowledge. As with cognitive and cognitive analytic therapy (Ryle, 1997), patients are encouraged to keep a diary or journal. More structured procedures may also be used, such as recording maladaptive thoughts, self-harming behavior, or mood, according to patient need and the stage of therapy.

The idea of self-knowledge and the role it plays in change is complex. A patient who received long-term treatment wrote later to say that although she had benefited from treatment and had learned much about herself, she was unsure what she had actually learned that was new to her. The matter was only resolved when she came across the following passage from T. S. Eliot's poem "Little Gidding":

> We shall not cease from exploration
> And the end of all our exploring
> Will be to arrive where we started
> And know the place for the first time. (1963, p. 222)

Most patients have some awareness of their problems, although they may be unable to articulate it fully. It is unusual for something totally new to appear during treatment. What seems to be involved in "know[ing] the place for the first time" is investment in the idea and an understanding of the implications of this knowledge. This focus changes something that was on the fringes of awareness into something that is a fully recognized and accepted part of self-experience. Shapiro (1989) described the process in this way: "The sort of self-understanding that is thought to be liberating or therapeutic, in fact, is generally understood to involve not new information so much as a rediscovery of what was in some sense already there. It is thought to involve a clarification of some aspect of mental or emotional life that had been unclear, unrecognized, or unconscious, yet had its effects" (p. 118). Shapiro also noted that therapeutic self-knowledge is not just intellectual knowledge of the kind produced by psychoeducational interventions (although such interventions may contribute to the process); rather, it involves changes in feelings and attitudes.

Knowledge about a maladaptive behavioral pattern, way of thinking, or trait focuses attention on the problem as the first step toward change. At the same time, it "changes the person's experience of himself [or herself]" (Shapiro, 1989, p.12). Awareness also leads to the realization that behavior has causes and consequences. Events that were thought to be unrelated are seen to be the consequences of one's own actions, and events that were considered unavoidable or inexplicable are seen to have origins and even a purpose. This increase in self-knowledge builds competency by improving feelings of *control and mastery*. Realization that the causes of many events lie within the self challenges the passivity associated with personality disorder, so that the person no longer feels him- or herself to be a pawn of circumstance but rather an actor in the drama of his or her life. In turn, this realization leads to another: that it is possible to behave differently and that problems can be solved. Choice replaces passive acceptance, and autonomy replaces helplessness. At the same time, the *self expands*, because events, qualities, and feelings that were poorly understood or divorced from the self are now incorporated into the self.

These changes lead to greater *differentiation* and *integration* of self-knowledge. The search for self-understanding forces clarification of self-experience that makes awareness of the self more detailed: Global impressions give rise to a more articulated understanding. A *more adaptive self system is synthesized* as therapy progresses and more links are made within self-knowledge. As Yalom (1975) pointed out:

> One way that self-understanding promotes change is that it encourages individuals to recognize, to integrate, and to give free expression to previously dissociated parts of themselves. When we deny or stifle parts of ourselves, we pay a heavy price—we feel a deep amorphous sense of re-

striction, we are "on guard," we are often troubled and puzzled by inner, yet alien, impulses demanding expression. When we reclaim these split-off parts, we experience a wholeness and a deep sense of liberation. (pp. 92–93)

Self-knowledge is related to *self-acceptance*. A hallmark of satisfactory adjustment is acceptance of one's personal qualities, with minimal conflict and distress, including those characteristics that one would like to change. This acceptance is rare in people with personality disorder. Almost without exception, patients seem at odds with themselves, locked in a continual struggle not to recognize or own important aspects of themselves and their experience. Even apparently obvious behaviors, such as self-harming actions, bulimic behavior, and substance abuse, may not be fully acknowledged let alone "owned" as self-generated.

Problems with self-acceptance limit self-knowledge. As one patient expressed it: "I have realized that acceptance and understanding go hand in hand. I used to think that acceptance would come from understanding. Now I know that's not the case. I can only begin to understand myself when I accept myself." Self-acceptance does indeed contribute to self-understanding, but simple, uncritical self-acceptance also can obstruct change. When people are too comfortable with themselves, there is little incentive to change. Nonetheless, self-understanding with too little self-acceptance can create a demoralized state that is paralyzing. The task is to promote self-acceptance while maintaining the motivation to change; this means helping individuals to accept, without self-condemnation, personal qualities that they find less than desirable—something that many personality disordered individuals find difficult. All too often insight leads to further self-criticism.

New Experiences

An important part of the generic framework is the provision of new experiences. The significance of new experiences versus insight in the change process has been controversial. Classical psychoanalytic approaches tended to assume that change results from insight achieved through interventions, especially those that capture "the urgency of the moment" by linking current events in therapy (the transference) to current and past events in the patient's life (Menninger, 1958; Strachey, 1934). Others have argued that intellectual insight alone is not sufficient and that change depends on "corrective emotional experiences," in which the therapist behaves differently from the patient's expectations, forcing changes to pathological beliefs and expectations (Alexander & French, 1946). Like many debates in the behavioral sciences, both positions contain elements of truth. As discussed earlier, insight in the form of self-knowledge is crucial, although insight in the traditional sense of uncovering unconscious processes may not be critical. However, the evidence also points to the importance of a therapeutic relationship that offers experiences that "correct" maladaptive cognitions and behaviors. When maladaptive schemata and associated patterns of relating are reenacted in treatment and the therapist behaves differently from the patient's expectations, the beliefs are disconfirmed and associated behaviors are weakened (Weiss, 1993). Given that personality disorder develops in the context of dysfunctional relationships, it is to be expected that experience of more functional ways of relating will be therapeutic. It seems that core maladaptive schemata are more likely to be changed through a therapeutic relationship that provides an ongoing corrective experience that disconfirms these beliefs than through interpretations and other interventions that seek to change them directly.

The psychodynamic tradition emphasizes the importance of new experiences within treatment, whereas cognitive and behavior therapy also use "homework" to encourage patients to continue self-exploration and attempt new behaviors between sessions. New experiences inside and outside therapy provide an opportunity to address fears and anxieties that previously felt overwhelming. Many behavioral and cognitive interventions bring about change by allowing patients to experience tolerable levels of anxiety and learn that their fears are unfounded. These techniques are often more effective when used in everyday situations. As Beutler and Harwood (2000) noted, "Therapeutic change is most likely when the patient is exposed to objects or targets of behavioral and emotional avoidance" (p. 18).

With personality disorder, encouragement to work on issues between sessions is consistent with the need to change maladaptive behaviors in everyday life and with the role of situational factors in maintaining maladaptive patterns. New experiences outside treatment tend to generalize treatment effects and reduce tendencies to attribute change only to therapeutic efforts (Andrews, 1990, 1993; Guidano, 1991b; Guidano & Liotti, 1983; Reeve, Inck, & Safran, 1993; Safran & Segal, 1990).

New Behavior

The ultimate goal of treatment is behavioral change, and most generic models incorporate specific interventions to promote the acquisition of new behaviors through skill development, graded exposure, and contingency management. A puzzling feature of the general psychotherapy literature, however, is the extent to which many therapies neglect directly promoting new behavior. Given the entrenched nature of personality pathology, direct interventions are required to inhibit old patterns, modify old habits, strengthen skills that are defective, and promote new skills. It is here that a need for an eclectic approach that draws upon a range of inter-

ventions from different schools of thought is most apparent. The delivery
of these interventions in a coordinated way that maintains the therapeutic
frame required to treat and manage core pathology is one of the challenges
of treating personality disorder.

COLLABORATIVE DESCRIPTION: THE WORK OF THERAPY

Theories of various therapies differ in the way they conceptualize the work
of therapy. Cognitive therapy uses collaborative empiricism and a Socratic
exchange. Classical psychoanalysis emphasizes free association, with a neutral therapist clarifying, confronting, and interpreting the patient's associations. Others have suggested that therapy adopt a more conversational
style. Constructivism, for example, uses the metaphor of therapy as "conversational elaboration" (Neimeyer, 1995, p. 18). The treatment of personality disorder requires an approach that facilitates therapeutic work while
minimizing the activation of reactive tendencies that may interfere with
treatment. This approach may be found in the ideas of guided exploration,
developed by theorists of cognitive therapy, and the collaborative reformulation approach proposed by Ryle (1997). This formulation suggests the
following principle:

> Basic Principle: The work of therapy is to facilitate a collaborative de-
> scription (1) of the patient's problems and psychopathology, and (2)
> the way these problems and psychopathology affect the patient's life
> and relationships.

Collaborative description is the primary vehicle for increasing self-knowledge.
The purpose is to help patients to recognize and understand how repetitive
patterns of action and experience contribute to their problems. As the
descriptive process unfolds and obstacles to self-knowledge are overcome, a
new understanding emerges that encourages the patient to contemplate
new ways of behaving.

Collaborative description combines an attitudinal stance on the part
of the therapist with an intervention strategy designed to facilitate and
guide the descriptive process. Along with the overarching goal of improving adaptation by building competency, collaborative description is a guiding principle that orientates the therapist to the way the goals of therapy
are to be achieved, how obstacles to treatment should be addressed, and
the way that other strategies should be implemented.

The therapist's role is to guide the process by asking for details when
descriptions are too global, seeking clarification when things are unclear,
and asking for examples to focus the descriptive process on specific events
and concrete behaviors. These interventions focus the patient's attention

on significant issues by (1) encouraging the patient to unpack the meaning of global descriptions so that the key components are apparent, and (2) highlighting those issues that are important for change. Rather like the student who highlights important parts of a text, the therapist unobtrusively underlines important parts of the patient's material. Hence the therapist not only elicits descriptions of problems but also shapes the patient's understanding by the questions asked (and not asked), by the issues selected to reflect back for further description, and by summary statements that reframe the patient's understanding. The result is a shared understanding that reframes patients' ideas about themselves and their lives and reformulates problems so that they are less distressing or lead to alternative courses of action. The goal is not a historical reconstruction of events but rather a detailed description of the way the person experiences, thinks about, and reacts to events, with the aim of reformulating aspects of this understanding that are the source of problems (Ryle, 1997). The new understanding is both a reconstruction and a creation. It is a reconstruction in that it uses the knowledge that the person has about his or her life and extends and reframes this knowledge, as necessary. It is a creation in that the process yields new understandings and synthesizes a more integrated "theory of the self."

The approach engages patients in a collaborative exercise that is the antithesis of the noncooperative, abusive, controlling, avoidant, or distant relationships that are familiar to most of them. This approach is equally valuable in treating the more reactive, confrontational behaviors of patients with emotional dysregulation and dissocial traits and the withdrawn and nonresponsive styles of those with the inhibited pattern. In each case, a direct challenge to basic patterns is avoided; instead the patient is drawn into ways of relating that counter the maladaptive expressions of these patterns. At the same time, a consistent focus on the content and process of thinking and experience—that is, on *"what* you think" and *"how* you think"—promotes more dispassionate self-appraisal and helps to counter derogatory self-talk.

It could be argued that this view of the work of therapy differs little from that of traditional psychodynamic psychotherapy, in which patients are encouraged to talk freely about the issues that are the focus of treatment, with the therapist commenting or interpreting as required, and that reframing interventions is merely interpretation with a different name. There is some validity to this argument. Moreover, some psychodynamic approaches conceptualize therapeutic endeavors in a similar way. As Feiner (2000) pointed out, within interpersonal psychoanalysis there has been a movement away from "labeling and explaining to a description of experience" (p. 22). Despite this similarity, there are differences in emphasis. The most important is in the *attribution of intention*. Interpretation usually involves attributing behavior to unconscious motives and impulses. In contrast, collaborative description covers the same material by exploring the antecedents and consequences of behavior, including its effects on others, without concern for "unconscious" processes or motives. Psychodynamic interpretation also seeks to uncover the origin of personality processes in past relationships, whereas here we are more concerned with how personality processes function in the present.

Collaborative description leads to a low-key form of therapy that fits well with a supportive, empathic therapeutic stance. Patients are encouraged to provide straightforward and matter-of-fact accounts of their problems and behaviors. It is also a nonpressuring, noncoercive approach that does not demand change. Instead, change is imperceptibly incorporated into the treatment process: The very act of describing and reframing experience leads inevitably to the idea that things could be different.

THE STAGES OF CHANGE

The next step in developing a framework for understanding change is to consider (1) how collaborative description may be applied in practice, and (2) the actual sequence through which behavior changes. One approach that is useful for this purpose is Prochaska and DiClemente's (1992) naturalistic descriptions of changes in addictive behavior (see also DiClemente, 1994; Prochaska et al., 1992, 1994). They described a six-stage process: precontemplation, contemplation, preparation, action, maintenance, and termination. When applying this model to changes in personality disorder, it is convenient to combine some stages, leaving a four-stage process. The first stage, *problem recognition*, involves recognizing and accepting problems and developing a commitment to change. This stage is followed by *exploration*, in which collaborative description is used to develop an understanding of a given problem and its associated feelings and thoughts. Attention is paid to the sequence of events leading to problem behavior and the consequences of these behaviors for the individual and others. Exploration covers both historical factors involved in the development of maladaptive patterns and contemporary cognitive and affective mechanisms underlying them. During the third stage, *acquisition of alternatives*, new ways of responding to situations and handling feelings and impulses are identified. This is essentially a problem-solving stage that seeks to find new solutions to old problems. In the process, new behaviors are learned and implemented. The final stage is one of *consolidation and generalization*; here steps are taken to ensure that new learning is strengthened and applied to everyday situations. An essential part of this stage involves acquiring the behaviors and skills required to prevent relapse when therapy is completed.

The following case vignette demonstrates how the approach may be used to understand change in drug misuse.

The patient, a single woman in her early 30s with the emotional dysregulation pattern and some dissocial traits, had a long psychiatric history, dating from the age of 14, when she began abusing drugs and alcohol, became highly promiscuous, and engaged in a variety of parasuicidal behaviors. Diagnostically, she met the criteria for DSM-IV borderline personality disorder and showed some antisocial (dissocial) traits. At the beginning of treatment with her current therapist, she denied problems with drug use. It soon became apparent, however, that she intermittently used analgesics excessively. These episodes usually coincided with self-mutilation. From a stage of change perspective, the patient was in the pretherapy stage of *nonrecognition*. Denial was maintained despite the development of serious medical problems caused by alcohol and substance abuse. The therapist continued to adopt a supportive but inquiring stance. Gradually, the patient acknowledged that analgesic abuse was a problem that she needed to change. The establishment of *preliminary awareness and problem recognition* was slow, and for a while the patient oscillated between recognition and denial. Eventually the link between drug use and medical problems was accepted, and the patient began to express concern about her general health and inability to control analgesic use. This concern gradually intensified into a commitment to change.

Exploration of the events associated with analgesic use was initially unsuccessful. The patient maintained that she did not know why she suddenly developed the urge to use drugs. When exploration consistently failed to identify triggering events, the therapist suggested that the patient record all instances of drug use. Doing so revealed that drug use was more frequent than initially acknowledged. This step was useful in itself because it provided a concrete record of analgesic abuse that was used to monitor change. Subsequently, it was suggested that the patient record her thoughts and feelings whenever she had the urge to take analgesics. One week later the patient mentioned that she had noted that the urge to take analgesics occurred when she felt panicky and empty. Although this realization was not surprising to the therapist, it was an illuminating one for the patient and led to further exploration of these feelings and the events that triggered them. In the process, she realized that the dysphoria often followed problems with a friend or acquaintance, which caused her to feel that she was alone and that no one cared about her. Gradually, the sequence of events culminating in drug misuse was established, leading to a modest increase in control. Equally importantly, it also led to an *exploration of alternative ways* of dealing with the dysphoria, which, in turn, eventually led to more adaptive ways of handling these feelings.

The next vignette shows how the stage of change approach may be used to modify maladaptive interpersonal behavior associated with an underlying trait, in this case, submissiveness. Although there are many aspects to this case, the vignette focuses only on submissiveness.

A 41-year-old woman with three teenage sons, over whom she had little control, was referred for treatment for longstanding symptoms of dysthymia and anxiety, major dependency problems, and chronic interpersonal problems, including recurrent relationships with abusive men. Diagnostically, she met the DSM-IV criteria for dependent personality disorder. A dimensional assessment highlighted submissiveness and insecure attachment. She described numerous subservient relationships with others, including parents, children, partners, and friends. She felt abused by everyone and referred to herself as a "doormat." Initially, the patient did not recognize the extent to which she was submissive or the way this pattern contributed to poor self-esteem and dysthymic symptoms. She was in the stage of *nonrecognition*.

As she discussed her problems in group therapy, a preliminary awareness of the submissiveness emerged when she noticed that her own needs were rarely met. She began to talk about being more assertive but was concerned about how others would react. Although this concern limited her commitment to change, she was motivated to change by the need to provide more effective supervision of her children. In one sense this response was another variant of the submissive pattern, in that she wanted to change for the sake of her sons. Nevertheless, it proved to be a powerful incentive and led to detailed *exploration* of the thoughts and feelings associated with submissiveness.

Growing awareness of the pattern increased her self-esteem because she was delighted that she could understand problems that had seemed incomprehensible. Recognition of the historical antecedents of this behavior in parental relationships provided an anchor of understanding that she used, in turn, to understand how she reacted to her own children. Her parents had been dominating and controlling, and she had responded with acquiescence. When she resisted their demands, she did so in an ineffective, passive way. She noted that she dealt with her children and partners similarly. As exploration continued, she recognized that she sacrificed her own needs for those of others and that this self-disregard enabled others to ignore her needs. She also had the strong belief that her needs were less important than those of others. She talked about the importance of placing others' needs before her own and sacrificing herself for others. This schema clearly played a central role in maintaining her subservient behaviors. She also recognized the consequences of being submissive and passive. Initially, she thought that these behaviors were reasonable ways to deal with others; later she recognized that such actions frustrated her own needs and caused her to feel neglected. Her tendency to externalize blame for her problems was replaced by the recognition that she contributed to her own sense of neglect and frustration. She began to note that often, when she believed she was doing the right thing by putting others' needs before her own, she felt worthless afterward. However, these feelings were usually quickly replaced by a sense of sacrifice for others. She also noted that fear of upsetting others and making them angry contributed to her tendency toward submissive behavior.

Recognition of the thoughts accompanying submissive acts gradually led to questions about whether she could behave differently. She began to dispute many of her thoughts and fears and to explore *alternative behaviors* and interpretations of events. She also began to consider saying "no" to some of her children's demands.

At about this time, a specific event occurred that was a further impetus for change. For many years she had wanted cosmetic surgery but repeatedly put it off because she felt that she should not spend money on herself. After discussing the topic extensively in the group, she decided to go ahead with it. Making this decision on her own behalf was a major change. When the treatment was completed, she was dissatisfied with the result. When she discussed her concerns with the surgeon, he dismissed them. She did not press the matter—a typical way of dealing with problems. By the time she got home, she was angry not only with him but with herself for not being more assertive. This response was also a major change. Furthermore, she decided to handle things differently. A follow-up appointment was planned, and she wrote a script for what she would like to say to the surgeon and the response she hoped he would make. She discussed the script with the group. This context provided an opportunity to role-play the anticipated meeting. The group also encouraged her to consider what she should do if the surgeon was dismissive again. When the meeting with the surgeon occurred, she was surprised that she could express herself in an assertive but nonprovocative way. She was also surprised at the surgeon's response. Not only did he listen to her complaints, he also agreed that he had been dismissive on the previous occasion and made suggestions to correct the problem. The outcome was better than she had hoped, and the event helped her to *consolidate and generalize* her gains.

The stages of change model provides a descriptive framework that imposes structure onto the complexities of change. The multiple problems presented by most cases often seem overwhelming, and it is often difficult for therapists to decide upon the most important issue to address at a given moment. Change, however, is a continuous process. Boundaries between stages are not always clear-cut and considerable movement often occurs across stages, even during a single session. Nevertheless, the model is a useful guide that helps therapists to select interventions by defining the tasks that need to be accomplished at each stage (Prochaska & DiClemente, 1992). For example, during the problem recognition stage the patient's task is to recognize specific issues that contribute to his or her difficulties and commit to change, while the therapist's task is to provide the therapeutic conditions that enable patients to feel sufficiently secure to recognize problems. The model suggests a further principle:

Basic Principle: Change occurs through a series of stages, and interventions should be appropriate to the stage of change that the patient is at with regard to a given problem.

Attempts to explore a problem before it is recognized as such by the patient, or to promote alternative behaviors before a problem is understood, are usually ineffective and often impair the treatment relationship. The model makes change more manageable by breaking problems into smaller parts. Instead of being confronted with the need to change well-entrenched behaviors, attention is focused on small steps that are less overwhelming for both patients and therapists.

The model is useful in managing both macro- and micro-levels of change. At the macro-level, where the focus is on repetitive maladaptive behavior patterns, considerable time may be spent on each stage; furthermore, attention moves back and forth across stages, as complex issues are explored from different perspectives. When treatment focuses on a single problem, the model can be used to describe the overall course of therapy, as occurs when treating addictions. The treatment of personality disorder, however, involves multiple problems. Each may be managed using this model. At any moment, the different problems may be at a different stage of change. The model is also useful in conceptualizing change in specific feelings, thoughts, or behaviors. At this micro-management level, minimal time may be spent on each stage, and several stages may be telescoped in a single intervention.

Problem Recognition

Most personality disordered individuals do not fully recognize the causes of their distress or the way they contribute to their problems and the turmoil around them. Problem recognition is limited because personality characteristics are ego-syntonic, that is, they are considered natural and unchangeable qualities. It is also be hindered by attributing responsibility for one's problems to other people, life circumstances, or upbringing. For these reasons, problem recognition always needs to be confirmed, even with obviously self-harming behavior. The therapist's task is to provide the support needed to acknowledge problems and offer sufficient explanation to enable patients to understand how their behavior contributes to their difficulties. This explanation usually involves some degree of reframing to help patients understand how the problem affects their lives. The patient's task is to recognize, acknowledge, and accept his or her problems and commit to change (see Table 4.1).

Problem recognition cannot be rushed: Change cannot occur until the need for change is accepted. Therapists sometimes forget this fact and push for change before a problem is fully acknowledged. When problems are not recognized or accepted, the only course is to continue providing support without pressuring the patient to change. Unfortunately, some therapists act as if denial is best dealt with through active confrontation. What is required, however, is a supportive confrontation that enables the patient "to see and accept reality, so that one can change accordingly" (Miller & Rollnick, 1991, p. 13). The therapist's function is to raise doubts in patients' minds about their denial and the validity of those ideas that hinder problem recognition. Unless this is done supportively, there is the danger that the therapist will be seen as critical or not understanding—perceptions that activate reactive and oppositional patterns. Casually and patiently inquiring about a problem and its effect on the patient and others is often sufficient to enable the patient to recognize and own the problem.

Problem recognition and ownership are not the only goals of this stage. Effective treatment requires the therapist to maximize the readiness to change (Sperry, 1999). Simple comments such as, "This seems to cause difficulties for you. Is this something that you want to change?" highlights the issue, in a nonthreatening and nonjudgmental way, as something to be addressed and builds motivation. Sometimes, however, more extensive work is required to address obstacles to commitment and the fear of change.

Exploration

During this stage knowledge about problems and repetitive maladaptive patterns and the factors that trigger and maintain them is increased through

TABLE 4.1. Problem Recognition

Goal:
- Identify problems as targets for change.

Patient's task:
- Recognize, acknowledge, and accept problem behavior.
- Commit to an effort to change.

Therapist's task:
- Provide the support and security needed to recognize problems and commit to change.
- Provide structured input and education to facilitate problem recognition.

collaborative description. The tasks and interventions involved are summarized in Table 4.2. The patient's task is to be open to exploration and collaborate in the process. This stance is often difficult for patients to achieve, because many problems are experienced as arising spontaneously. Thus the process of exploration often begins by helping patients to recognize events that trigger maladaptive responses. The therapist's task is to clarify events leading to these behaviors and their consequences and to deal with obstacles to self-exploration. In addition, the therapist needs to ensure that exploration proceeds at an appropriate pace and that the patient is not harmed by hasty self-revelation or ruminative introspection.

Creating Connections within Descriptions

To have self-knowledge is to understand, intuitively, the relationships among what is happening to you, what you are experiencing, and what you do. Hence a key intervention is to promote recognition of maladaptive patterns by *linking and connecting* events, experiences, actions, and consequences that previously seemed unrelated. This linkage brings meaning and order to experience and promotes integration. The antecedents–behavior–consequences model (A-B-C model) used in behavioral and cognitive therapy is a useful way to organize this process, regardless of the theoretical orientation of the therapist. The model involves a simple de-

TABLE 4.2. Exploration

Goal:
- Increase self-knowledge.

Patient's task:
- Be open to self-exploration.
- Engage in the collaborative description of problems.

Therapist's task:
- Help the patient to recognize sequences of events leading to problem behaviors and the consequences of these actions.
- Manage the process of descriptive exploration to ensure it proceeds at an appropriate but nonthreatening pace.
- Address obstacles to self-exploration and self-understanding.

Strategies and interventions:
- Create connections within descriptions.
- Reframe descriptive material.
- Focus on molar and molecular aspects of dysfunctional behavior.
- Promote self-observation and self-monitoring.
- Identify environmental contingencies that maintain dysfunctional behaviors.
- Explore obstacles to exploration and the acquisition of self-knowledge.

scriptive process that is neither intrusive nor threatening. Structured methods, such as diaries and daily records of problem behaviors, fit readily into this framework.

The purpose of exploring antecedents is to identify the sequence of events leading to maladaptive responses. Antecedents may be remote "causes" lying in the patient's distant past or more contemporary in origin, or external or internal to the person. In general, the emphasis is on understanding proximal causes. Attention is paid to events in the present that trigger problem behaviors and the cognitive mechanisms that mediate these actions. Attention is also paid to the longer-term consequences of these behaviors for self and others because many patients only consider the immediate effects. This limitation is most apparent with self-mutilation—these acts produce immediate relief, and most patients are unconcerned about longer-term consequences.

Linking is not confined to the temporal sequence of antecedents, behavior, and consequences. It is also important to connect feelings, cognitions, and behaviors. For many patients, discontinuities exist within experience. With emotionally dysregulated or borderline individuals, intense affects lead rapidly to action, so that they rarely reflect on the connection between affect and action, or on the cognitions that precede action. Attention to these components helps to slow the tendency to leap into action and begins to establish the basis for control. With inhibited or schizoid–avoidant individuals, affects are separated from thought and action; hence considerable attention is devoted to gaining access to feelings so that these patients can *feel* that their thoughts and actions are genuine.

Descriptive Reframing

A second element of exploration is to reframe or restructure the meaning attributed to experience. Change is assumed to result from understanding and challenging the way personality processes operate in the present, rather than from insight into the origins of beliefs, feelings, and actions. Reframing changes the way events are perceived and alters their significance for the self; it also stimulates further exploration. Reframing statements are unsettling because they offer a new perspective. To be accepted, they need to arise from the immediate content of therapy and be offered in the context of an effective relationship in a way that is not affectively or cognitively overwhelming.

Reframing statements may be simple responses to a specific event or more complex responses that are the result of a lengthy exploration. The following vignette illustrates the former:

> Assessment of a patient with severe emotional dysregulation had been complicated by the cancellation of several interviews because

the patient was hospitalized with self-inflicted injuries. When discussing the arrangements for therapy, the therapist noted that frequent admissions to the hospital would make it difficult to provide the help that the patient was requesting and needed. The patient responded by saying that she knew that she was a bad person for doing these things. Indeed, her family doctor had told her that he was not prepared to keep her as a patient if she continued to injure herself. The patient added that she would understand if the therapist wanted to draw up a contract in which she agreed not to hurt herself and that treatment would end if she did it again. The therapist noted that she had entered a similar agreement with other therapists, and that it had not worked. She agreed but reiterated that she would understand if the therapist insisted, because she was bad for acting in this way. The therapist commented that it seemed that she cut herself not because she was a bad person but because she could not find a better way to end the painful feelings. The patient was surprised by the remark and began to discuss ways in which she could avoid hospital admissions and attend regularly.

This simple reframe provided an alternative perspective on self-harm that reduced the pressure the patient felt to justify herself and freed her to explore options.

The second example demonstrates a reframing statement that occurred after lengthy exploration:

The patient had been in therapy for some months for the treatment of major depression and problems associated with an inhibited or schizoid–avoidant pattern. A recurrent theme in therapy was the patient's difficulty in deciding upon a direction for his life, including a career. The problem was difficult to resolve because nothing seemed real—everything lacked authenticity, even his feelings and wants. This unreality caused intense despondency that contributed to the depressive symptoms. Difficulty establishing a sense of identity and determining a life course had been discussed for some time. Part of the difficulty was that the patient always felt criticized by himself and others. No matter what he did or wanted, there was always a nagging inner voice that criticized his decisions and actions. He recognized that the self-criticism related to childhood feelings that his parents never truly valued anything he did but rather continually criticized his performance and abilities. His father had been especially critical, telling his son that he would never be as good as he himself. The patient assumed that his father must be right. This assumption allowed the boy to continue loving his father and believing that his father loved him, despite the cruel things the father said. He also thought that his father would not be able to cope if his opinions were challenged. In some way that he did not fully understand, the family behaved as if the father were extremely vulnerable.

During the session in question, the patient mentioned that he had felt criticized by a casual friend who had stayed with him the previous weekend. His friend was married and had a job. He had been critical of everything that the patient did and wanted to do. During the previous few weeks, the patient had made several decisions, including some career choices, and he had taken important steps to realize these goals. His friend criticized both the decisions and the steps. The patient was devastated and became acutely depressed. He felt that his acquaintance must be right and that he had got it all wrong. He added that he could not disagree with his friend because that might upset him. The therapist offered the simple reframe that the patient always seemed to be prepared to sacrifice his ideas for those of other people, even if that meant devaluing his own thoughts and ideas. The patient paused and said, "I give in to everyone." A few moments later, he added, "I have suddenly realized: *This* is the cause of my problems." This realization led to a discussion of how he sacrificed his self-esteem for the good of others. He recalled discussions in previous sessions about his father, and how he had accepted what his father had said as right because it seemed to be the best thing *for his father*. During the next few sessions, this statement was explored at length, along with work the patient did between sessions on identifying everyday incidents where he automatically accepted what others said, regardless of his own views. He came to recognize that this way of thinking undermined his self-esteem and, more importantly, his belief in himself and his ability to establish a sense of identity.

The Molar and Molecular Components of Dysfunctional Behavior

Repetitive behavior patterns are explored and changed using a two-step strategy: (1) ensure recognition of the global pattern, and (2) explore the specific behaviors through which the pattern is expressed. This strategy combines the psychodynamic approach of identifying broad patterns of relating with the behavior therapy focus on detailed behavioral analysis of specific acts and causal chains leading to problem behavior. Change begins when a global pattern is recognized. This recognition connects diverse experiences and behaviors and changes the way events are experienced. But change lies in the details. It depends upon recognizing the specific ways that these patterns are expressed in everyday life. Consider the submissive patient discussed earlier. An understanding of this pattern helped the patient to understand how submissiveness affected her life and relationships. But the idea is rather abstract, and it was difficult for the patient to figure out how to act differently. By encouraging the patient to identify the specific ways in which she acted submissively, the pattern was decomposed into progressively more specific features (see Figure 4.1). One component of submissiveness in this patient was the tendency to put other people before herself. This behavior involved (1) acceding to others demands, (2) difficulty expressing and satisfying her own needs, and (3) problems expressing her opinion. Specific examples of these tendencies became the targets for change. For example, when the patient would meet a friend socially, she was encouraged to say what she would like to do occasionally, rather than always deferring to the friend's suggestions, or to say no sometimes to an unreasonable request from a family member. Such specific changes are more likely to be successful and less threatening than trying to change a global pattern. Not many successes are needed to modulate the pattern.

The following vignette illustrates work on the two levels:

A patient who had been in combined group and individual therapy for just over a year arrived for an individual session, enraged about the group that she had just attended. She had been looking forward to the group because several problems had arisen that she wanted to discuss and she thought that she would receive support. However, people talked about their own problems, and no one asked how she was feeling. As the group progressed, she became increasingly angry but remained silent. About 20 minutes before the end, one member noted that she had been quiet and wondered whether there was something that she wanted to talk about. The patient said that she had nothing to say.

The therapist asked what had happened next. Apparently everyone continued to talk about their problems. When the therapist wondered about her reaction, the patient said that she was so mad at being ignored that she was not prepared to talk to people who

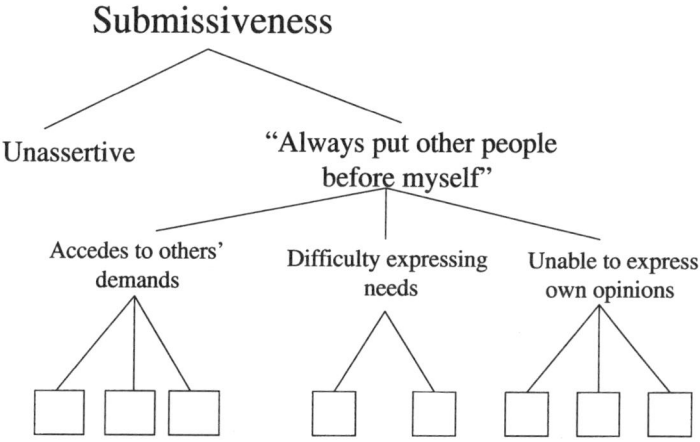

FIGURE 4.1. Components of submissiveness.

treated her in that way. The therapist wondered who lost out in this situation. Angrily, the patient replied that she did. The others did not care. Her silence gave them more time to talk about themselves. After a moment's reflection, she asked, "Do you think I am passive–aggressive?" The therapist wondered whether this kind of situation happened frequently. This question led to an extensive discussion of other instances. The therapist then asked whether this was a problem and whether she wanted to do anything about it. The patient noted that this behavior complicated all her relationships and that she would probably get on much better with people if she stopped acting in this way. She could only express anger and resentment in a passive, indirect manner, which led to the breakup of many relationships.

Recognition of the pattern helped the patient to understand many events both in her current and past life. But it was only when she began to notice this behavior in everyday life and discussed these examples in depth in treatment that change began to occur. Instead of noting more dramatic examples that led to intense anger, she began recognizing the nuances of this behavior and the specific ways it influenced everyday interactions. A focus on incidents that did not arouse strong feelings made it easier to recognize the pattern, challenge associated thoughts, and act differently. Over time she began to understand that she could be assertive without creating problems, and that she could let other people know about her thoughts, feelings, and wants without untoward consequences.

This example illustrates the value of working at molar and molecular levels simultaneously. Acknowledgment of the passive–aggressive pattern enabled the patient to understand some common relationship problems that had previously been blamed on others. The therapist's query about whether this was something that she wanted to change established a commitment to change. Exploration of the situations that triggered this behavior and its consequences increased feelings of control and provided the basis for considering alternatives actions. However, change ultimately depended on recognizing how the pattern was expressed in everyday situations.

Promoting Self-Observation and Self-Monitoring

Improved self-observation and self-monitoring skills are important consequences of exploration. Self-monitoring should be distinguished from self-awareness. Self-awareness occurs when attention is focused on an aspect of the self (Wicklund, 1975; Wicklund & Duval, 1971). Self-monitoring combines *awareness* of an aspect of the self with an *evaluation* of the experience. The distinction between self-awareness and self-monitoring is pertinent to understanding self-experience in personality disorder. Many individuals with personality disorder are exquisitely self-aware and experience things intensely but have difficulty reflecting on this experience. Instead, they suppress knowledge of the experience, ruminate over it, or leap impulsively from experience to action. The challenge is to encourage patients to be curious about their own minds and reflect on the nature, causes, and consequences of their experience. This curiosity establishes a reflective loop that increases self-regulation and sets the stage for more effective goal-directed behavior. Goal attainment depends upon the ability to monitor the effects of one's actions (Carver & Scheier, 1998). Most of the time people are trying to reach particular goals, whether these are long-term goals such as career plans, short-term goals such as going to the movies, personal goals such as learning tennis, or interpersonal goals such as eliciting care. Success depends on monitoring progress and modifying behavior to ensure goal attainment. With many simple goals, monitoring is automatic, but complex goals require conscious evaluation. This kind of self-monitoring is difficult for many patients, especially when intense affects are involved, because their attention then focuses on the experience rather than on evaluation.

Self-monitoring skills are promoted by encouraging patients to reflect on their experiences during treatment and through mindfulness or attention control training (Linehan, 1993; Teasdale, Segal, & Williams, 1995). A longer-term objective is to encourage patients to incorporate into their coping repertoire the techniques and skills that the therapist uses to understand and analyze problems. This incorporation is facilitated by focusing on improved self-observation, with comments such as:

> "You seem to be recognizing how you react."
> "You seem to be finding it easier to recognize your patterns."
> "You seem to be able to stand back more and take a look at what is going on."
> "Rather than just reacting, you seem to have developed the ability to step back and try to understand what is happening and why you are reacting in this way."

Self-monitoring is also enhanced by keeping a journal to record the occurrence of problematic behaviors and thoughts and the feelings, thoughts, and actions associated with everyday events. To be effective for this purpose, the journal should be a vehicle for reflecting on experiences rather than simply emoting.

Identifying Maintenance Factors

A key part of exploration is to identify factors that help to maintain problems. In Chapter 3, it was noted that cyclical maladaptive interpersonal patterns are maintained by internal factors, such as selective attention to information, and external factors, such as other people's reactions that confirm these patterns. Patients do not always recognize, however, how other people reinforce their behavior. Change requires that these reinforcing factors are identified and modified.

Obstacles to Exploration

The path to self-knowledge is often blocked by self-deception strategies and personality characteristics, including cognitive styles that limit self-understanding. Avoidance is common in patients with personality disorder (Young, 1990, 1994). Self-knowledge is actively suppressed by distraction and diverting attention from painful affects and experiences. It is common for patients to say, "I don't want to think about that" or "I don't want to talk about that." In most circumstances, however, the patient is not aware of the avoidance. Self-deception strategies may be managed using classical defense interpretations based on the triangle of conflict (Ezriel, 1952; Malan, 1979), in which the therapist confronts defensive behavior and comments on the anxiety that evokes it with the intent of uncovering hidden feelings. Figure 4.2 shows a more general version of the model, which applies to the self-deceptive behaviors that limit self-experience and obstruct the development of self-knowledge. Suppression, avoidance, and distraction are among the many behaviors used to limit self-understanding and avoid the fear, shame, guilt, or pain that is believed will result from acknowledging, thinking about, or revealing what is being avoided.

An important question is how self-deception is best managed. In some dynamic therapies an *anxiety-provoking approach* is used, in which defenses

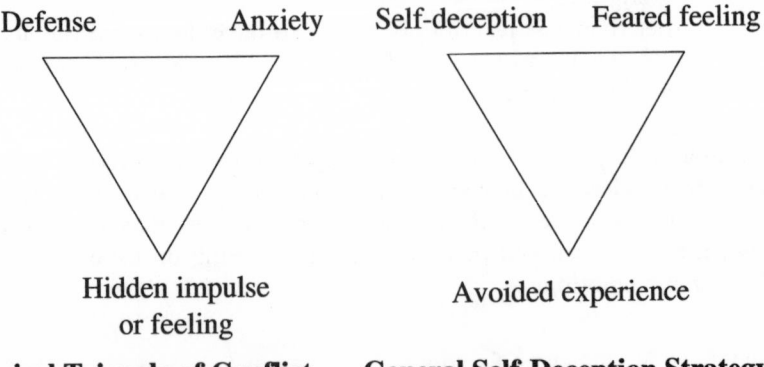

Classical Triangle of Conflict   **General Self-Deception Strategy**

FIGURE 4.2. Triangle of conflict and self-deception strategies.

are actively confronted and interpreted. This approach tends to cause problems when treating personality disordered patients. The anxiety aroused increases behavioral disorganization, and the challenge involved tends to activate reactive patterns in emotionally dysregulated and dissocial patients and to feel intrusive and overwhelming, leading to further withdrawal, in inhibited patients. An *affect-regulating approach*, which helps patients to deal with warded-off experience in tolerable amounts, is more effective (McCullough & Vaillant, 1997). In this approach the avoidance is noted and the patient invited to join the therapist in observing his or her own behavior. For example: "I have noticed that whenever we begin to discuss your anger with your mother, you quickly start talking about something else. Have you noticed this?" Such interventions invite collaboration in self-observation that can be extended by asking about the worse aspects of their fears, shame, or pain (McCullough & Vaillant, 1997). The result is a supportive and encouraging exploration of the feared consequences of disclosure.

Other personality characteristics may also obstruct exploration. Affective lability, for example, may produce an intense and volatile emotional climate that is not conducive to exploration and reflection. Global and diffuse ways of thinking, as characterized by the hysterical cognitive style (Shapiro, 1965), make it difficult to focus on the details of experience. Similarly, a self-invalidating cognitive style hinders exploration because affected individuals continually doubt their experience.

Acquisition of Alternative Behaviors

The development of alternative behaviors is a critical stage that warrants more attention than it typically receives from many therapies. Although exploration using the A-B-C model automatically facilitates the identification of alternative behaviors, the transition from understanding to behavioral change is not easy. Most clinicians have encountered patients who believe that therapy will not be helpful because they are already aware of the reasons for their difficulties but cannot translate understanding into behavioral change. The patient's task is to be open to change and to identify and apply alternative behaviors (Table 4.3). The therapist's tasks are to ensure that the understanding achieved through exploration leads to change and to maintain the commitment to change.

Achieving change involves attitudinal and behavioral components. The attitudinal component usually requires addressing the fear of change and anxiety about the consequences of acting differently. The behavioral component includes the acquisition of new responses and skills and the inhibition of old behaviors. Considerable therapist activity is often required to support and validate new developments. This role is readily accepted by therapists of more eclectic, cognitive, or behavioral orientations. Psycho-

TABLE 4.3. Acquisition of Alternative Behaviors

Goal:
- Identify and implement alternative behaviors.

Patient's task:
- Be open to change.
- Identify alternative responses.
- Apply new learning.

Therapist's task:
- Ensure that self-understanding is translated into behavior change.
- Maintain the commitment to change.
- Address obstacles to change.

Strategies and interventions:
- Generate alternative responses.
- Maintain motivation to change.
- Inhibit old patterns.
- Provide skill training.

dynamic therapists also have noted that many aspects of personality disturbance are best modified by a noninterpretative stance that supports new
experiences and actions (Buie & Adler, 1982; Gunderson, 1984), and that
therapists should encourage the patient to explore new interests and ways
of relating to the world during the later stages and be prepared to discuss
these activities in detail (Masterson, 1976).

Generating Alternatives

The acquisition of alternatives is a *problem-solving stage* that is managed
with considerable attention to process. Patients need to acquire new skills
in analyzing problems and flexibility in considering alternatives. Problem
solving can often be handled in a direct way, though sometimes a lighter
touch is required, in which patients are encouraged to "play" with the idea
of doing things differently. This approach often helps to reduce fears of
change and the feeling of pressure to act differently. When we play, we
can tell ourselves that we do not really mean it. This fantasy quality lets
patients try out things without the worries that occur when actions are really meant. However, many patients have difficulty playing and have little
sense of fun or pleasure. Hence this stage provides an opportunity to encourage spontaneity, to experiment, and to enjoy the idea of doing things
differently. This idea also recognizes the significance of a supportive relationship. As attachment theory makes clear, young children are only able
to play and explore their environments effectively when they feel secure.
Similarly in therapy, patients can only make full use of the opportunity to

explore problems freely and contemplate or play with alternatives when they feel secure and supported.

Maintaining Motivation to Change

For many patients, the challenge of implementing change is a frustrating one. The feeling of being stuck decreases self-esteem, increases self-blame, and tends to reactivate maladaptive patterns. The therapist's challenge is to acknowledge and validate fears and frustrations while maintaining hope and motivation. Old patterns are familiar, and the patient knows what to expect even though they cause problems and distress. Change creates uncertainty and anxiety because it requires patients to relinquish major assumptions about self and others, on which they have based their lives.

Motivation is often easier to maintain and change is more likely when patients feel that they can change gradually rather than all at once. The *gradual substitution of progressively more adaptive behaviors* is an effective way to modify various forms of dysfunctional behavior, including self-harming acts (see Chapter 8) and maladaptive trait expressions (see Chapter 12). For instance, it is difficult to relinquish self-harming behaviors that reduce distress until more adaptive ways to manage distress are learned. Change initially may focus on reducing the frequency of these acts or delaying their onset rather than ceasing them altogether. It may also involve encouraging patients to seek help from a crisis service or an emergency room, without engaging in self-harm. Subsequently, patients may be helped to manage distress and postpone seeking help until the next appointment. In effect, patients gradually substitute more adaptive ways of dealing with crises until they acquire the skills needed to manage their distress and problems without engaging in self-harm. Similar sequences of substitution can be developed to deal with other behaviors, such as maladaptive traits.

Inhibiting Old Patterns

Maladaptive thoughts, feelings, and actions often occur so rapidly and automatically that it is difficult, in the moment, to apply new learning. Hence strategies are required to inhibit habitual responses long enough for the individual to reflect upon the situation and deploy new responses (Benjamin, 1993). Perhaps the simplest way to inhibit an old pattern is to use *a direct approach that relies upon the therapist's authority to inhibit an action*. Although this type of intervention may cause problems for the alliance, the approach is justified when the patient engages in serious self-harming behaviors. For example, a patient who had been in therapy for several years continued to have unprotected sex with casual partners because she could not refuse their demands. Although she had discussed alternative ways of handling such situations many times, she could not use them when the need arose. After one incident that had been particularly dangerous, the therapist commented, "You can't keep doing this without serious consequences." The word *can't*, with its prohibitive connotations, was used to emphasize risk. Under some circumstances, such interventions may increase acting-out behavior or provoke anger. However, interventions are influenced by context. In this case, there was a strong alliance and the patient perceived the comment as an expression of concern. When she was next in a similar situation, she recalled the therapist's words—which created sufficient distance and control within her to allow her to apply newly acquired assertiveness skills. She continued using this memory until she became comfortable setting limits on her own, without the need to recall the therapist's comment.

Changing impulsive behaviors such as self-harming acts is often difficult because the strong feelings that trigger these acts prevent the use of new coping behaviors. In these cases, *distracting activities* may reduce feelings sufficiently to inhibit an old pattern and allow the patient to mobilize coping skills. A variety of activities that can be used with minimal thought—such as exercise, seeking the company of a friend, or watching a movie—can be identified in advance and applied the moment the impulse to self-harm arises. In most cases, a combination of cognitive, behavioral, and pharmacological interventions is needed to create *a delay between the triggering stimulus and the resulting response.*

Teaching New Skills

Change often requires the use of skills that are poorly developed or absent or that the individual is not comfortable using. Under these circumstances, skill training or strengthening is an important therapeutic task (Linehan, 1993). Two kinds of skill deficits occur in people who have personality disorder. *Instrumental deficits* involve the skills needed to manage emotions and impulses or solve interpersonal problems, such as affect regulation, assertiveness, social, and communication skills. These deficits can usually be remedied by appropriate training. The other deficit is more complex. In many patients, instrumental deficits reflect fundamental *problems of a procedural nature* that are part of the core pathology—patients lack an intuitive understanding of what behaviors are appropriate or expected in given situations. These deficits are more difficult to remedy, and skill training appears to have limited effect.

Consolidation and Generalization

Changes of the magnitude involved in treating personality disorder take time to consolidate. Change is usually gradual (Piper & Joyce, 2001); behaviors fluctuate and dysfunctional patterns return, especially at times of stress and as termination approaches. Change will be sustained only if (1) new coping strategies continue to be used when treatment ends, and (2) new behaviors are consolidated into habitual action patterns that are generalized to everyday situations. The tasks and interventions associated with this stage are summarized in Table 4.4.

The Importance of Repetition

Faced with the many challenges of treating personality pathology, it is easy to overlook the value of simple repetition in consolidating change. Repetition is required to help patients recognize the many different ways maladaptive patterns are expressed and to strengthen new skills and coping strategies. Considerable therapist tolerance is required to cope with reversals and the persistence of old patterns. When frustrated by the degree of repetition required, it is often helpful for therapists to recall the many times that maladaptive behaviors were reinforced over the years and that the reinforcement of more adaptive responses in treatment is meager in comparison.

A problem with repetition is that it may increase the patient's frustrations with the slow pace of change and evoke resentment if interventions are perceived as stereotyped, critical, and invalidating, or as a sign that the therapist has lost interest. An effective therapeutic alliance reduces the chances of interventions being misperceived in this way. It also often helpful to incorporate a psychoeducational component to explain that the behavior in question was learned over a considerable period of time and, like any habit, it is difficult to change. For some patients, however, repeti-

---

TABLE 4.4. Consolidation and Generalization

Goal:
  • Consolidate change and generalize new learning to everyday events outside therapy.

Patient's task:
  • Apply new learning to everyday life.

Therapist's task:
  • Ensure transfer of training to everyday life.
  • Strengthen the skills required to maintain change.
  • Address obstacles to consolidation and generalization.

Strategies and interventions:
  • Provide repetition to consolidate change.
  • Apply new learning to specific, everyday situations.
  • Develop maintenance strategies.
  • Ensure appropriate attribution of change.

---

tion is reassuring. One patient who engaged in repetitive suicidal and parasuicidal behavior talked about suicide as if it were a reversible state. Reality testing was improved when the therapist commented, "Death is forever." The patient found the repetition of this phrase in treatment comforting, and she repeated it to herself whenever she thought about suicide.

Applying New Learning to Specific Situations

Generalization is facilitated by encouraging patients to apply new learning to specific situations. Real-life situations provide an opportunity to discuss the details of new behaviors and deal with problems encountered when acting differently. With anxiety-provoking situations, it may be necessary to *rehearse* these scenarios, either in imagination or via role playing in the session, so that patients can fine-tune their behavior. In the example of the submissive patient described earlier, discussion of a specific problem situation—interaction with her plastic surgeon—increased the patient's understanding of the pattern and her confidence in acting differently. Change was facilitated by developing a script for a desired interaction with the surgeon, which was then role played in the group. Subsequently, change was consolidated by the group's persistent interest in hearing about the patient's results from acting more assertively.

Developing Maintenance Strategies

Skills such as self-understanding and problem analysis, affect and impulse regulation, self-monitoring, self-validation, and problem solving are critical for enduring change. As therapy moves into the later stages, these skills should be reviewed and the patient helped to recognize how to apply them in future. Particular attention also should be paid to habitual self-deception mechanisms so that the patient is alerted to the way these contribute to problems. Coping mechanisms that are critical for the individual can be highlighted and problems in their application discussed. This approach provides an opportunity to anticipate problems that the patient is likely to encounter in the future, so that strategies can be developed for the patient to use should problems arise.

Attribution of Change

An important factor in maintaining behavioral change is the individual's explanation of the change process. Research on healthy subjects shows that changes attributed to internal factors are more likely to be maintained than changes attributed to external factors (Schoeneman & Curry, 1990; Sonne & Janoff, 1979). Also, subjects reporting successful change are more likely to refer to internal control mechanisms and less likely to refer to ex-

ternal obstacles (Heatherton & Nichols, 1994a, 1994b). This pattern suggests that attributing change to one's own efforts—to personal effectiveness, agency, and internal control—helps to maintain change (Weiner,
1985). Individuals who believe that they overcame a problem through
their own efforts create a self-fulfilling prophecy that may help to maintain
the change (Heatherton & Nichols, 1994b). This finding suggests that patients should be encouraged to take realistic credit for any changes that
they make, and that attempts to minimize the significance of change or attribute it to the therapist or other external factors should be curtailed.
This focus helps the patient to "own" the changes that have occurred
(Horvath & Greenberg, 1994) and promotes self-esteem and attributions
of self-efficacy. If used consistently throughout treatment, it also helps to
diffuse excessive dependency. Nevertheless, the therapist's contribution
also needs to be acknowledged. Achieving this balance between self and
therapist attributions facilitates the consolidation of cooperative behavior—
an objective of therapy—and offsets the dangers inherent in the patient
believing that "I had to do it all by myself" (Horvath & Greenberg, 1994,
p. 4).

Stages of Change: Additional Principles

Several additional issues are pertinent to implementing the stages of change
approach: (1) the importance of addressing problems from multiple perspectives, (2) emphasizing the role of cognitions, (3) capitalizing on specific events, and (4) evaluating the role of transference interpretations.

Utilizing Multiple Perspectives

It is useful to focus on problems from multiple perspectives to minimize
the potential stalemate caused by the fact that most maladaptive patterns
are well entrenched and most interventions have limited efficacy. The
availability of an array of interventions tends to reduce resistance to
change and the activation of reactive behaviors that may occur when a
given intervention is used persistently. As Horowitz and Marmar (1985)
noted, persistently challenging obstacles to change usually evokes further
resistance in patients, and also tends to provoke patients to perceive the
therapist malevolently and as authoritarian. In contrast, the use of multiple interventions is often less threatening and anxiety provoking, provided
the interventions are "held" within a coherent framework.

Emphasizing Cognitions

Although interventions are drawn from different schools, emphasis is placed
upon understanding the cognitive processes underlying maladaptive behav-

ior: how patients perceive and understand themselves, other people, and their situation. Attention is paid to the origin of these processes *only if it is necessary to understand contemporary functioning and validate significant experiences*. An emphasis on cognitions reflects the importance that most therapies place on understanding how maladaptive cognitions initiate and sustain symptoms and problems. It also reflects evidence that patients with personality disorder respond better to the more structured behavioral and cognitive treatments (Hardy et al., 1995; Shea, Widiger, & Klein, 1992).

A cognitive approach is an effective way to manage the different patterns of personality disorder; it provides the structure patients with the emotional dysregulation or borderline pattern need to contain chaotic feelings and impulses, and it is consistent with an affect-regulating, as opposed to an affect-ventilating, strategy, which appears to be more effective especially early in treatment. Patients with the inhibited or schizoid–avoidant pattern also find a cognitive approach less threatening, because it provides structure without being intrusive. This nonintrusiveness is more likely to foster the therapeutic alliance than methods that push for affect expression. Similarly, compulsive patients find a cognitive approach more consistent with their preference for structure, and it reduces their fear that they will lose control if they express their feelings.

Capitalizing on Specific Events

Studies of nonclinical subjects indicate that the decision to change is often triggered by specific events that cause them to see their situation differently (Heatherton & Nichols, 1994a). As noted, change is a source of conflict for many, and the benefits of change are weighed against the costs of change. Specific events often motivate the individual to reexamine the situation and alter the relative weights of changing versus staying the same (Miller & Rolnick, 1991). This shift toward change is illustrated by the following vignette:

> The patient, a 28-year-old single mother with a long history of impulsive and acting-out behavior, had been in treatment with her present therapist for just under a year, although she had previously received extensive therapy. During this time little had changed. High levels of affective lability created major difficulties in therapy and everyday life. On one occasion, the patient arrived for therapy in an extremely angry and reactive state. Within minutes of beginning the session, she jumped from her chair, swept everything off the therapist's desk, and stormed from the office. Everything happened so quickly that the therapist had little opportunity to react. Subsequent attempts at contact failed.
>
> Three years later the patient contacted the therapist for an appointment. The subsequent meeting was illuminating. The interview

began with the patient asking whether the therapist recalled the previous incident, which indeed he did. She then explained what had happened afterward. As she walked across the car park after storming out of the office, she suddenly stopped and told herself that she could not continue to behave or live in this way. The realization was powerful and transforming. On the spot she decided not to seek further treatment but to change nonetheless. Although the ensuing 3 years had been difficult, she had radically changed her lifestyle. She had discarded friendships that contributed to her problems and found a job, and she had managed to work nearly full-time for the last 2 years. Now she felt ready for more challenging work. The reason for contacting the therapist was to seek advice about this next step and to ask the therapist to provide a medical report to help her obtain further training.

This vignette is interesting because it is an unusual illustration of a real-life event triggering quantum change in a person with a personality disorder (Miller & C'de Baca, 2001). The incentive to change requires a sense of discontentment with one's life or some aspect of oneself (Baumeister, 1991, 1994). Without feeling that things are not the way one would like them to be, there is little commitment to change. When these events occur, they serve as powerful enhancers of the commitment to change.

Evaluating Transference Interpretations

A critical issue for treatment is the role of transference interpretations in the change process. Although psychodynamic interventions form only part of the repertoire of interventions proposed here, the significance placed on transference interpretations in psychodynamic models of change forces us to consider their use. Unfortunately, information on the relationship between transference interpretations and the therapeutic alliance and outcome is based largely on studies of short-term individual therapy. These studies initially suggested that the frequency of transference interpretations is positively related to outcome (Malan, 1979; Marziali & Sullivan, 1980). Later studies using better methodology did not support this conclusion (Marziali, 1984; Piper, Marrache, & Koenig, 1986). Instead, it has been found that the relationship between transference interpretations and outcome depends on patient characteristics, especially the quality of object relationships (Connolly et al., 1999). In patients with poor object relationships, high levels of transference interpretation are associated with a poorer alliance and outcome (Ogrodniczuk, Piper, Joyce, & McCallum, 1999). Although these findings apply to quality of object relationships rather than personality disorder, the characteristics defining poor object relationships are similar to those used to define personality disorder (see Chapter 2).

They are also consistent with suggestions that transference interpretation should be used cautiously with those who have difficulty reflecting on their personal relationships (Gabbard et al., 1994). Thus current evidence suggests that minimal use should be made of transference interpretations when treating personality disorder. Given this conclusion, it is important to understand what is meant by a *transference interpretation*.

Transference interpretations address the patient's reaction to the therapist and the extent to which that reaction was determined by the patient's previous relationships (Piper, 1993). The term also refers to dynamic processes such as wishes, anxieties, and defenses. It does not include interventions that clarify the patient's relationship to the therapist—for example, a simple description of the relationship. Hence the proposal that transference interpretations be minimized does not mean that the therapist should not refer to the relationship; indeed, there is considerable value to doing so. Such interventions, however, should be confined to describing and clarifying how the patient relates to the therapist and should minimize attributing the pattern to unconscious processes and motives.

Transference interpretations probably have an adverse effect on patients with severely impaired interpersonal functioning because such individuals have difficulty using the therapeutic relationship as a vehicle for understanding their problems (Ogrodniczuk et al., 1999). These patients usually want to develop a relationship with their therapist, or they are fearful of that relationship, or there is a conflict between the want and the fear. In these circumstances, transference interpretations interfere with the bond between patient and therapist. An interpretative focus may also generate anxiety or lead the patient to conclude that the therapist is being critical. Both reactions place a strain on the relationship, which leads to the patient's disengagement (Ogrodniczuk et al., 1999). It is also possible that therapists focus on the transference more when therapy is not progressing satisfactorily and when the therapeutic alliance is impaired. With personality disordered patients, doing so appears to make the problem worse.

However, it may be appropriate to handle positive and negative reactions to the therapist differently. Positive feelings may be used to build the alliance. As Buie and Adler (1982) noted, a positive transference can be allowed to change through what Kohut (1971) referred to as "optimal disillusionment." As treatment proceeds, the patient notices discrepancies between his or her idealized views and the therapist's actual behavior. Small failures by the therapist gradually transform an idealized perception into a more realistic impression that incorporates positive *and* negative elements. Each little disappointment with the therapist, provided it is not overwhelming, helps patients to modulate idealized views. The therapist can facilitate this process by openly discussing these "failures." Negative transference, on the other hand, requires more direct attention, especially when it threatens to disrupt therapy. The emphasis should be on clarifying negative feelings and supporting the patient in expressing them, rather than interpreting them in the traditional sense.

COMMENT

This chapter provides a broad overview of change processes from a generic perspective that is intended to bring order and structure to a complex arena. A generic approach is adopted because the evidence suggests that the nonspecific component makes the greatest contribution to change; an approach based on generic mechanisms promises to provide the most effective way to manage and treat core pathology. Two principles are introduced that are consistent with this emphasis. First, the work of therapy is viewed as a process of collaborative description, wherein patient and therapist work together to understand the structures and processes contributing to the dysfunctional behavior. Second, the stages of change approach is used to organize the management of specific problems, ranging from self-harming behavior to maladaptive interpersonal patterns. In subsequent chapters these ideas are extended to include a framework for understanding the overall structure of treatment.

CHAPTER 5

Assessment

Comprehensive treatment planning requires a detailed assessment to establish a diagnosis of personality disorder, evaluate personality patterns, and describe problems across the six domains of psychopathology—symptoms, situational factors, affect and impulse regulation, traits, interpersonal behaviors, and self system—that will become the targets for change. The information obtained is used to formulate the individual's psychopathology and the circumstances that led to current problems and to construct a treatment plan and negotiate the treatment contract.

OVERVIEW OF THE ASSESSMENT PROCESS

Assessment typically requires two or three interviews. Although this length may be considered excessive in some settings, the reality is, it takes time to assess complex disorders. In the long run, it is more cost-effective to conduct a careful assessment than engage in therapy when many issues are unclear. The exception is an emergency evaluation of a crisis state involving serious self-harming and suicidal behavior or serious Axis I symptoms. Here a more focused assessment is appropriate to provide sufficient information to take action that ensures the patient's safety and manage immediate problems.

As with any mental disorder, assessment begins with a detailed psychiatric history and mental state examination. Because history and examination are standard procedures, they are discussed further. Subsequent interviews are used to expand the developmental history by obtaining more detailed information about:

Parental and family relationships
Reactions to key developmental events and transitions
Significant losses or separations, including relocations
Preliminary assessment of incidents of trauma and deprivation
Peer relationships
Important memories

Subsequent interviews are also used for more systematic evaluation of personality. The latter part of assessment is devoted to discussing the formulation with the patient and establishing the treatment contract.

Attention to Process

The assessment process offers opportunities to begin establishing the conditions for treatment by building credibility, forging positive expectations about treatment, beginning to establish a working relationship, and preparing patients for therapy. To achieve these objectives, the process of the interview needs to be monitored and any difficulties addressed immediately, even if the more structured aspects of assessment have to be suspended. Difficulties often arise in this early stage because many patients distrust perceived authority figures and come for assessment burdened with negative expectations formed during earlier experiences with the mental health system, as illustrated by the following vignette:

A 25-year-old woman attended an outpatient clinic for assessment. The only information available to the assessing clinician was that she had a psychiatric history dating from her early teens, and that she self-mutilated frequently. Initial inquiry about the problems that led to the referral elicited a sullen response and few details. After a few minutes, the interviewer commented that she looked uncomfortable and seemed to be experiencing difficulty with the interview. He added that he needed her help if he was to offer constructive suggestions for treatment. The patient became more animated. She said that she did not think that the interviewer was really interested or wanted to talk to her. She added that she certainly did not want to be there and, anyway, she enjoyed being obnoxious to psychiatrists. The clinician wondered whether that was because of bad experiences in the past. The patient said that she had never found psychiatrists to be helpful and, in fact, that they always treated her badly. The clinician asked when that "bad treatment" first happened. The patient explained that in her mid-teens, she was admitted to a hospital where the staff were critical and judgmental. The interviewer commented that he could understand why that unpleasant experience was having such a big impact upon her now. Nevertheless, he needed her help if he was to be able to suggest ways to help her.

This vignette indicates the importance of flexibility during assessment. Patients often present with considerable baggage, so that it is important to avoid giving the impression of following a fixed assessment protocol or having preconceived ideas about their difficulties. It also helps if the interviewer shares appropriate information about his or her developing understanding of the patient's problems and asks for the patient's reaction. Structuring the interaction in this way communicates the idea that treatment is an active collaboration. For this reason, it is helpful to ask, "What would you like to get out of our meeting?" at some point during the first interview.

Structured Assessment Instruments

It is often useful to supplement clinical interviews with structured assessment instruments. These instruments offer an economical way to obtain additional information on symptoms, traits, coping behaviors, interpersonal problems, and self-functioning (MacKenzie, 1994, 2001, 2002). Several measures are discussed later that the clinician may wish to consider. Structured measures are particularly useful in correcting biases that may occur when clinicians make intuitive assessments of personality rather than assess diagnostic features (Blashfield & Herkov, 1996; MacKenzie, 1994; Morey & Ochoa, 1989); they also provide systematic information with which to assess progress and evaluate treatment. Questionnaires may be completed between interviews in the office or at home. The results should be available for the last assessment session and incorporated into the formulation.

Clinicians are sometimes concerned that questionnaires will adversely affect the treatment relationship. This rarely happens if the interviewer explains that the information gained will be helpful to treatment and that the patient will be given the results. Many patients appreciate the information provided by questionnaires and find that the process focuses their attention on critical issues. Problems arise when the patient feels that the information is being collected for the therapist's benefit or only for research purposes.

DIAGNOSIS OF PERSONALITY DISORDER

The diagnosis and assessment of personality disorder is approached in two steps (Cloninger, 2000; Livesley, 1998, 2003; Livesley et al., 1994). First, evaluate the presence of personality disorder based on general diagnostic criteria, such as those proposed by DSM-IV and ICD-10, or the adaptive failure definition described in Chapter 2. Second, assess individual differences in personality disorder, using either DSM-IV or ICD-10 diagnoses,

or a dimensional model such as the four patterns and component traits discussed in Chapter 2. It is useful to evaluate the presence of personality disorder *per se* because this is more stable than diagnoses of specific categories
of disorder (David & Pilkonis, 1996). The two-step process also provides
more information for treatment planning.

Although the DSM-IV general criteria for a personality disorder (see
Table 5.1) describe important features common to all cases, ultimately
they are not helpful in establishing a diagnosis because they are poorly defined and difficult to evaluate reliably. For example, specific problems with
"interpersonal functioning" are not specified. Moreover, the criterion set
does not provide the information on core pathology needed for treatment
planning. For these reasons, the criteria based on the adaptive failure definition are adopted here. Many clinicians, however, will likely be more
comfortable basing their diagnoses on the DSM. This preference is consistent with the current approach to treatment, although it should be supplemented with an evaluation of the core pathology that is needed to plan
the overall approach.

Personality disorder was defined in Chapter 2 as the failure to estab-

---

TABLE 5.1. The DSM-IV General Criteria for Personality Disorder

A. An enduring pattern of inner experience and behavior that deviates markedly from
the expectations of the individual's culture. This pattern is manifested in two (or
more) of the following areas:

(1) cognition (i.e., ways of perceiving and interpreting the self, other people, and
events)
(2) affectivity (i.e., the range, intensity, lability, and appropriateness of emotional
response)
(3) interpersonal functioning
(4) impulse control

B. The enduring pattern is inflexible and pervasive across a broad range of personal
and social situations.

C. The enduring pattern leads to clinically significant distress or impairment in social,
occupational, or other important areas of functioning.

D. The pattern is stable and of long duration and its onset can be traced back at least
to adolescence or early adulthood.

E. The enduring pattern is not better accounted for as a manifestation or
consequence of another mental disorder.

F. The enduring pattern is not due to the direct physiological effects of a substance
(e.g., a drug of abuse, a medication) or a general medical condition (e.g., head
trauma).

Note. From American Psychiatric Association (1994, p. 633). Copyright 1994 by the American Psychiatric Association. Reprinted by permission.

lish: (1) an adaptive self-system; (2) the capacity for intimacy and attachment; or (3) the ability to function effectively at a societal level. Diagnosis is based on the presence of one or more of these features. Although these criteria may also seem vague, they can be specified in ways that lead to reliable assessment (Livesley, 1998). Table 5.2 provides a detailed description of each feature. A standard history generally provides considerable information on which to base a clinical evaluation of these features. For example, general details of social and interpersonal behavior are pertinent to assessing capacity for intimacy and whether the individual is capable of cooperation and functioning effectively in society. Initial assessment can be supplemented by more systematic evaluation, based on the features listed in Table 5.2 and the patient's self-description, resulting in a clinical evaluation of whether problems with the self and interpersonal and societal functioning are indicative of personality disorder.

Assessing Self-Functioning

It is useful to begin an evaluation of the self system by asking the patient to provide a self-description. Simple instructions provide the most information. For example: "We have talked about your problems and your life. It would be helpful now if you could tell me a little more about yourself. Who are you? What sort of person are you? What are your main qualities? What do you think about yourself?" Sufficient time should be allowed to produce a description before seeking elaboration and clarification; usually only a few minutes are needed. This task is fairly difficult for most patients because they rarely access knowledge about themselves in this way. Nevertheless, most can produce a brief sketch of themselves.

Diagnostic information is provided by the way the person goes about the task and the degree of differentiation, integration, and self-directedness revealed by the resulting description. Information is also provided on the contents of the self; these contents can be used later to assess personality patterns and traits and other domains of the personality system. The patient's approach to the task provides preliminary information on the *differentiation* of self-knowledge. Those with a poorly differentiated self find the task almost incomprehensible and often comment that they do not know what to say. One articulate patient with well-established intellectual interests looked bewildered when asked to describe himself. He fell silent and then said, "I don't know what to say. I do not know who I am, and I am not sure of anything about myself. I can't say what I am like or what characteristics I have." Even with encouragement, he could only note one or two interests.

Information on differentiation is also provided by the number of personal qualities described and references to different aspects of personality, such as traits, motives, interests, and values. Poor differentiation is indicated by descriptions containing only a few items and little reference to

TABLE 5.2. Core Features of Personality Disorder

1. Self pathology
   I. Structural problems
      A. Problems of differentiation
         1. Poorly delineated interpersonal boundaries: difficulty differentiating self from others; allows others to define self experience; confuses others' feelings with own; frequently experiences others' comments as intrusive
         2. Lack of self clarity/certainty: difficulty identifying and describing feelings and other experiences; uncertainty about personal qualities and characteristics, including values, beliefs, and identity
         3. Sense of inner emptiness
         4. Context-dependent self-definition: sense of self depends on who he or she is with; monitors others carefully to decide how he or she should feel and act
         5. Poorly differentiated images of other people

      B. Problems of integration
         1. Lack of historicity and continuity: feels as if he or she does not have a past; difficulty recalling impressions of self only a few years ago; self-images unstable and change from day to day
         2. Fragmentary self-representations: inconsistent and contradictory images and feelings about the self; lacks a sense of wholeness; feels fragmented; opinions and feelings about another person change frequently
         3. Self-state disjunctions: feels as if there are several different self-states; people tell them that they change so much that it sometimes seems as if they are a different person
         4. Real self–false self disjunction: feels as if the "real me" is trapped inside and not able to get out; does not let people see the "real me"; when he or she talks about self, it feels as if he or she is describing someone else

      C. Consequences of structural problems
         1. Lack of authenticity: feelings and experiences feel unreal and not genuine; feels like a fake or sham
         2. Defective sense of self: sense of being flawed, as if something is fundamentally wrong with self
         3. Poorly developed understanding of human behavior: does not understand other people at an intuitive level; does not have a good sense of how to relate to other people

   II. Conative problems
      A. Lack of autonomy and agency: unable to influence events or control own life and destiny
      B. Lack of meaning, purpose, and direction: lacks a clear sense of direction; feels actions are purposeless and pointless
      C. Low self-directedness: has difficulty with setting and attaining rewarding personal goals; derives little satisfaction from goal attainment; has difficulty integrating goals with other parts of self

(*continued*)

TABLE 5.2. (*continued*)

2. Interpersonal problems

    A. Fragmentary person representations: images of other people are unstable and fragmentary; opinions and feelings about others change frequently and rapidly

    B. Intimacy: impaired capacity for close intimate relationships of mutuality

    C. Attachment: lacks the capacity to form attachment relationships and to function adaptively in attachment relationships; avoids attachments; unable to tolerate someone being dependent on him or her

    D. Affiliation: inability to establish affiliative relationships; disinterested in social contact; solitary and spends most time alone; inability to establish friendships

3. Societal problems

    A. Impaired capacity for prosocial behavior: problems with cooperative and socialized behavior

    B. Not altruistic; would never sacrifice self to help someone else; avoids helping other people

    C. Exploitative: does not see anything wrong with taking advantage of someone who is easily conned

    D. Prepared to engage in illegal activity

---

personality characteristics, or reliance on global evaluative terms such as "nice" or "good" without explanation or qualification. For example:

> "I think that I am a nice person. I am moody. I live alone. I can't find a job; I am unemployed. I have a cat that I am very fond of. I don't know what else to say about myself. There is nothing else about me."

In contrast, someone with a more adequately differentiated self might note:

> "I am a temperamental person with a quick temper, so that it does not take much to arouse me. But most of the time, I am happy. When I get angry, I regret it afterward because I am sympathetic to people and like to help others. I work hard and have a quick mind. I want to be a teacher because I like children and want a job that makes me feel useful and that I am applying my abilities. I enjoy being different from other people and doing my own thing. I hate being one of a crowd, although I am very sociable and have lots of friends. I used to be religious and went to church regularly, but I don't now. Sometimes I worry a lot and when I'm anxious, I talk a lot, and this gives people a bad impression."

This description is qualitatively different from the first; the descriptive items are more differentiated and cover multiple aspects of self-functioning. There is also seems to be greater clarity and certainty about the characteristics mentioned. The degree of clarity and certainty can be tested by questioning the basis for ascribing these qualities to the self.

The other important aspect of differentiation is the formation of effective interpersonal boundaries. Self-descriptions do not usually provide information on this issue. Sometimes the history provides clues about the extent to which the individual is influenced by others and is able to maintain interpersonal distance. In many cases, however, boundary problems only come to light with systematic inquiry, based on the features listed in Table 5.2.

The second feature of the self that holds diagnostic significance is that of integration and cohesiveness. The self-descriptions of individuals with adaptive self systems are not merely lists of attributes. Instead, they are organized ways that attempt to (1) indicate which qualities are most important, and (2) explain or qualify these qualities. The second description above contains simple qualifying terms that modify our understanding of the person's moodiness and hints at how this affects other qualities, such as concern for others. It also reveals a little about the way traits and abilities have influenced career decisions. These are the linguistic reflections of an underlying unity and coherence to the self. If we were to press the person for more details, we could test the extent of this coherence.

When the description contains few indications of integration, additional questions are needed about the fragmentation of the self and self-state and real self–false self disjunctions to ensure that the problem is actually due to integration deficits and not difficulty articulating self-experience (see Table 5.2) (In Chapter 13, a more detailed way to evaluate self-states, for use in treating core pathology, is described.) When the description contains apparently or potentially inconsistent information, such as describing the self as aggressive and also concerned about others, the apparent discrepancy is drawn to the patient's attention to see if the problem is recognized and attempts made to reconcile the apparent incongruity. If this elaboration does not occur, the individual is asked to clarify how these qualities affect each other and how they go together. It is not the presence of apparently inconsistent qualities that has diagnostic significance but the individual's ability to reconcile them.

The final aspect of the self that is important for diagnosis is the capacity for self-directedness. Again, a standard history interview usually provides information on the capacity to set meaningful long-term goals and pursue them effectively. Preliminary inferences can be checked by exploring the features noted in Table 5.2.

For diagnostic purposes, significant problems in any of the three properties of the self—differentiation, integration, and self-directedness—is sufficient to warrant a diagnosis of personality disorder. However, the three components are not totally distinct, and most cases have problems in each area.

The following are typical examples of self descriptions:

A man in his late 30s, with inhibited or schizoid–avoidant traits, provided the following self-description: "I don't have many ideas about myself. I have no idea what I want. I don't really know who I am or what I want to be. Nothing really matters to me. How can it—I never know what I want, I have no purpose. I have always drifted and lived a day-to-day existence. I don't know what to do with people. I can't talk to anyone. I don't know what to say. It upsets my family. They want more from me, but I don't know what it is." Further discussion revealed difficulties expressing and understanding feelings. He thought that his family wanted a connection with him, but he did not know what this really meant. Emotions were a mystery to him. There were many times when he did not know what people expected from him or how he should behave. He thought that he simply did not understand people and their reactions.

This description illustrates the core features of self pathology—the poorly developed sense of self, the lack of an intuitive understanding of the most basic features of human behavior, the lack of coherence to self-knowledge, and lack of self-directedness. It also provides pertinent information for evaluating other life tasks, since it reveals difficulties with intimacy and attachment.

Another man with inhibited traits described the same problems more succinctly. He said: "I don't know who I am. I simply drift through life. Nothing really affects me, and no one has really touched me." He went on to compare himself to a glass ball floating through space: nothing that came in contact stuck, it just slipped off, and the ball was hollow. Another patient expressed the same ideas in this way: "*I* is a fallacy of sorts. *I* is an infinitely deconstructionable conglomeration of shreds and patches, the mental picture of being 'under erasure,' as always having an X marked through it. *I* is a piece of abstraction; it is a kind of tense numbness or void where I seem to willingly hide but am almost unable to extract myself from."

A somewhat different self-description was provided by a 42-year-old woman with emotional dysregulation traits: "I don't know what to say. It's difficult. My ideas change all the time. Everything is a series of snapshots. I don't know where I am in them. Sometimes I feel all right and I'm able to cope well, but not really. Then it all comes crashing down. I don't know why. I can't think, so I give up. I am not sure about anything else."

Here we also see poor differentiation of the self, with little understanding of personal qualities and great uncertainty and lack of authenticity about self-experience. There are also suggestions of integration problems, with distinct self-states that appear to be disconnected. Subsequent exploration revealed that the patient felt fragmented, as if she had different aspects to the self that were separate from each other. The description also implied the presence of traits such as cognitive dysregulation (the tendency for thinking to become disorganized when stressed).

> A 39-year-old unemployed patient, with strong narcissistic traits, few relationships, and a long history of unsuccessful treatment, described herself in inflated terms: "I am a very intelligent and capable person. It is difficult for therapists to deal with me because I am so bright and well informed. They are afraid of me. I am also a very moral person—my parents raised me that way. I am very grateful to them for this. Others are not like me. . . . " The description continued by reiterating these points.

This description reveals a relatively poorly differentiated self structure, although it sometimes appeared masked by the patient's articulateness. However, it is a one-dimensional view of the self that conveys the impression of cohesion because few qualities are described.

Each of these accounts reveals serious problems with the structure of the self. The features reflected in the descriptions differ, but all show evidence of a failure to develop a clearly defined and integrated self that is able to exert an organizing effect on the individual's behavior.

Assessing Interpersonal and Societal Functioning

As with core self pathology, information on interpersonal and societal functioning in the history provided is often sufficient for diagnosis. This is certainly the case with intimacy and attachment problems. Difficulty in establishing lasting relationships is usually apparent from routine questions about past and current relationships. These questions also elicit information on attachment and the extent to which the individual is capable of forming adult attachments. When necessary, initial impressions can be checked using questions based on those in Table 5.2.

One aspect of interpersonal functioning that requires more direct evaluation is the capacity to form integrated representations of others. Even here the interview often provides preliminary material. In the process of gathering routine information about parents and significant others, it is useful to ask about what sort of person each one is, much as the patient was asked to furnish a self-description. The descriptions can be examined to evaluate the extent to which impressions are integrated. Any suggestion of discrepancies or inconsistent images can be explored to determine whether the individual can integrate them. For example, when discussing Mother, the patient may describe her as extremely warm and caring yet later refer to incidents when she was neglectful or punitive. These apparently inconsistent impressions can be brought to the patient's attention and he or she asked to explain them. As with distinct self-images, the important issue is whether a higher-order explanation that integrates these differences can be offered. Of course, Mother may have been so inconsistent in her behavior that integration is not possible. Individuals with the capacity to form integrated representations usually recognize the problem and offer an explanation.

Finally, the capacity for prosocial and cooperative behavior is also usually apparent from standard interview material. Additional questions can be based on items in Table 5.2.

The evaluation of adaptive failure is a crucial component of assessment that has major implications for treatment planning because core pathology is an important indicator of severity; and the more severe the disorder, the greater the reliance on supportive and structured interventions. It is interesting to note the parallel with Kernberg's model of borderline personality organization, which also emphasizes the importance of assessing the structural or organizational component of personality (Clarkin et al., 1999).

The definition of personality disorder as adaptive failure is probably more stringent that the DSM-IV criteria. Epidemiological studies report that the prevalence of personality disorder in the general population is 10% or higher (Mattia & Zimmerman, 2001; Merikangas & Weissman, 1986; Torgersen, Kringlen, & Cramer, 2001). This is a high figure, which suggests that the DSM criteria may not differentiate between personality disorder and maladaptive traits. It is likely that many individuals diagnosed with personality disorder in these studies would not be considered personality disordered using the criteria of adaptive failure.

Differentiation from Other Mental Disorders

It is important to rule out the possibility that presenting problems are solely due to an Axis I disorder because of differences in outcome and treatment. Although classifying personality disorders on a separate axis creates the impression that they are fundamentally different from other mental disorders, this is not the case (Livesley, 2003). In practice, it is often difficult to determine whether some symptoms are due to personality disorder or part of an Axis I disorder. Differentiation begins by evaluating the extent to which the patient meets criteria for personality disorder. Un-

fortunately, neither the DSM-IV criteria nor the criteria for adaptive failure are specific to personality disorder. The features of adaptive failure are
more specific and directly related to personality disorder; however, these
features also can occur with a serious Axis I disorder. For this reason, personality disorder should not be diagnosed in the presence of a pervasive
condition such as a cognitive or schizophrenic disorder. The criteria are
more effective in differentiating personality disorder from nonpsychotic
disorders. To be indicative of personality disorder, the defining features
should be *longstanding* and *pervasive*; they should have been present since
adolescence or early adulthood and affect broad sectors of the individual's
life and functioning.

Failure to apply these conditions can lead to the diagnosis of personality disorder when only an Axis I diagnosis is appropriate, and conversely,
to the diagnosis of an Axis I disorder when only personality disorder is
present. The *misdiagnosis of personality disorder* when an Axis I diagnosis
alone is appropriate is probably infrequent, because most clinicians appear
biased toward diagnosing Axis I disorders. The problem commonly occurs
when the patient shows features that clinicians associate with personality
disorder. For example, self-harming behavior, especially in young women,
increases the probability of a personality disorder diagnosis (usually borderline personality disorder), regardless of the other features that are present
(Blashfield & Herkov, 1996; Morey & Ochoa, 1989). Misdiagnosis also occurs when an Axis I disorder does not respond, as expected, to treatment.
A consideration of personality disorder is appropriate in these circumstances because comorbid personality disorder may indeed reduce the effectiveness of Axis I treatment (Reich & Green, 1991; Reich & Vasile, 1993;
Tyrer, Gunderson, Lyons, & Tohen, 1997). However, a diagnosis of personality disorder should always be based on the presence of defining features, not merely unresponsiveness to treatment. In both instances, attention to *core pathology* and the *pervasiveness and duration of personality
features* is usually sufficient to avoid misdiagnosis, as illustrated by the following case.

> Gillian was in her mid-30s, and married with three children, when
> she presented at a hospital emergency department following an over-
> dose of tranquilizers prescribed for stress. The initial assessment re-
> vealed strong suicidal ideation, low mood, tearfulness, insomnia, loss
> of appetite, weight loss, decreased interests, and decreased concentra-
> tion. Gillian also reported difficulty coping with her children, the
> youngest of whom was only several months old. She had been well
> until approximately 2 months after the birth of her last child. Gillian
> was diagnosed as having a major depressive disorder and admitted to
> the hospital. Following discharge several weeks later, the symptoms
> continued. Over the next year, Gillian was hospitalized several times
> for suicidal ideation and behavior.

During the last admission, the diagnosis was changed to borderline personality disorder, and the mood symptoms were attributed to affective lability. On discharge, Gillian was referred for treatment of borderline personality disorder. Further assessment revealed that, apart from suicidal behavior and possibly mood symptoms, Gillian did not meet any criteria for borderline personality disorder, nor did she show any defining features of personality disorder. She had functioned effectively throughout her adult life until a year earlier. Her upbringing had been stressful due to family problems. Nevertheless, she completed her college education and found employment at an institution, where she progressed rapidly to a responsible executive position. She had a well-defined sense of self and a clear sense of direction and purpose to her life. Her marriage was stable, and she enjoyed a close relationship with a supportive husband. She had also coped with raising children until after the birth of her third child. She had a wide range of social relationships and even maintained close friendships made during adolescence. Previously, her affects had been stable. If anything, she had been a little overcontrolled in that she liked everything to be organized and ordered and tended to deal with stress and difficulties by adopting a mildly obsessional style. The diagnosis was changed to major depressive disorder, and it was noted that compulsive traits played a role in the clinical picture.

A more common problem is the *failure to diagnose personality disorder* and to attribute clinical features to an Axis I disorder. This probably occurs because many clinicians believe that Axis I disorders are more treatable and find a personality disorder diagnosis pejorative. Common problems are the diagnosis of a mood disorder rather than personality disorder and, probably even more common, the failure to diagnose comorbid personality disorder. Differentiation of personality and mood disorders is often difficult. They frequently co-occur (Charney, Nelson, & Quinlan, 1981; Downs, Swerdlow, & Zisook, 1992), leading to the suggestion that some personality disorders, most notably borderline personality disorder, are merely variants of mood disorders (Akiskal, 1991, 1994, 1995; Akiskal et al., 1985). Family studies, however, do not support this contention (Nigg & Goldsmith, 1994). Presentations of personality disorder often include symptoms such as dysphoria, general distress, and depression that resemble the diagnostic criteria for major depressive disorder. Differentiation is further complicated by the inclusion of mood symptoms in the criteria for some DSM-IV personality disorders. As MacKenzie (1997) pointed out, there is also considerable scope for bias in assessing criteria for mood disorder, because criteria such as "depressed mood most of the day" are highly subjective. Such symptoms may be features of mood disorder or manifestations of the affective lability or despondency associated with personality disorder. The failure to diagnose comorbid personality disorder is illustrated by the following case.

Patricia presented in her late 30s with symptoms of low mood, insomnia, weight loss, lethargy, fleeting suicidal thoughts, difficulty coping, which prevented her from working, and dissatisfaction with her life. Mood symptoms had been worse during the last year, although she said that she had always felt "a little depressed." She was diagnosed as having a major depressive disorder. All her problems were attributed to the mood disorder, including longstanding interpersonal difficulties and problems establishing a sense of direction and purpose to her life. Although she presented as sociable, Patricia had never had a lasting relationship. She had been in several relationships over the years, but none had lasted for more than a few weeks. Typically, she became involved with people, only to withdraw when she felt overwhelmed by their needs. She said that she preferred to be alone but was ambivalent. She maintained that she would be content spending the rest of her life alone; however, she had difficulty dealing with loneliness. Patricia also described longstanding employment problems. She completed college after considerable difficulty. Subsequently, she was unemployed for some time and then held a series of casual jobs, each lasting only a few months. From adolescence onward she had struggled with discovering what she wanted to do with her life. She had difficulty describing who she was and what sort of person she believed herself to be. She talked of feeling empty and that she was a sham. She thought that the smooth demeanor that she presented to other people was just a facade, and that there was nothing of her real self in her relationships with others.

Failure to respond to antidepressant medication led to a request for a further evaluation, which indicated that Patricia showed the self pathology and interpersonal difficulties diagnostic of personality disorder. Using the DSM-IV system, she met the criteria for major depressive episode and avoidant personality disorder. Using the current dimensional system, she had personality disorder and the inhibited (schizoid–avoidant) pattern.

Depressive disorders are not the only mood disorders that are difficult to differentiate from personality disorder. Problems also arise with bipolar II disorder, which is a relatively common comorbid disorder. It is important not to miss the diagnosis of personality disorder either as the primary diagnosis or as a comorbid condition, because the treatment of patients with a comorbid personality disorder differs from that of patients with a pure Axis I condition. The management of patients with comorbid personality disorder is primarily the management of personality disorder. Interventions to treat the Axis I disorder may be thought of as specific interventions that are delivered in the context of attending to the management of core pathology.

A diagnosis of personality disorder may also be missed when the presence of quasipsychotic features lead to the diagnosis of a psychotic disorder. Typical features are feeling confused, difficulty thinking and processing information, perceptual aberrations such as illusions, and paranoid symptoms that may involve mildly delusional thoughts, such as transient ideas that other people are talking about them. Differentiation from psychotic disorders is not usually difficult, however, because symptoms are more transient, less pervasive, and are not associated with the loss of insight that typically occurs with psychotic conditions. A similar problem occurs when the "inner voices" experienced by some severely personality disordered individuals leads them to report "hearing voices." These "voices" are pseudohallucinations that differ from the typical auditory hallucinations experienced by patients with schizophrenia, in that the patient does not usually attribute them to an outside source, and they usually involve a single voice that sometimes can be linked to the voice of an abusive person from his or her past. With personality disorder such symptoms are usually transient and not associated with the deterioration typically observed in patients with schizophrenia. Persistence beyond the immediate crisis or for more than a week or so is usually reason to review the diagnosis in patients who do not have schizotypal personality disorder.

An additional diagnostic problem is the *failure to diagnose a comorbid Axis I disorder*. Most patients with personality disorder have a substantial array of Axis I symptoms (Dolan-Sewell, Krueger, & Shea, 2001; Oldham et al., 1995) and from 66% (Dahl, 1986) to 97% (Alnaes & Torgersen, 1988) meet criteria for an Axis I disorder. The prevalence of personality disorder among patients with an Axis I disorder ranges from 13% (Fabrega, Pilkonis, Mezzich, Ahn, & Shea, 1990) to 91% (Alnaes & Torgersen, 1988). The range of disorders that are commonly comorbid with personality disorder is extensive: the mood and anxiety disorders discussed earlier, and substance abuse disorders, most notably with Cluster B disorders; across studies 57.4% of patients with personality disorder also had a substance disorder diagnosis (Trull, Sher, Mink-Brown, Durbin, & Burr, 2000).

Since the features of personality disorder overlap with Axis I symptoms, it is often difficult to determine whether the presenting symptoms reflect an Axis I disorder, personality disorder, or both. Every effort should be made to arrive at an accurate diagnosis to ensure adequate treatment of any Axis I disorder. Improvement in Axis I symptoms often leads to substantial improvement in personality functioning. In addition, comorbid disorders increase the risk of suicidal behavior (Soloff, Lynch, & Kelly, 2002). In many cases, however, it is difficult to differentiate Axis I and Axis II features. Under these circumstances, a general rule is to incorporate interventions to treat symptom clusters that respond to specific pharmacological or psychotherapeutic interventions into the treatment plan. (This issue is discussed further in Chapter 8.)

ASSESSMENT OF SPECIFIC PERSONALITY PATTERNS

Although an understanding of core features is fundamental to treating personality disorder, we also need to assess individual differences in personality traits to tailor therapy to personality as well as psychopathology. Traits influence responses to psychological interventions. For example, patients with high scores on conscientiousness seem to prefer more structured interventions (MacKenzie, 1994, 2002; Miller, 1991; Sanderson & Clarkin, 1994, 2002), and the trait of psychological mindedness predicts treatment response (McCallum & Piper, 1997). We also need to evaluate trait structure because maladaptive traits, such as affective lability, dependency, and impulsivity, are intrinsic aspects of most clinical presentations that are often the target of specific interventions. As noted earlier, individual differences may be described using DSM-IV or ICD-10 diagnoses or dimensional models of personality disorder traits.

DSM-IV Diagnoses

Given the familiarity of most clinicians with the DSM-IV, the different personality disorders will be mentioned only briefly. The 10 personality disorder diagnoses listed on Axis II are organized into three clusters:

Cluster A: paranoid, schizoid, and schizotypal
Cluster B: antisocial, borderline, histrionic, and narcissistic
Cluster C: avoidant, compulsive, and dependent

An additional diagnosis of personality disorder not otherwise specified is included to describe patients with personality disorder who do not meet the criteria for any given disorder. Clusters are based loosely on Eysenck's three dimensions of personality—psychoticism, extroversion, and neuroticism—which suggests that the authors of recent editions of DSM recognize that a small number of broad dimensions underlie categories of personality disorder.

Many criticisms have been leveled at the DSM-IV. For example, the reliability of diagnoses is variable. Although agreement among clinicians is often satisfactory, diagnostic stability is a major problem (David & Pilkonis, 1996; Grilo & McGlashan,1999). The validity of most diagnoses is not fully established. Investigations of the way the features of personality disorder co-occur in actual patients fail to find patterns that resemble DSM-IV diagnoses (Ekselius, Lindstrom, von Knorring, Bodlund, & Kullgren, 1994). In many ways the system fails to meet the requirements for a satisfactory classification. However, our concern is whether the DSM-IV is adequate for treatment planning. Here there are also major problems.

A DSM diagnosis provides little information that can be used for planning purposes. There is little evidence that specific personality disorder diagnoses predict treatment outcome, except in the most general sense, nor do they help in selecting interventions. Even the authors of the DSM-IV note that the system is inadequate for this purpose. Indeed, Beutler and Clarkin (1990) maintained that diagnosis generally has failed to provide the basis for selecting interventions. Most interventions are designed to treat specific clusters of behaviors or symptoms rather than global diagnostic categories (Sanderson & Clarkin, 1994, 2002), and outcome studies show that these features, rather than disorders *per se*, respond to treatment (see Chapter 3). An additional problem is that each DSM diagnosis consists of a cluster of traits, and patients with the same diagnosis often have very different features (Shea, 1995) that may require different combinations of interventions.

There is also the problem that actual patients bear little resemblance to DSM-IV personality diagnoses. Most patients do not fit a single category but rather meet the criteria for several diagnoses (Widiger et al., 1991). In some studies, *personality disorder not otherwise specified* is the most common diagnosis. This finding suggests that actual patients show more complex combinations of features than are recognized by DSM-IV. Also the DSM-IV does not appear to have diagnoses representative of some common personality problems: Many patients being treated for personality pathology (defined as enduring maladaptive patterns of thought, feeling, motivation, and behavior leading to dysfunction or distress) cannot be diagnosed on Axis II (Westen & Arkowitz-Westen, 1998). Given these limitations of DSM-IV and ICD-10 categorical diagnoses, both in terms of evidential support and value in treatment planning, attention has focused increasingly on dimensional models that can provide detailed information needed to plan the overall approach to treatment and select specific interventions.

Dimensional Models

Dimensional models have several advantages for an evidence-based approach. Reviews of the research literature show that they are more consistent with evidence on the way personality disorder is organized (Livesley et al., 1994; Widiger, 1993). The higher-order patterns reflect the genetic architecture of personality and hence represent fundamental differences in personality structure. The hierarchical organization of traits provides a systematic and yet parsimonious way to evaluate personality. The clinician can focus on the higher-order dimensions when an understanding of the broader aspects of personality functioning is sufficient, or on the lower-order dimensions when more detailed assessment is needed. Trait models also encourage clinicians to consider all aspects of personality, assets as well as liabilities, not just the limited range of maladaptive features forming the criteria for specific disorders. Patients find a dimensional approach more acceptable. Traits terms are more akin to everyday language of personality description. This familiarity minimizes the problem of labeling that occurs with categorical diagnoses; many patients are concerned about being "pigeonholed," especially because the more prevalent Axis II diagnoses are considered pejorative. Trait descriptions also help patients understand the connection between their personality and their problems, which often makes them feel more involved in the assessment process.

Dimensional assessments facilitate treatment planning. The broader patterns help to determine the general therapeutic approach, and they are further useful in anticipating the kinds of problems that may be encountered during treatment, especially connected with the treatment relationship. Specific traits are useful in identifying important themes and targets for change. Lastly, incorporating a trait approach into perspectives of therapeutic change tempers clinicians' expectations of the extent to which treatment is likely to lead to change (MacKenzie, 1997).

Assessing Traits and Personality Patterns

Traits can be assessed using self-report questionnaires or through clinical assessment. Two kinds of questionnaires are available: measures designed to assess normative personality, and measures based on clinical concepts. The most useful measures of normative traits are based on the five-factor approach, such as the Neuroticism Extraversion Openness–Personality Inventory—Revised (NEO-PI-R; Costa & McCrae, 1992). This widely used measure has a factor structure that is stable across clinical and nonclinical samples and different cultural groups. The scale provides scores on the five domains and the six facet scales forming each domain (see Chapter 2). The latter are helpful in selecting interventions. A limitation of the instrument is that scale names do not resemble clinical concepts because they are based on normal personality. Furthermore, clinically important traits such as cognitive dysregulation are not included, and others such as interpersonal traits are poorly represented. In addition, the NEO-PI-R does not discriminate well within clinical groups. Because the measure was designed for use with general population subjects, patients' scores tend to accumulate at the extremes of dimensions, so that it is not always possible to differentiate between patients with high scores, even though these differences may be clinically important.

An alternative is to use a measure developed from clinical concepts to assess personality disorder traits, such as the Schedule for Non-Adaptive and Adaptive Personality (SNAP; Clark, 1993) or the Dimensional Assessment of Personality Pathology (DAPP; Livesley & Jackson, in press). However, as noted in Chapter 2, there are significant parallels between normal and disordered personality. The evidence suggests that personality disorder traits merge with normative personality structures, and there is broad agreement that individual differences in personality disorder can be represented by four higher-order dimensions: emotional dysregulation (borderline) pattern, inhibited (schizoid–avoidant) pattern, dissocial (psychopathic) pattern, and compulsive (obsessive–compulsive) pattern. This model is used to discuss individual differences in personality disorder. Table 5.3 defines the 16 basic traits that form the four patterns. Three of the main patterns are described by two core traits that essentially define the pattern and other traits that are usually associated with the pattern. In the case of emotional dysregulation, two further traits, suspiciousness and narcissism, are noted as additional traits that are less strongly associated with the pattern; they are found in some analyses and not others. When present, they influence the expression of other traits in the pattern. Narcissism is also a feature of the dissocial or psychopathic pattern. The fourth pattern, compulsivity, describes a much narrower set of behaviors than the other patterns and is represented by a single trait.

Clinical Assessment of Personality Dimensions

The higher-order patterns and associated traits may also be assessed clinically. This type of assessment may take several forms, the simplest of which is to focus only on the four patterns, since these have immediate implications for management. The first step is to evaluate the core traits for each pattern. The core traits are:

> Emotional dysregulation: affective lability and anxiousness
> Inhibitedness: intimacy problems and restricted expression
> Dissocial behavior: callousness and rejection

Compulsivity is evaluated by the presence of orderliness and conscientiousness. The definitions provided in Table 5.3 are used as guides informing the kind of questions that may be asked to evaluate each trait. Thus, an evaluation of anxiousness would be based on self-descriptions as a lifelong worrier (*trait* as opposed to *state* anxiety), tendencies to brood and ruminate over minor worries and embarrassments, intense guilt even about thoughts that were not acted upon, and difficulty making decisions due to worry. Similarly, an evaluation of affective lability would be based on evidence of rapid and unpredictable mood changes occurring in response to minimal stimulation, intense or extreme emotional responses, hypersensitivity, intense labile anger or rage, and extreme irritability. When one or both core traits are considered clinically significant, in the sense that they contribute to problems and symptoms, the other traits forming the pattern are assessed; otherwise, assessment moves to the next pattern. For example, evidence of the presence of a high level of affective lability and/or anxiousness would lead to an assessment of the other traits forming emotional

TABLE 5.3. Traits Delineating the Four Patterns of Personality Disorder

Emotional dysregulation

Core traits

Anxiousness	Trait anxiety, guilt proneness, indecisiveness, rumination
Affective lability	Affective instability and overreactivity, generalized hypersensitivity, labile anger, irritability

Other traits

Cognitive dysregulation	Depersonalization, schizotypal cognition, brief stress psychosis
Submissiveness	Subservience, suggestibility, need for advice and reassurance
Anxious attachment	Separation protest, secure base seeking, proximity seeking, feared loss, inability to tolerate solitude
Social avoidance	Low affiliation, defective social skills, social apprehensiveness, fearful of interpersonal hurt, desire for improved affiliative relationships
Oppositionality	Passivity, oppositional, lack of organization

Additional traits

Narcissism	Need for adulation, attention seeking, grandiosity
Suspiciousness	Hypervigilance, suspiciousness

Inhibitedness

Core traits

Intimacy problems	Desire for improved attachment, inhibited sexuality, avoidant attachment
Restricted expression	Reluctant self-disclosure, restricted expression of anger, restricted affective expression, restricted expression of positive sentiments, self-reliance

Other traits

Social avoidance	Low affiliation, defective social skills

Dissocial behavior

Core traits

Callousness	Contemptuousness, egocentrism, exploitation, interpersonal irresponsibility, lack of empathy, remorselessness, sadism
Rejection	Rigid cognitive style, judgmental, interpersonal hostility, dominance

Other traits

Conduct problems	Interpersonal violence, juvenile antisocial behavior, addictive behavior, failure to adopt social norms
Stimulus seeking	Sensation seeking, recklessness, impulsivity
Narcissism	Need for adulation, attention seeking, grandiosity

Compulsivity

Compulsivity	Orderliness, precision, conscientiousness

dysregulation. This kind of evaluation can be completed rapidly, using a few well-formed questions. More detailed evaluation of other traits could occur during treatment.

A more detailed approach is to use the 16 traits as a checklist that is completed during assessment, much as DSM-IV diagnostic criteria are assessed, supplemented as needed by questions based on items listed in Table 5.3. Clinical assessment using this approach correlates well with more detailed evaluation of these traits using a questionnaire. The information obtained provides a profile of the 16 traits. This information can also be combined to provide an overall evaluation of each pattern. However, a pattern would not be considered present, using this method, if the patient did not show clinically significant levels of a core trait. The value of a more comprehensive clinical evaluation is that it provides a systematic account of personality traits and hence identifies strengths as well as problems.

> Natasha was a single mother with two children who presented at the age of 38 with a long history of psychiatric problems that primarily involved affective lability, frequent interpersonal crises, a long history of abusive relationships with men, including the partner with whom she was currently living, and repetitive self-harming acts involving overdoses of drugs and cutting. Physical and sexual abuse had occurred throughout childhood and adolescence. She was furious about the way her life had turned out. She blamed her partners for her problems, complaining that none had been understanding or supportive. The DSM-IV diagnosis was borderline personality disorder with dependent and narcissistic traits.
>
> Personality evaluation showed clinically significant features of anxiousness, a core trait of emotional dysregulation. She had high levels of trait anxiety ("I'm a worrier; I worry about everything and always have"), guilt proneness ("I feel guilty about everything, even silly little things"), rumination ("When I am worried, everything goes round and round in my mind and I can't stop it"), and indecisiveness ("When I am worried about something, it's hard to decide what to do; I keep changing my mind").
>
> Affective lability was also high. Natasha complained of frequent and unpredictable mood changes (I'm moody; my moods are up and down for no reason"), intense emotional expression ("I am very emotional; everything affects me"), and hypersensitivity ("Sometimes everything is too intense; I just want to switch everything off"). She was also filled with rage ("I get so furious I can't control myself") and highly irritable.
>
> Evaluation of other traits in the emotional dysregulation pattern revealed high levels of submissiveness. She found it hard to be assertive ("I always do what others want; I am a doormat; I can't say 'no' "), she always sought advice, support, and reassurance ("I always

ask others what I should do, even when I know what's best for me"), and was very suggestible ("I can be talked into anything").

Questions about cognitive dysregulation suggested a moderate level of this trait. When distressed her thoughts became "a little fuzzy—I just can't think, and this makes me more worried and upset," but there was no evidence of more severe manifestations such as depersonalization/derealization or quasipsychotic symptoms. There was also a modest level of narcissism.

The other traits forming this pattern were not considered clinically significant. Evaluation of the other higher-order patterns only yielded evidence of modest levels of compulsivity in the form of concern for order ("I am a neat freak") and conscientiousness (several times during the assessment, she commented on the importance of keeping one's word or promises and that she liked to be punctual because she did not like to keep people waiting).

This patient clearly had the emotional dysregulation or borderline pattern. This diagnosis suggested the need to help Natasha learn how to contain affects and develop improved self-management of emotions. The high levels of submissiveness explained recurrent problems with interpersonal relationships and suggested that the modulation of this trait was likely to be an important focus of treatment. The moderate level of cognitive dysregulation indicated the importance of an affect-regulating approach that avoids overwhelming information-processing and self-control mechanisms with elicited emotions. The moderate level of compulsivity was discussed with her as an asset that would be beneficial to her treatment by helping her to persist in dealing with problems and develop a more satisfying lifestyle.

The above example illustrates an important point about dimensional models: Many patients do not show all the traits that compose a higher-order pattern. Furthermore, the higher-order patterns are not mutually exclusive; some patients have high levels of two or more of these patterns, such as inhibitedness and dissocial behavior, or, as in the above example, high emotional dysregulation and modest compulsivity. For this reason, each pattern should be assessed. In addition, some individuals meet the criteria for personality disorder but do not fit any pattern and have high levels of specific traits. For example, a person may meet the criteria for personality disorder and only show high levels of suspiciousness. In DSM-IV terms, such a patient would be considered to have a paranoid personality disorder. With the current approach, the patient would be diagnosed as having personality disorder, and the specific trait of suspiciousness would be noted. Similarly, some individuals with personality disorder may score highly on narcissism but not necessarily on other dimensions. In other cases, several traits may be elevated without meeting the requirement of any pattern; for example, extreme levels of submissiveness, insecure attachment, and narcissism. The value of using a dimensional system is that it allows the clinician to capture the almost protean variations in personality disorder without the procrustean effort of forcing patients into a diagnostic category that ill-fits them.

ASSESSMENT OF THE PERSONALITY SYSTEM

Evaluation of core pathology and trait constellations does not complete the assessment of personality. We also need to consider other personality domains that have an immediate bearing on treatment planning: symptoms, interpersonal patterns, and situational factors.

Symptoms

In addition to evaluating Axis I disorders, attention also should be paid to the symptomatic components of personality disorder: psychological distress, self-harming behaviors, dysphoria, cognitive disorganization, cognitive–perceptual symptoms, dissociative behavior, and neuropsychological symptoms. Each symptom cluster has implications for treatment planning. Typically, symptoms are assessed during the first interview as part of a systematic review of the person's mental state.

Parasuicidal and Suicidal Behavior

An important assessment task is to evaluate the short-term and long-term risk of suicidal, parasuicidal, and other self-harming behaviors. These acts are most prevalent with emotional dysregulation and dissocial patterns: Increasing emotional arousal reduces coping, leading to impulsive actions. Over 70% of patients with borderline personality disorder have a history of suicide attempts (Soloff et al., 2002; Soloff, Lynch, Kelly, Malone, & Mann, 2000; Zisook, Goff, Sledge, & Schuchter, 1994). Since self-harm and other impulsive acts reduce dysphoria, they become learned ways of coping with distress.

It is easy to underestimate suicide risk in patients with chronic suicidal and parasuicidal ideation. However, follow-up studies show that 5–10% of patients with borderline personality disorder commit suicide (McGlashan, 1986; Paris, Brown, & Nowlis, 1987; Paris, Nowlis, & Brown, 1988, 1989; Perry, 1993; Stone, 1990, 1993). Fewer longitudinal studies have been reported on other personality disorders. Risk appears to be lower for antisocial personality disorder (Perry, 1993). However, the presence of antisocial (dissocial) traits in patients with borderline personality increases the risk of suicidal behavior (Soloff et al., 2002). Clinical observation suggests that the inhibited or schizoid–avoidant pattern also involves substantial risk.

Deliberate self-harm is a common and serious problem; 1% of individuals who harm themselves commit suicide in the following year, and up to 10% commit suicide at some time (Gunnell & Frankel, 1994). Parasuicidal behavior is especially common among patients with borderline personality disorder; the incidence ranges from 46% to 92% across studies (Clarkin, Widiger, Fances, Hurt, & Gilmore, 1983; Cowdry, Pickar, & Davis, 1985; Dulit, Fyer, Leon, Brodsky, & Frances, 1994; Friedman, Aronoff, Clarkin, Corn, & Hurt, 1983; Fyer, Frances, Sullivan, Hurt, & Clarkin, 1988; Mehlum, Vaglum, & Karterud, 1994; Shearer, Peter, Quaytman, & Wadman, 1988; Soloff, Lis, Kelly, Cornelius, & Ulrich, 1994). Parasuicidal behavior is believed to be less frequent in other forms of personality disorder, although fewer reports are available.

In patients with borderline personality disorder, self-harming acts are related to severity of the condition (Soloff et al., 1994; Yeomans, Hull, & Clarkin, 1994). These patients have more Axis I pathology, such as buliminia, anorexia nervosa, major depression (Dulit et al., 1994), increased paranoia, hypervigilance, and resentfulness (Yeomans et al., 1994) than those who do not. They are also younger, more symptomatic, make more suicidal threats and attempts, have more serious suicidal ideation, and report more depression, depersonalization, delusions, and other schizotypal symptoms than those who do not self-mutilate (Soloff et al., 1994). Self-injurious behavior is associated with sexual abuse and dissociative behavior (Zweig-Frank, Paris, & Guzder, 1994), obsessionality (Gardner & Gardner, 1995), and obsessive–compulsive symptoms (McKay, Kulchycky, & Danyko, 2000).

Assessment of parasuicidal and suicidal behavior would be improved by a set of risk factors that indicated those who are most at risk of suicide. Unfortunately, such determinants do not exist at present. Although many factors are associated with these behaviors (Bongar, 1991; Linehan & Shearin, 1988; Maris, Berman, Maltsberger, & Yufit, 1992), those studied have limited predictive value (Paris, Nowlis, & Brown, 1989). Consequently, evaluation of risk is largely a matter of clinical judgment. Parasuicidal and suicidal behavior are both increased by losses, reduced social support, hopelessness, depressed mood, previous parasuicidal behavior, and drug and alcohol use. Additional factors contributing to increased suicide risk are bereavement, family history of suicide, increasing age, intense anxiety and panic attacks, insomnia, and previous history of parasuicidal behavior. Additional risk factors for parasuicidal behavior are separations and disrupted relationships, a hostile family context, a rigid but impulsive cognitive style, and interpersonal friction and conflict. Parasuicidal behaviors are more common in women than in men; the reverse applies to suicide. Parasuicidal behavior itself is an important risk factor for suicide. For this reason, these acts should always be taken seriously. In crisis situations, drug and alcohol misuse are also important risk factors.

In the case of specific diagnoses, the risk of suicidal behavior in patients with borderline personality disorder is increased by comorbid depressive disorder, antisocial traits (dissocial behavior), hopelessness, and severity of borderline pathology. The occurrence and severity of sexual, but not physical, abuse also increases risk; the odds of a sexually abused patient attempting suicide in adulthood are 10 times greater than for individuals who have not been abused (Soloff et al., 2002). Childhood abuse, especially sexual abuse, also increases suicidal ideation and parasuicide independently of diagnosis (Briere & Runtz, 1986; Briere & Ziadi, 1989; Romans, Martin, Anderson, Herbsion, & Mullen, 1995). Antisocial personality is also associated with suicide (Stone, 1989).

When evaluating suicide risk in patients with personality disorder and substantial mood symptoms, an important differential diagnosis is whether current suicidal ideation and behavior are primarily a consequence of a mood disorder or personality pathology; each has different implications for treatment planning and immediate management. When a mood disorder is determined to be a significant contributor, immediate steps, including inpatient treatment, may be needed to ensure safety.

Perceptual–Cognitive Symptoms

Perceptual–cognitive symptoms define schizotypal personality disorder and are common in borderline personality disorder, occurring in about 75% of patients (Chopra & Beatson, 1986; Frances, Clarkin, Gilmore, Hurt, & Brown, 1984; George & Soloff, 1986; Pope, Jonas, Hudson, Cohen, & Tohen, 1985; Silk, Lohr, Westen, & Goodrich, 1989; Zanarini, Gunderson, & Frankenburg, 1990), and are also associated with inhibited and dissocial patterns. These symptoms run the spectrum from a tendency for thinking to become disorganized when stressed to quasipsychotic features such as ideas of reference and paranoid thoughts. This symptomatic component of cognitive dysregulation is a valuable indicator of the patient's capacity to tolerate the emotional arousal and stress that are often unavoidable parts of treatment. The presence of strong tendencies toward cognitive disorganization indicates the need to adopt a more supportive approach that minimizes emotional expression, especially in the early stages of treatment; they also give an indication of the problems that are likely to occur in crises and hence enable the clinician to anticipate the management of these situations. The occurrence of these symptoms may indicate the need for pharmacological treatment.

Dissociation

Dissociative behaviors are common in this population. Most theorists agree that dissociation is "the failure to integrate or associate information and experience in a normally expectable fashion" (Putnam, 1997, p. 7). The

DSM-IV (American Psychiatric Association, 1994), for example, defines dissociation as "a disruption in the usually integrated functions of consciousness, memory, identity, or perception of the environment" (p. 477). The most benign dissociative phenomenon is the sense of absorption, a mild form of depersonalization, which occurs in a substantial percentage of the normal population when a person is engrossed in a task and loses sense of time and surroundings. The most severe are amnesic episodes that characterize dissociative disorders but also occur with personality disorder. Between these extremes are depersonalization and derealization. *Depersonalization* refers to the sense of being detached from experiences occurring at the time—a common reaction to a traumatic event. *Derealization* refers to experiences in which the world around one seems unreal.

These symptoms have similar implications for treatment as the perceptual–cognitive symptoms. Especially problematic is the occurrence of severe episodes in which the patient becomes unresponsive to the point of immobilization and muteness. An understanding of the extent to which these symptoms occur enables the therapist to plan for their management, should they occur during treatment.

When evaluating dissociative behavior, it is also helpful to gain a preliminary assessment of any symptoms indicative of trauma: reexperiencing, hyperarousal, and avoidance. Caution, however, is needed in exploring trauma themes (or any other theme that is likely to be intensely distressing and hence potentially destabilizing). Our concern is with getting the information needed for planning therapy rather than exploring all eventualities; at this stage it is especially important to manage emotional arousal carefully.

Neuropsychological Symptoms

A common clinical observation is that a small but significant number of patients with severe personality disorder have a history of minor head injury or one suggestive of minimal brain dysfunction. There is some evidence to support this observation in patients with borderline personality disorder (Andrulonis et al., 1981; Van Reekum et al., 1993). The presence of neuropsychological problems complicates treatment, but in many cases it is difficult to assess the clinical significance of these features.

The impact of minimal brain dysfunction on personality functioning is readily understandable. Many basic components of personality, such as self and interpersonal systems and self-regulation, depend on the ability to integrate perceptual, cognitive, emotional, and behavioral information to form coherent representations of self and others. The power to differentiate among types of information and to combine information into hierarchical structures is an integral part of adaptive behavior that requires intact neuropsychological structures. Adaptive functioning also requires the capacity to regulate and inhibit affect and impulse expression; this is also affected by neuropsychological deficits. It is likely that factors influencing the capacity to integrate information and self-regulation will be implicated in the etiology of personality disorder, suggesting that attention should be paid to the possibility of neuropsychological problems. In such cases, treatment should include strategies to improve impulse control and regulation.

It should also be noted that there is some debate about the connection between borderline personality and adult attention deficit disorder (Wender, 1995). It is not clear whether these problems are also associated with other personality patterns.

Interpersonal System

In planning treatment, is it helpful to take into account salient interpersonal pathology. The most important features are maladaptive schemata, cyclical maladaptive patterns of interpersonal behavior, and quality of object relations.

Maladaptive Schemata and Cyclical Maladaptive Interpersonal Patterns

A goal of medium- and longer-term therapy is to change maladaptive schemata and interpersonal behavior. An important aspect of assessment is to identify these schemata and patterns and develop an understanding of the ways in which they are maintained. This aspect of assessment not only begins to identify targets for change but also gives an indication of the various ways the patient is likely to relate to the therapist and the problems that are likely to be encountered if these patterns are activated in treatment.

A full evaluation of maladaptive self and interpersonal schemata is difficult to accomplish during a few assessment interviews; many schemata and interpersonal patterns only become apparent during treatment, when they begin to influence the relationship with the therapist. It is, however, helpful to identify core maladaptive schemata that were influenced by adversity, such as those concerning attachment, abandonment, and trust, because these will influence treatment from the beginning. Various sources of information may be used for this purpose, including the nature of the presenting problems and the way they are described, information about critical developmental epochs and events, reactions to losses and separation, descriptions of relationships, and precipitants of crises. During treatment, additional information is provided by events recollected, reactions to the therapist and within-therapy events such as therapist absences, ruptures in the alliance, and failures of validation. Structured assessment methods are also available, such as the Schema Questionnaire (Young, 1994).

Linked to maladaptive schemata are maladaptive interpersonal patterns involving a cycle of events beginning with (1) a state within the person (a want, wish, goal, or expectation) that gives rise to (2) actions that, in turn, (3) evoke responses from others, which (4) are interpreted by the first person who acts accordingly. Thus the cycle continues. To take a simple example, a person may want someone to listen to his or her problems and to show interest and concern. This wish may remain unexpressed because the person may feel that the other person should know without being told. Instead, the person may remain silent or feign disinterest, despite the underlying need. Others may interpret these behavioral cues as indications that the person is coping satisfactorily, in response to which they act accordingly—whereupon the person becomes frustrated that his or her needs were not met—a perception that confirms the underlying expectation that others are not interested, do not care, or are not reliable.

In clinical practice, these patterns are usually identified during assessment and confirmed in treatment. The information used to identify maladaptive schemata also typically provides information on characteristic patterns. Additional information can be obtained by administering systematic assessment methods, such as the Core Conflictual Relationship Theme (Luborsky, 1977, 1997a, 1997b), Cyclical Maladaptive Pattern (Schacht et al., 1984), and interpersonal circumplex (Leary, 1957). Often, however, it is sufficient to supplement the standard history by asking patients to provide anecdotes of specific events with designated individuals, such as mother, father, siblings, and friends, when describing their relationships with significant others. This is essentially the procedure used by the Core Conflictual Relationship Theme method. Asking patients to describe specific events with significant others follows naturally from asking them to describe themselves and significant others, creating flow and coherence to the assessment process. If the interviewer listens to these narratives with the idea of maladaptive patterns in mind, key themes can usually be identified; for example, a wish for care and support followed by an experience of rejection by the other person and a response by the self of discouragement and despondency, or demands for help followed by hostile rejection of what is offered.

An alternative way to describe cyclical maladaptive interpersonal patterns is through information obtained from measures based on the interpersonal circumplex (Leary, 1957). An extensive literature suggests that interpersonal behavior may be explained using two independent dimensions: *affiliation*, which ranges from loving and caring to cold, rejecting, and nonrevealing behaviors; and *control*, which ranges from domineering and controlling to submissive behaviors. Two measures are in common use: the Inventory of Interpersonal Problems (Horowitz, Rosenberg, Baer, Ureno, & Villasenor, 1988), and the Structural Analysis of Social Behavior (SASB; Benjamin, 1988). The SASB incorporates the idea of *complementarity*, which is useful in understanding maladaptive relationships (even if the SASB is not used). Benjamin suggests that a relationship shows complementarity when both members focus on the same individual in the relationship and both show the same amounts of affiliative and control–emancipation behaviors. Consider two individuals, A and B. Complementarity exists in their relationship when A blames and criticizes B, and B reacts with resentment and sulkiness. B may then internalize this relationship and react by blaming him- or herself. This idea often illuminates maladaptive patterns and enables patients to understand how their actions affect others and the way others treat them. For example, an extremely submissive individual who has difficulty with asserting his or her own wants can be helped to recognize how submissiveness elicits the reciprocal response of control, a pattern that is common among submissive individuals who self-mutilate. Similarly, abuse and attack from another may lead to fear and recoil in the patient, followed by self-blame. Or being ignored by another may result in withdrawal and self-neglect. As Benjamin (1993) noted, these patterns are essentially self-fulfilling prophecies—an idea that was also captured in the description of the cyclical maladaptive pattern.

Quality of Object Relationships

A different aspect of interpersonal behavior that is important in treatment planning is the quality of object relationships; patients with poor capacity for object relationships respond better to supportive interventions. The standard evaluation typically ascertains the capacity to relate to others and whether there is evidence of a sustained quality to relationships in adulthood.

The Quality of Object Relations Scale (Azim, Piper, Segal, Nixon, & Duncan, 1991) may be used if more systematic assessment is needed. This scale, which assesses patients on five levels of object relationship (derived from psychoanalytic concepts), has been shown to predict outcome. Each level is described in terms of characteristic behaviors, capacity for regulating affect and self-esteem, and definition of identity or self. The *primitive* level involves overattachment and hypersensitivity to loss. Typical affects include rage, fear of annihilation, and intense feelings of emptiness. Self-esteem is regulated by idealization and devaluation and strong reliance on others. The self is characterized by unstable representations. The next level, *searching*, involves seeking and losing substitute others. This state is associated with intense craving/longing and infatuation and disappointment. Self-esteem depends upon the availability of others, and the self is defined by the presence of relationships. Object relationships at the *controlling* level are characterized by passive or active possessive and controlling acts, with associated feelings of anger and ambivalence. Self-esteem is maintained through control and possession, and identity depends on control over others. At the *triangular* level, object relationships are characterized by competitiveness. Affects involve fear of success, anxiety, and guilt over intimacy. Self-esteem is dependent upon comparisons between self and others, and identity depends upon a sense of success or triumph over other people. Finally, the *mature* level demonstrates an equitable, give-and-take quality to relationships. Affects are appropriate in depth, and loss and separation can be tolerated. Self-esteem is based upon realistic evaluation of self and others and identity is derived from equity and mutuality in relationships. Most patients with personality disorder function at levels one or two and only a few at level three.

Psychological Mindedness

In addition to the traits discussed earlier, it is also useful to evaluate *psychological mindedness*—the capacity to understand and utilize psychological explanations of behavior (McCallum & Piper, 1997; Piper, McCallum, & Azim, 1992)—because patients with low levels of this trait have difficulty using psychological interventions and require a more focused behavioral approach. Highly psychologically minded individuals are able to form a complex understanding of human behavior and offer more complex explanations of their own and other people's actions. Those with low levels may appreciate the existence of internal psychological experiences but find it difficult to describe them effectively—a characteristic seen in patients with alexithymia. Others may have difficulty understanding important components of mental life, especially feelings, and therefore have difficulty understanding what others really mean when they talk about feelings; this constellation was described earlier as a feature of core self pathology. Less extreme levels of psychological mindedness involve recognition of internal states but limited awareness of the factors that produce them.

Situational Factors

Traditionally, clinical descriptions of personality disorder have concentrated on the role that internal structure and dynamics play in maintaining maladaptive patterns. When environmental factors are incorporated into formulations, they are usually either historical events that are thought to have influenced development, or contemporary stressors. Less attention is given to how the current environment initiates and maintains dysfunctional behavior. As noted in Chapter 3, however, people seek out environments that are consistent with their personality; environmental factors then enhance the stability of personality by constraining the behavioral options available to the person and reinforcing basic tendencies. Because environmental contingencies are important in maintaining some behaviors, they may constitute important obstacles to change. Hence assessment needs to take into account patients' social context, the way other people in their lives act to maintain maladaptive behavior, and the extent to which significant others are likely to support initiatives to change. If necessary, plans can be made to help the patient deal with situational and relationship issues contributing to his or her problems, and to involve others in the treatment process.

FORMULATION

The endpoint of assessment is a formulation that organizes complex and often contradictory biological, psychological, and social information into a descriptive account of the major facts of the patient's life and personality that explains current problems and psychopathology and defines the problems and themes that will be the focus of treatment (Eells, 1997). This description should consist of statements made in everyday language that are close to observable behavior and actual statements made by the patient. It is desirable to avoid theoretical speculation and jargon. This suggestion contrasts with the traditional psychodynamic formulation that emphasizes a theoretical conceptualization of the case (Perry, Cooper, & Michels, 1987).

Reliance on theory for guidance is minimized because a comprehensive theory of personality disorder is not available; furthermore, a willingness to draw from several theories can facilitate a comprehensive understanding of the patient and the creation of a multifaceted treatment plan. Avoidance of theory also helps to ensure that the formulation is closely tied to observable behavior, making it easier to translate into specific interventions. A totally atheoretical account, however, is neither feasible nor desirable. The clinician's understanding of personality disorder and its etiology inevitably influences the way facts are selected, investigated, and organized into an explanatory narrative. The aim, however, is to achieve this overview with minimal assumptions and inferences.

Although it is not possible to adopt a standardized format that is appropriate to all situations, a comprehensive formulation typically includes (1) vulnerability factors, including genetic predisposition and concomitant Axis I pathology; (2) a description of the strengths and liabilities of the personality system; (3) an account of salient aspects of life history; and (4) a critical evaluation of the way these different factors interact to give rise to current problems and psychopathology and the factors that maintain these problems. A formulation should also identify the major problems that are the target for change, interventions that are likely to be effective, and behaviors that are likely to interfere with treatment. This narrative serves as both a guide to planning treatment and selecting interventions and the blueprint to help the patient develop a new understanding or "theory" of the self. This blueprint is not fixed during assessment but regarded as a set of hypotheses that is modified as new information emerges during treatment.

Several authors suggest that the formulation should be written (Perry et al., 1987; Ryle, 1997). A written account forces the clinician to evaluate the information critically and to be clear and concise. It is also readily available and can refresh one's memory of the central issues. A written formulation can also be shared with the patient. Ryle (1997) advocates writing a "reformulation" letter that links the patient's problems to his or her history. This formulation is usually discussed, written out, and then given to the patient. It is discussed further, and revised if necessary, during the last assessment session. A written formulation helps to focus the patient's attention on critical issues. Revising the initial formulation following on a discussion with the patient models openness and emphasizes the collaborative nature of treatment. The formulation also brings order to experiences, which may reduce the chaos felt by many patients. Of course, there is the danger that the patient may be overwhelmed by the information. Sometimes this possibility may warrant the editing of the main formulation before sharing it with the patient, deleting hypotheses and ideas that may be too anxiety-provoking. Nevertheless, the patient needs to be given sufficient information to form the basis for establishing a treatment contract.

CHAPTER 6

Treatment Planning and the Treatment Contract

With multiple-problem disorders, detailed treatment planning is not possible as it is with more circumscribed disorders that can be treated using a defined protocol. It is possible, however, to identify the broad strategies and some of the specific interventions that are likely to be required, and to anticipate problems that may emerge during treatment and make plans for managing them. It is useful to discuss these issues when establishing the treatment contract, so that the patient understands what to expect from treatment and how he or she can contribute to the process. It is also useful to plot the major strategies that will be used; doing so helps to ensure a more consistent treatment process by minimizing the extent to which major treatment decisions are influenced by moment-to-moment changes in psychopathology. The more specific interventions that may be discussed with the patient are addressed in later chapters (8–13). Here broader issues are considered, such as of the extent to which generic supportive interventions will be supplemented by other interventions, the sequence in which different problems may be addressed, and the treatment contract.

TREATMENT PLANNING

Treatment planning involves five broad decisions (Frances, Clarkin, & Perry, 1984; Sanderson & Clarkin, 2002) regarding (1) treatment setting:

inpatient, partial hospitalization or day hospital, or outpatient; (2) treatment format: individual, group, family therapy, or some combination; (3) major strategies and techniques to be used throughout treatment, and the sequence of interventions; these decisions include selection of theoretical models, such as psychodynamic, cognitive-behavioral, or psychoanalytic; (4) duration and frequency of treatment: whether crisis intervention, short-term, or long-term therapy is indicated, and the frequency of appointments; (5) decisions about the use of medication and the way medication will be combined with other interventions. Together, these five categories provide a comprehensive way to plan treatment that is consistent with the tailored approach advocated.

It is assumed that clinically meaningful changes in personality pathology (i.e., involving more than symptomatic relief) are likely to require longer-term treatment and that this is best managed through outpatient treatment, although empirical evidence on these points is lacking. Throughout this volume, treatment is presented as if delivered through individual therapy format, because this is easier to describe. However, the approach is readily applied to group treatment. Perhaps the best format is a combination of group and individual treatment (see Chapter 14). Again, empirical evidence is lacking. The intermittent use of conjoint sessions is also consistent with the approach (MacFarlane, in press). The use of medication is discussed in Chapter 8.

Partial hospitalization programs are effective in managing severely disturbed patients (Azim, 2001; Bateman & Fonagy, 1999, 2001; Piper, Rosie, Azim, & Joyce, 1993). It is suggested that their role be confined largely to that of managing patients in decompensated or crisis states, a contingency that is discussed when considering the management of crises (Chapter 8). Although a variety of longer-term inpatient and residential programs has been described, there is no evidence that they are more successful than outpatient treatment and are not considered a treatment option here. Short-term hospitalization is a common occurrence for these patients, with dubious benefits. Admission is best avoided, when possible; if not possible, the period should be brief: 24–72 hours. This circumstance is also discussed in Chapter 8. Residential community programs have been developed to treat the more extreme forms of dissocial or psychopathic behavior usually under the auspices of forensic services; evidence of their efficacy is mixed. Furthermore, the treatment of extreme levels of psychopathy is outside the scope of this volume.

Since an eclectic approach is adopted, the selection of treatment model is not relevant. Instead, attention is focused on the relative use of so-called expressive or exploratory interventions and supportive techniques, and the sequence in which issues and problems are addressed. Duration and frequency of treatment are discussed as these relate to the goals of therapy and the treatment contract.

Intervention Strategy: The Expressive versus Supportive Therapy Debate

The literature on treating personality disorder, especially borderline personality disorder and organization, was dominated for some time by debate over the best approach. Recommendations ranged from psychoanalysis to psychoanalytic psychotherapy to lower-frequency and less-intensive supportive treatment. An important issue in this debate is the relative importance of expressive versus supportive interventions. Although definitions vary, expressive therapy generally uses standard psychodynamic interventions of clarification, confrontation, and interpretation to uncover unconscious wishes, fears, conflicts, and defenses. Change is assumed to arise from exploration and interpretation of a patient's relationship with a therapist (Clarkin et al., 1999; Horwitz et al., 1996; Luborsky, 1984). In contrast, supportive therapy is concerned with promoting adaptive functioning through emotional support and a therapeutic relationship and structure that helps patients to work toward their goals.

Although much of this debate is only pertinent to psychodynamic therapy, the expressive–supportive distinction is relevant to the current approach because it captures important dimensions of therapist behavior that influence outcome. A key distinction is that supportive interventions are *relationship-based*—the therapeutic relationship and interventions based on the relationship are the primary vehicles for effecting change—whereas expressive interventions are more directly *change focused*—they seek to increase and change self-knowledge and maladaptive patterns. The latter were referred to earlier as specific interventions. Because they focus directly on change, these interventions are more likely to be experienced as challenging and intrusive. Hence, they need to be used more cautiously when treating people with severe personality disorder.

In psychodynamic therapy, expressive and supportive interventions are considered poles of a continuum, as if they were opposing forms of intervention. Presumably, extensive support is inconsistent with exploration because it influences therapist neutrality and the development of the transference. Since these considerations are not relevant to the current model of change, relationship-based and change-focused interventions are considered to be separate rather than opposing dimensions. As discussed in Chapter 2, the goal is to maximize relationship-based interventions because these make the greatest contribution to change and offer the most effective way to manage core pathology. An important treatment decision is the extent to which change-focused interventions should also be used. This issue can be considered with reference to Figure 6.1. Given the priority of generic interventions, therapeutic activity should fall within the right-hand quadrants of Figure 6.1. The question we need to consider is what determines whether interventions should fall in the upper or lower right-hand quadrants.

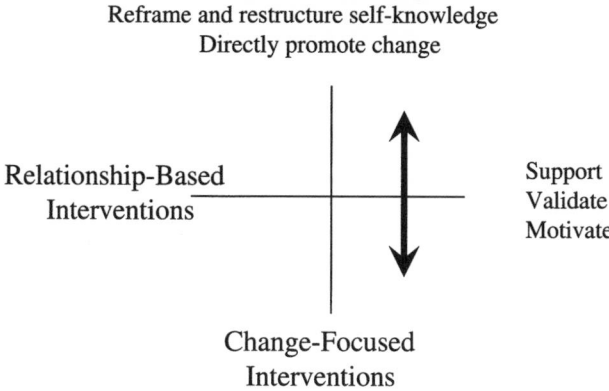

Increase self-knowledge
Reframe and restructure self-knowledge
Directly promote change

Relationship-Based
Interventions

Support
Validate
Motivate

Change-Focused
Interventions

FIGURE 6.1. Relationship-based and change-focused intervention strategies.

Indications and Contraindications for Change-Focused Interventions

Throughout treatment, decisions on the use of change-focused interventions are based on strategic considerations of the patient's ability to tolerate and benefit from potentially more stressful interventions and tactical considerations about the appropriateness of change-focused interventions at that moment in treatment.

Strategic Considerations. Three sets of enduring patient characteristics have a bearing on the overall use of change-focused interventions: mental state, developmental factors, and personality characteristics (see Table 6.1). The significance of *mental state symptoms* related to Axis I pathology and personality disorder lies in the extent to which they influence the patient's ability to tolerate the stress and challenge that often accompanies a change-focused approach. In the short term, these interventions are contraindicated when the patient's functioning is affected by a concurrent Axis I disorder. In the long term, predisposition to a severe Axis I disorder may also be a reason to minimize their use. For example, a patient with severe personality disorder and a bipolar disorder who becomes psychotic when stressed would be treated primarily using relationship-based and structured techniques (plus medication). Symptoms more directly related to personality disorder, such as dissociative and regressive behaviors, and some cognitive–perceptual symptoms that are stress-induced are also a reason for exercising caution about using interventions that are likely to evoke strong emotions, especially in the earlier stages of treatment. Similar considerations apply when the clinical picture is complicated by neuropsychological problems, because change-focused interventions place more demands on information-processing mechanisms and

TABLE 6.1. Relative Indications and Contraindications for
Change-Focused Interventions

Strategic factors

1. Mental state
   a. Severe Axis I disorder
   b. Neuropsychological dysfunction

2. Developmental factors
   a. Severe physical, emotional, or sexual abuse
   b. Severe deprivation or privation

3. Personality factors
   a. Severity of core pathology
   b. Extremity of personality pattern
   c. Psychological mindedness
   d. Externalization of responsibility
   e. Affect and impulse control
   f. Quality of object relationships

Tactical factors

1. Quality of the treatment relationship and rapport
2. Motivation
3. Level of affect arousal
4. Level of impulse control
5. Capacity to process information

may exceed the individual's capacity to process information and regulate
affects and impulses.

Developmental factors that may indicate more exclusive use of relationship-based interventions are abuse and severe deprivation or privation, although none is an absolute contraindication. Important considerations are
(1) the patient's capacity to tolerate stress and affect arousal, and (2) the
degree of deficit pathology present. In general, a history of trauma and
deprivation suggests caution, at least until the individual's capacity to
manage affects and impulses is fully evaluated or the self-management of
emotions and impulses improves. A further caution: therapists often overestimate the capacity to tolerate affects in abused patients who are articulate and verbally intelligent.

Personality factors that have a bearing on the use of change-focused interventions include severity of core pathology, extremity of personality
pattern, and the presence of specific traits. In general, the greater the severity of core self pathology (based on the features discussed in the previous chapter), the greater the reliance placed on supportive and structured
interventions. Extreme levels of the personality patterns, with the possible
exception of compulsivity, also create problems in tolerating the challenge

of change-focused interventions, especially when there is also severe deprivation and trauma. A critical issue here is the degree to which the individual can tolerate affect expression.

As noted earlier, a degree of psychological mindedness is required to understand and use reframing interventions. When this attribute is not present, there is little benefit to be derived from an extensive exploration of psychopathology and a change-focused approach. Such interventions tend to affect the treatment relationship adversely and exacerbate impulsivity. Linked to low psychological mindedness is the tendency to attribute the causes of problems to external factors. Patients who are not psychologically minded tend to externalize responsibility for their problems and often react adversely to change-focused interventions—initially because such interventions imply that at least some of the factors contributing to difficulties are internal to the individual. Quality of object relationships also influences ability to make use of an active interventional strategy. Patients with poorly developed object relationships do better with a more supportive approach (Piper et al., 1991).

The factors noted can be used as a checklist. The more factors that are present, the more caution should be exercised about using change-focused interventions, at least in the early stages of therapy, until affect tolerance and affect and impulse regulation improve sufficiently to permit greater use of a more challenging strategy.

Tactical Considerations. At any moment in treatment, the decision to use a more specific intervention is influenced by an assessment of the therapeutic process and patient variables. Throughout treatment, specific interventions are only used when the therapeutic alliance, the bond between patient and therapist, and rapport are favorable. Patient factors that have a bearing on moment-to-moment selection of interventions include level of motivation and affect arousal. Although motivation has some trait-like qualities, it is also changes throughout treatment. Patients need to be adequately motivated to use more specific interventions. If this motivation is not present, it is often better to focus on the relationship and on building motivation than attempting interventions that may be ineffective or even cause further deterioration in the alliance. High levels of affect arousal tend to be destabilizing; in effect, they reduce the person's ability to manage and use cognitive information. Consequently, there is little value in using complex interventions when the patient is in a highly emotional state. It is more useful to focus on containment and affect regulation (see Chapter 8).

Domains of Psychopathology and Treatment Planning

A second aspect of treatment planning concerns the anticipated duration of treatment and the sequence for addressing different domains of problems and psychopathology. These issues are closely related to stability of personality pathology.

Stability of Personality Pathology and Treatment Planning

It was suggested in Chapter 3 that personality pathology varies in stability. Symptoms fluctuate naturally and appear to be the most amenable to change. An intermediate level of stability is formed by affect and impulse control, cyclical maladaptive interpersonal patterns, aspects of triggering situations that are closely linked to personality characteristics, dysfunctional cognitive styles, self-attitudes (including self-esteem), and maladaptive expressions of traits. Although more stable than symptoms, they are relatively amenable to change. Core self and interpersonal pathology involving the deficits associated with adaptive failure form the most stable aspects of personality.

This hierarchy forms a useful guide in treatment planning (see Table 6.2) because it establishes an approximate sequence for tackling problems that has implications for duration of treatment. The goal of brief treatments such as crisis management, which typically last four to eight sessions in an ambulatory setting or a day or two in an inpatient unit, is to return the patient to the previous level of functioning as quickly as possible. The focus is on symptomatic improvement and containment of affects and

---

TABLE 6.2. Hierarchy of Change: Implications for Planning Therapy

Crisis management

Approximate duration: Inpatient treatment 1–2 days; ambulatory treatment 4 to 8 sessions

Focus: To return the patient to previous level of functioning, with associated symptomatic and situational change

Shorter-term therapies and early stages of longer-term therapy

Approximate duration: 15–30 sessions

Focus: Symptoms including parasuicidal acts; triggering situations; associated maladaptive interpersonal patterns and personality characteristics; consequences of trauma; maladaptive cognitive styles

Longer-term therapy

Approximate duration: 30 sessions to several years

Focus: Enduring maladaptive interpersonal patterns; core self and interpersonal problems

---

impulses. With shorter-term treatment (15–30 sessions) and the earlier phases of longer-term treatment, the focus extends to problems at the second level of the hierarchy. Initially, interventions are focused on those aspects of psychopathology that directly influence symptoms and the eruption of crises: namely, self-regulation of affects and impulses and triggering events. Later the focus widens to include maladaptive interpersonal patterns, the maladaptive characteristic expressions of dispositional traits, and maladaptive cognitive styles. Change involving the core features of personality disorder—the development of a more adaptive self structure and integrated representations of others is the goal of longer-term therapy. It often takes several years or more to achieve meaningful changes; even then, problems often remain.

These guidelines are general. The treatment of personality disorder is in its infancy, and we are only beginning to explore the efficacy of various interventions. It may be that techniques will emerge to change core features in shorter periods of time.

Sequence of Interventions

Information on the stability of personality and psychopathology also forms the basis for planning the sequence in which problems are addressed and interventions implemented. This sequence gives an overall structure to treatment and provides a framework for integrating different kinds of specific, change-focused interventions. Treatment is divided into five phases: safety, containment, control and regulation, exploration and change, and integration and synthesis (see Table 6.3). The first phase is characterized by interventions that ensure the *safety* of the patient and others when the patient is in a crisis state. Achieving this may involve admitting the patient for inpatient treatment or other similar interventions to provide the structure and support needed until the crisis resolves. The goal of the next phase, *containment*, is to settle crisis behavior, contain impulses and affects, and restore behavioral control. This phase of treatment is also part of crisis management, and usually the two phases merge imperceptibly. These early phases are more concerned with management of symptoms and crisis behavior than treatment per se. Containment is primarily achieved through the use of general treatment strategies, with a heavy reliance on support, validation, and empathic understanding, supplemented by medication as necessary.

The third stage, *control and regulation*, begins during crisis management but continues after the immediate crisis has settled. Here the goals are to reduce symptoms and help the patient acquire the skills needed to manage and control affects and impulses, including suicidal and parasuicidal behavior. These skills compensate for the deficiencies in self-regulatory mechanisms arising from genetic predisposition and psycho-

TABLE 6.3. Phases in Treating Personality Disorder: Intervention Strategies

1. *Safety*: Interventions to ensure safety of patient and others

2. *Containment*: Interventions based primarily on general therapeutic strategies to contain affective and behavioral instability, supplemented with medication as necessary

3. *Control and regulation*: Behavioral, cognitive, and pharmacological interventions to reduce symptoms and improve self-regulation of affects and impulses

4. *Exploration and change*: Cognitive, interpersonal, and psychodynamic interventions to change the cognitive, affective, and situational factors contributing to problem behavior

5. *Integration and synthesis*: Interventions designed to address core pathology and forge a new sense of self and more integrated and adaptive self and interpersonal systems

social adversity. Most patients, even those with more inhibited traits, have difficulty controlling and tolerating affect. Affects tend to escalate, leading to impulsive and parasuicidal acts that are intended to reduce the dysphoria. The development of affect tolerance and affect management skills is a prerequisite to controlling these behaviors. During this phase, the general treatment strategies continue to provide the core interventions, supplemented by a combination of behavioral, cognitive, and pharmacological interventions. These more structured strategies work well at this stage of treatment; the evidence suggests that they are effective in reducing self-harm and promoting emotional regulation. They are also less demanding than other change-focused interventions that require greater exploration. Once these self-management skills have been acquired, attention is given to treating the consequences of trauma and adversity that contribute to self-harming behavior.

Facilitating changes in specific dysfunctional behaviors, such as deliberate self-harm, occurs during the control and regulation phase of treatment, using the stage of change model discussed in Chapter 4. However, less emphasis is placed on exploration than in later phases of treatment, to avoid the potentially destabilizing effects of intense emotional arousal. Exploration of self-harming behavior and associated affects is confined initially to delineating the sequence of events that triggers self-harm. Once this sequence has been identified, cognitive-behavioral strategies are used to control self-harming acts and manage associated dysphoria, and medication is used to manage impulsivity and mood symptoms.

As affect regulation and tolerance are acquired, treatment moves imperceptibly into the phase of *exploration and change*. Here there is greater emphasis on exploring psychopathology. The issues addressed during this phase typically include maladaptive schemata associated with self-harming behavior, maladaptive interpersonal behavior patterns, dysfunctional cognitive styles (such as self-invalidating and catastrophic thinking), and maladaptive trait-based behaviors. This phase is the work of medium- to longer-term treatment and it requires a combination of cognitive, interpersonal, and psychodynamic interventions. Again, the stages of change model is used to manage changes in targeted behaviors. The process begins by identifying a specific behavioral problem and establishing a commitment to change. Subsequently, the sequence of events leading to these behaviors, and their effects on the individual and his or her relationships are explored to varying degrees, according to the nature of the problem and the extent to which change-focused interventions are considered appropriate. Gradually, the exploration of issues gives way to a consideration of alternative ways of acting and the application of new learning, inside and outside treatment.

The third and fourth stages (control–regulation and exploration–change) involve the traditional work of therapy. The goal is to identify, understand, and change maladaptive behavior, including feelings and cognitions. The process may be thought of as one of substitutive change, in which maladaptive thoughts, feelings, and behavior are replaced with more adaptive alternatives. In contrast, the final phase of treatment is one of *integration and synthesis*, involving the development of more adaptive self and interpersonal systems. These tasks are primarily the work of long-term treatment. Here the goal is to integrate the fragmented components of personality and self functioning and to synthesize new personality structures, especially more effective interpersonal boundaries, a more coherent self, more integrated representations of others, and the capacity for self-directedness. These changes are not primarily effected through analysis and resolution of maladaptive and conflicted ways of being but rather through the development of new personality processes and structures. Clinical evidence suggests that such changes are more difficult to achieve and usually require long-term treatment.

This sequence brings order and structure to the treatment process. Along with the stages of change model and the distinction between general and specific interventions, the sequence provides the therapist with a map that broadly charts the course of treatment. Having such a map minimizes the confusion most clinicians experience when faced with multiple problems and pathology and the need to manage multiple interventions from different therapeutic approaches. However, the sequence is not intended to be rigid or fixed. In practice, treatment rarely follows a neat, consistent path, and overlap among phases of treatment is the norm. Nevertheless, the sequence is a useful guide for planning therapy and determining the order in which major themes will be tackled.

ESTABLISHING THE TREATMENT CONTRACT

Ideas about relationship-focused and change-focused interventions, the duration of treatment, and the sequence of interventions, along with a detailed understanding of problems and psychopathology, form a context for working with the patient to establish a mutually acceptable treatment contract. This is also the time to introduce a psychoeducational component by explaining a little about the nature of personality problems, the way therapy works, and the patient's and therapist's roles in the process.

The treatment contract "defines the purpose, format, terms, and limits of the enterprise" (Orlinsky & Howard, 1986, p. 312). As with most treatments, an integrated, tailored approach requires an explicit therapeutic contract. The contract helps to structure the therapeutic relationship and treatment process and contributes toward the creation of a safe environment that can contain self-destructive acts and maladaptive interpersonal behavior. Such a contract has three components: therapeutic goals, the treatment agreement, and pretherapy education. *Goals* structure treatment by defining therapeutic tasks, thereby delineating treatment boundaries; the *treatment agreement* defines the spatial and temporal aspects of these boundaries; and *pretherapy education* defines patient and therapist roles in achieving treatment goals. As Borden (1979) noted, the bond, tasks, and goals of therapy are interdependent, and the strength of the treatment alliance depends on the level of agreement between patient and therapist about the goals and tasks of treatment. Discussion of the therapeutic contract helps to forge the idea that treatment is a collaborative process, for which patient and therapist share responsibility.

Most forms of treatment, including Kernberg's psychodynamic model, cognitive therapy, and Linehan's approach, emphasize the value of an explicit therapeutic contract. Only the relationship management approach of Dawson (1988; Dawson & MacMillan, 1993) does not establish a contract. Even here a form of contract is used for inpatient treatment. Clarkin and colleagues' (1999) description of Kernberg's approach emphasizes a contract that clarifies the roles of therapist and patient and establishes a therapeutic framework that permits interpretation of any deviations from the frame. The task is then to understand these deviations and confront the impact that they have on therapy. This approach is also applied to impulsive and parasuicidal behaviors. The patient is not expected to cease these actions; rather, the therapist attempts to understand this behavior, encourages the patient to consider alternative ways to obtain help, and confronts the negative effect of such actions on treatment.

Linehan's (1993) position is similar, although the theoretical rationale is different (Hurt, Clarkin, Monroe-Blum, & Marziali, 1992). An explicit contract is established that specifies the practical arrangements for treatment, which is invariably time-limited, with the opportunity to continue depending on progress. There is also a substantial psychoeducational component that includes an explanation of the causes of parasuicidal behavior. As with Kernberg's approach, the patient is not expected to refrain from self-destructive and parasuicidal behavior. However, patients engaging in suicidal or self-harming behaviors must agree not to kill themselves while in dialectical behavior therapy, and agree that reducing or eliminating such behavior is a goal toward which they are willing to work (Linehan, 1993; Robins et al., 2001).

Establishing Treatment Goals

The first step in developing a treatment contract, after discussing the formulation, is to agree upon treatment goals. These goals reflect what the patient hopes to achieve in therapy, as modulated by the therapist's understanding of what can be accomplished realistically, given the patient's problems and resources and the treatment options available. When considering goals, it is useful to distinguish between broad treatment goals that guide the therapist and collaborative goals established with the patient.

General Goals

Treatment is guided by the basic principle that the *general goal is to improve adaptation* (Chapter 2). As Kroll (1988) noted, the ultimate goal for most therapies is to build competency in as many areas as possible. This goal orients the therapist to the overall objectives of treatment. More concrete goals are required, however, to conduct treatment and select interventions. These goals can be specified in relation to the six domains of psychopathology (see Chapter 2): (1) reduce symptoms and improve competency in managing symptoms; (2) develop more adaptive ways to manage situational problems; (3) build competence in managing and regulating affects and impulses; (4) develop more adaptive ways to use and express basic traits; (5) improve interpersonal skills and develop more adaptive ways of relating; (6) promote more adaptive solutions to universal life tasks by developing more integrated and coherent self and interpersonal systems.

These goals provide a framework for working with patients to establish collaborative treatment goals. Within each domain, one or more specific goals may be identified. For example, the symptom domain may give rise to such goals as (1) finding alternative ways to manage dysphoria, (2) improving mood, and (3) increasing control over dissociative behavior. Not all general goals, however, are relevant to all therapies. Sometimes treatment may focus on specific issues, such as the resolution of an immediate crisis. Even under these circumstances, however, the general goal of improving adaptation by building competence provides a frame of reference that reminds the therapist of the possibilities and limitations of treatment.

Setting Collaborative Goals

Collaborative goals should be *clearly defined, specific, realistic, attainable*, and *positively worded*. During the joint process of negotiating the treatment contract and goals, the therapist explores what the patient wants to achieve and helps the patient to express these wants as realistic and attainable goals. This may be a brief process or more prolonged, if patients are unclear about their goals or have unrealistic expectations that need to be shaped into a more attainable form.

It is desirable to formulate goals in a positive way, whenever possible, to avoid conveying the impression that the task of therapy is to address the patient's shortcomings. Hence it is preferable to talk of learning new ways to relate to people rather than relinquishing maladaptive patterns. Positive phrasing is experienced as validating and less critical. It also builds hope by implicitly recognizing the patient's potential.

Therapists often pay too little attention to working with the patient to establish treatment goals. This inattention may occur because the therapist (1) lacks a framework by which to organize clinical information into realistic goals, or (2) is reluctant to confront unrealistic expectations. Reluctance to set goals may also arise from the philosophical position that therapy is a growth process to be facilitated rather than directed, or that defining outcomes violates patients' rights to decide on the direction of their development. Most contemporary approaches to treatment, however, recognize that several advantages accrue from goal setting: Goals help to organize the treatment process, and they help patients focus on specific problems—a step that often initiates change (Borden, 1994).

When working with people who have personality disorder, goals, like a shared formulation, help to structure and contain behavioral reactivity. The process of goal setting often transforms an overwhelming sense that everything is wrong into a relieved agreement regarding a discrete set of attainable targets. It also encourages the recognition that therapy is not something that is passively received but rather requires the patient's active participation. This insight begins to correct tendencies to externalize problems and fosters a less passive stance about the ability to control one's life. In the process, motivation and commitment to treatment are increased. Working together to identify problems is an important first step in forming a treatment alliance and building a collaborative relationship (Gaston, 1990).

Establishing Realistic and Specific Goals

The initial goals should reflect realistic targets, given the severity of the patient's problems and available resources. They should also be specific and measurable, so that it is readily apparent to patient and therapist whether the goal has been achieved. Goal attainment can then be used to enhance the alliance and build a commitment to change. The establishment of specific *modest* goals helps to ensure success. For example, in the beginning, the goal of *reducing* deliberate self-harm is more likely to be achieved than the goal of *ceasing* to self-harm.

Unfortunately, patients and therapists often share unrealistic expectations about what can be accomplished. Therapists often want to accomplish too much and have difficulty in helping patients modulate their expectations. For example, perusal of the goals for brief crisis admission to inpatient units for patients with severe emotional dysregulation (borderline) pathology revealed such goals as "resolving problems with anger" or "developing better relationships." Similarly, in community mental health settings where the treatment options are limited to weekly appointments for several months, goals may include helping the patient "develop a sense of identity" or "the capacity for intimacy." Since such goals are unrealistic given the expected duration of treatment, they establish the conditions for failure. Therapists, finding little progress in attaining such goals, become frustrated, unduly pessimistic about outcome, and may even feel incompetent. Such feelings are easily projected onto patients, who are then held responsible for the lack of progress. As patients recognize that they are not progressing as expected, self-blame increases and the therapeutic relationship deteriorates. Unrealistic expectations also tend to feed the widespread belief among some mental health professionals that personality disorder is untreatable.

Goal setting begins by encouraging the patient to compile a list of problems that he or she would like to address. Discussion of these problems in ways that shape them into attainable goals begins to establish *collaborative description* as the vehicle for therapeutic work. It also focuses attention on specific problems rather than diffuse and global difficulties. All too often patients are unclear about their goals or couch them in general terms that are difficult to achieve.

A patient in her early 30s was referred by her family doctor for assessment and treatment of longstanding personality problems. The patient described herself as sad and unhappy and noted that she had felt that way for as long as she could remember, certainly since early adolescence. Her moods were variable and changed without apparent cause. When distressed, she would burn herself because she felt so angry about what had happened that she had to punish herself. She described herself as very sensitive to the way she was treated by others and often felt rejected and alone. Although she had several friends and was sociable, her relationships tended to be stormy. There had been many men in her life, but the relationships never lasted. She had had a disturbed adolescence and ran away from home repeatedly, eventually leaving at the age of 16. For several years, she lived a somewhat peripheral life and was even homeless for a while. She now felt intense guilt and shame about those years. In her early

20s she settled down a little, found employment, and moved into an apartment on her own. Since then, she has moved from job to job but generally managed to remain employed until a few months earlier, when she had been too distressed to work.

Over the years she has seen many psychiatrists and psychologists, but therapy "never worked out," and in each case she terminated treatment after a few months. Toward the end of the first interview, the clinician broached the question of what she wanted to achieve in treatment. She said that life was terrible—it always had been—and she wanted to change it. When asked more about this desire, she said it was obvious what was wrong—in fact, there was nothing *right* about her life, everything had to change. It was apparent that little would be achieved in pressing for further details at that time, and it was suggested that she think about some of the specific things that she would like to change and to make a list that could be discussed next time. When the assessment was completed and the formulation discussed, the issue of what she would like to achieve in treatment was again raised. The patient said that she had thought about it a little, but it seemed so obvious that everything was wrong, so there was no need to think about what she wanted to change—she wanted to change everything about her life.

When the therapist asked about what she had wanted from the previous therapies, the patient gave the same answer. Discussion of her experiences in previous treatments indicated that she had approached them in the same way. She wanted to change her life totally and quickly became disheartened and disillusioned when radical changes did not occur. In each case she simply stopped attending because there seemed little point.

This vignette illustrates the importance of setting attainable goals and how they contribute to the alliance. Because the patient set a broad, vague goal, she never felt that she accomplished anything. Small improvements were not valued as successes or taken as indications that change was possible but rather as reminders of what had still to be achieved. To establish viable treatment that did not repeat previous failures, it was necessary to break up her major goal into attainable components. The patient resisted this step partly because she was fixated on quantum change and partly because the establishment of a global goal protected her from the greater pain of looking at specific problems that could be changed. The problem was dealt with by accepting the broad goal and concentrating on the things that she thought would indicate that her life was better. At the same time, the therapist noted that she seemed to feel that treatment was impossible and was pessimistic about the outcome. The patient agreed, noting that she was such a mess that it seemed overwhelming. This comment provided an opportunity to suggest that it *is* overwhelming to believe that everything has to change at once rather than step by step. Gradually she began to talk about the shame of hurting herself and how she wished that her feelings were less labile, all the while continuing to protest that *everything* was wrong. Initial goals were established that involved reducing self-harm, learning to manage her affective lability, and finding alternative ways to deal with anger and dysphoria without engaging in deliberate self-harm. She also said that she wanted to deal with the shame she felt over the things that she had done in her teenage years. As therapy progressed, new goals were set for addressing relationship problems and difficulties with parents.

Although treatment cannot begin until agreement has been reached on immediate treatment goals and practical arrangements for therapy, not all goals need be specified at the outset. Preliminary goals may simply involve working on controlling parasuicidal behavior with the understanding that other goals may be considered once this goal is achieved. Or, agreement may be reached to work on a specific goal while attempting to identify other longer-term goals. The important point is to establish initial targets for collaborative work. Changes to the contract are negotiated later as issues are clarified and new problems emerge. The following vignettes illustrate the kinds of goals that are appropriate for this approach.

A man, age 32, who was living a solitary lifestyle due to inhibited traits, sought treatment for the anxiety symptoms and because his family was concerned that he did not have many relationships outside of his work situation. He was employed in the computer and software industry, and he worked mainly on his own. He did not have any close friends, nor did he really want relationships, but he did admit that he would like to feel more comfortable talking to his coworkers. He was very clear about his goals for treatment. He wanted help with the anxiety symptoms and with the discomfort he felt with others. He also wanted help with dealing with his family. As these matters were discussed, it was apparent that he did not want to socialize. He preferred a solitary lifestyle, enjoyed being alone, and had a wide range of pursuits. The collaborative goals established for time-limited treatment were: reduce anxiety; explore ways to feel more comfortable interacting with coworkers and address his fears about these contacts, especially when feelings were involved; and help him feel more comfortable with the lifestyle that that he had chosen, which meant learning ways to deal with his family.

A woman, age 39, expressed her desire for help in dealing with self-harming acts and mixed feelings of anxiety and depression. She had secretly cut herself for 20 years. Although she had sought help repeatedly in the past, nothing had really changed. Recently, the self-harm had increased in frequency and severity. These changes appeared to occur shortly after she discovered that one of her children had similar problems. The patient felt intense guilt and responsibility, believing that her daughter's problems were due to abuse inflicted by a previous partner some years earlier. Her daughter was only 8 or 9 at the time, and she thought she should have protected her better. The daughter's problems had also activated memories of abuse she had suffered for many years as a child. Assessment revealed multiple additional problems, including dissociative behavior and transient psychotic episodes. Personality assessment revealed high scores on most traits associated with the emotional dysregulation pattern, except submissiveness, and high scores on compulsivity.

The patient had a long list of things that she wanted to accomplish, including stopping self-harm, overcoming the depression, stopping dissociating, avoiding psychotic episodes, stopping flashbacks of abusive events, dealing with problems of abuse, learning how to control her life better, and behaving in a more perfectionistic way so that she could stop worrying about not doing things well enough. This list was given shape by asking her to cite her most pressing problems. The patient thought that self-harm was the most pressing because it had increased recently and was causing new difficulties at home, when she could no longer keep it secret. She also wanted to talk about the abuse but became distressed and dissociated to the point of being unresponsive for the rest of the session.

When the subject of treatment was discussed again in the next session, she brought up the issue of abuse again in the context of depressive symptoms. The therapist noted her desire to learn to deal with urges to self-mutilate and the problems she was having managing her feelings and wondered aloud whether the patient would like to deal with these feelings first, because of the many difficulties they were causing. The patient agreed that this seemed like a good idea but added that she also needed to talk about the abuse. The therapist agreed that addressing the abuse was important but noted how it was also very distressing and wondered how the patient would feel about talking about the way the abuse contributed to the self-harm, leaving work on actual events until she was feeling more in control and able to manage the feelings aroused. The patient thought that this was a good idea; she was worried about what had happened during the previous session and wondered what she could do about dissociating. The therapist responded by agreeing that the dissociative behavior also seemed important and wondered whether they could look at what triggered it at the same time they talked about the things that caused her to harm herself.

This collaborative discussion ended with agreement that self-harming acts, dissociative behavior, and the mood problems would be the immediate focus of attention and that the initial goal was to reduce the frequency of these acts as the first step toward stopping them. Later, when the patient felt ready, they would deal with the problems caused by abuse. The patient thought that this was a good plan. She noted that no one had ever suggested a detailed plan before, but she thought that it was a good idea because it provided a focus on which to concentrate. She added that she would also like to talk about how to deal with her daughter, who was having similar problems. The therapist suggested that the patient raise the matter whenever she was concerned.

Obstacles to Goal Setting

It is often difficult to establish treatment goals due to problems with collaboration, fears about committing to treatment, and a general difficulty in setting goals due to problems with self-directedness that is part of the core pathology. It is not surprising, therefore, that in one study only one-third of borderline patients had reached an agreement with their therapists about treatment goals and methods after 1 month of treatment, and only one-quarter were actively collaborating with their therapists in working on these goals (Frank, 1992). These findings suggest that careful attention should be paid to goal setting and establishing the treatment contract, and that the process is often a protracted one.

Goal setting may also be a challenge with patients who are primarily focused on symptoms and symptom relief and unaware of the personality problems that contribute to their difficulties. In these circumstances, during the discussion of goals it is useful to build in ideas about looking at the factors that contribute to the distress, so that the patient begins to incorporate these ideas. If necessary, additional goals may be identified later as the patient becomes aware of other factors. This process is illustrated by the case of Natasha, whose personality profile was described in the previous chapter.

> Natasha presented in a crisis state with intense dysphoria and self-harming behavior; she attributed her distress to the fact that "everyone is against me." She had little understanding of the way her actions contributed to the interpersonal situations to which she was reacting. Natasha's initial goals were to receive treatment for the dysphoria and to learn to deal with the distress caused by others without resorting to self-harm. When treatment goals were discussed, it was difficult for her to move beyond these objectives. Tendency to externalize responsibility and blame prevented her from recognizing how she contributed to problems with others. Because it was too soon to address this style, treatment initially was focused on the dysphoria and self-harm. As therapy progressed and an effective alliance formed, Natasha began to recognize how she externalized responsibility and how this behavior contributed to the interpersonal situations that she found so distressing. As a result, additional goals were established that involved understanding and changing dysfunctional cognitive styles, interpersonal patterns, and a submissive, passive–aggressive stance. This phase of Natasha's treatment is discussed in Chapter 11. Later still, she became concerned about how nothing felt real or authentic and about the lack of direction in her life.

These perceptions were used to discuss new goals directed toward developing greater self-directedness (see Chapter 13).

Goals and Integrative Functioning

Thus far treatment goals have been discussed largely in the context of the treatment alliance and the effect of goal setting on the relationship and the patient's approach to treatment. However, another aspect of goal setting that is specific to treating patients with personality disorder concerns the way goals integrate personality functioning by organizing and directing behavior. As Carver and Scheier (1998) noted, "the self is partly the person's goals" (p. 100). Moreover, the ability to establish and work toward goals is an important achievement of an adaptive self system. Goal setting as part of establishing a treatment contract should also be viewed within this context. Most individuals with personality problems have difficulty establishing goals. The resulting absence of goals contributes to a sense of meaninglessness and to the feeling of being directionless. The establishment of treatment goals serves to organize and focus the work of treatment. It also serves as a model that can be extended to other aspects of life. In a small but important way, goal setting promotes integration and begins the task of creating meaning and direction in the person's experience and behavior.

Treatment Agreement

The contract includes the practical arrangements for therapy, including appointment times, frequency and duration of sessions, and the duration of treatment. These arrangements establish the literal structure and boundaries of treatment. Although most therapists recognize the importance of these matters, it is surprising how often they are neglected when treating patients with personality disorder. The initial discussion about treatment should include details of the length of each session to avoid the potential problems that can occur, for example, when the therapist concludes a session after 45 minutes when the patient was expecting a full hour. Whereas these straightforward matters are readily clarified with less dysfunctional patients, such misunderstandings can take on greater significance with severely personality disordered patients, and are more disruptive of the treatment alliance.

When discussing practical arrangements for treatment, it is also useful to discuss the way vacations and professional leave will be handled. Patients should be advised that they will be informed well in advance of therapist absences. When longer-term treatment is planned, it is often possible to provide information at the outset about therapist availability for many months ahead. This overview contributes to a sense of stability and consistency and affirms the therapist's commitment to treatment.

Some events occurring during treatment can be predicted, such as crises, requests for additional appointments or to prolong a particular session, and telephone calls between appointments. Hence it is helpful to decide in advance how these issues will be handled to ensure that they are handled in ways that are consistent with the frame. It is also useful for the patient to be aware of these arrangements ahead of time. Developing explicit guidelines for dealing with these occurrences is not a matter of adopting rote responses; rather, it is an attempt to establish a set of principles to guide clinical decisions and reduce the chances of responding inappropriately, under pressure of events or the influence of countertransference. Discussion of these issues when establishing the treatment contract helps the patient to anticipate possible problems and establishes an understanding that can be referred to later, if problems arise.

Discussion of the frequency of sessions is a convenient time to broach the topic of therapist availability between sessions in the event of an emergency. The position taken depends upon the therapist's professional situation and the severity of the patient's condition. This matter should be discussed before treatment, not after problems have emerged. Sometimes the therapist's professional circumstances prevent him or her from being available between sessions, in which case a plan should be developed for the patient to follow in an emergency, such as attending an emergency room at a local general hospital, contacting an agency that undertakes crisis intervention, contacting a support group, or visiting the family doctor. When it is possible for the patient to contact the therapist, the therapist should outline the ways in which he or she will be available and how the patient should initiate contact. In addition to making the arrangements explicit, these matters need to be discussed in a way that does not convey an unrealistic impression of availability, encourage excessive contact between sessions, or imply that crises are inevitable or that the patient will not be able to manage them.

The contract should also include an understanding of the likely duration of treatment. In some settings a limited number of sessions may be available. If these constraints apply, they should be discussed frankly from the outset and treatment goals should be established with these limitations in mind. Any discussion of the duration of therapy should include a realistic discussion of the time required to effect major changes in personality disorder. Many patients (and some health-care organizations) are attracted by short-term interventions. Patients need to realize, however, that although rapid progress may occur in dealing with some problems, long-term therapy is often required to effect lasting change in core problems. Even cognitive therapists, who normally advocate short-term therapy, suggest that 1 to 3 years is required to treat more severe conditions such as borderline personality disorder (Layden et al., 1993). Some patients do not realize that their current problems are reflections of underlying problems and hence have unrealistic expectations of the duration of treatment. Others realize, however, that their problems are lifelong and hence are unlikely to change quickly or easily. Such patients are often reassured by a frank discussion of time issues, and many are content to have found a therapist who recognizes the need for longer-tem treatment, something that they have intuitively felt they needed.

Pretherapy Education

The final component of contract setting is psychoeducation. The goals are to educate the patient (and, if necessary, significant others) about the nature of personality disorder and provide information about the way therapy works, the way treatment goals will be achieved, and the roles of patient and therapist in the change process. Although psychoeducational programs have a well-established role in the treatment of various conditions, their use in treating of personality disorder has received less attention (Ruiz-Sancho, Smith, & Gunderson, 2001). In addition to providing information about therapy, two forms of education about personality disorder seem promising. The first is instruction about the *nature and origins of personality difficulties*. Most patients are puzzled by the complexity of their problems and feelings and their inability to get their lives in order. A brief explanation of the origins of personality disorder makes their experience more explicable. It also allows patients to understand the reasons for the treatment plan and enables them to make more informed decisions about embarking on treatment. The realization that problems are explicable builds hope and contributes to an effective treatment relationship. It is useful to include information about the genetic basis of key traits so that patients understand that these characteristics are part of their biology—information that often helps to reduce self-blame. Care should be taken, however, not to create the impression that these characteristics cannot be changed. Instead, ideas about learning to use these traits effectively and to express them in more adaptive ways should be discussed. This is the initial stage of education that will be an ongoing part of therapy. Pretherapy education, however, needs to be provided judiciously, as is the case with inclusion of psychoeducational material, because a didactic style tends to activate resistance and reactive responses, as has been shown to be the case in family therapy for patients with addiction problems (Patterson & Forgatch, 1985).

The second form of education about personality disorder is *information on mental processes and interpersonal behavior*. Brief information about the patient's problems may be helpful when discussing treatment, but more detailed explanation is probably best left until later. The kinds of explanations offered will differ according to the patient's problems and current state. Typically reference is made to the way past events have influenced the way the patient thinks about self and others and the way these thoughts affect mood and emotions. Brief explanations may also be offered about long-term effects of trauma and the factors that contribute to self-harm, when applicable, and about the way maladaptive interpersonal patterns operate. The idea is not to provide detailed instruction about the nature of personality disorder. Rather, the goal is three-pronged: to (1) convey the impression that problems are explicable, (2) stimulate curiosity about the mental processes that contribute to the presenting problems, and (3) encourage self-observation and self-appraisal.

Another goal of psychoeducation at this stage, as noted, is to provide information about treatment. This process begins with a discussion of the formulation and the establishment of goals. A commitment to treatment is enhanced with information about the way treatment works, the sorts of benefits the patient may expect, and the contributions of the patient and clinician to the process. All too often, patients are enrolled in treatment with little information of what is expected of them or their role in the process. This lack of information creates (1) uncertainty and anxiety, which hinder the formation of an effective alliance, and (2) the conditions that activate maladaptive patterns and reactive affects. It is better to manage patients with personality disorder in ways that minimize opportunities for problems to arise than to struggle with the consequences of these problems. Discussions about treatment should emphasize its collaborative nature, so that the patient fully understands this aspect of the process.

Information about treatment and the nature of the individual's difficulties form the basis for discussing treatment options. The clinician is being consulted as an expert; hence it is important to convey clear information about the treatment available and to offer an opinion about what is likely to be helpful. These recommendations should be offered in a collaborative manner and the patient's opinion and reactions sought and discussed, to avoid creating the impression that treatment is all the clinician's idea and the patient is merely complying with recommendations.

Obstacles to Contract Setting

Establishing a treatment contract is not always straightforward, and many patients resist the process. Problems typically occur when the severely disturbed patient is in a crisis, during which it may be difficult for him or her to process information. Even under these circumstances, however, a contract should be discussed. This contract may be very simple; for example, meeting for a short time to address an immediate problem. Other patients may feel they are too distressed and disorganized to attend for treatment regularly. This type of response is best dealt with by offering support and validation while confronting reality, as illustrated in the following vignette.

A patient with a long history of severe self-harming behaviors and several treatment failures due to irregular attendance claimed that she might not be able to attend therapy regularly and on time because she was new to the city and was unable to find her way around. In addition, she said that she was often too distressed to make the journey. As a solution to the problem, she suggested that the therapist meet her somewhere nearer to where she lived. The therapist agreed that it was hard to find one's way around a new city, particularly when feeling unwell. He added that it was not possible to help her unless she attended for treatment. He agreed that it would be convenient if he had an office nearer her home, but this was not the case. He then went on to note that regular attendance had also been a problem with previous courses of treatment, and that regular sessions were essential for treatment to be successful.

Another difficulty encountered when discussing the treatment contract occurs when patients have fixed ideas about the causes of their problems and how to remedy them. For example, a patient may insist that "I must have been abused," and he or she may need to "uncover memories of what happened." These ideas are especially problematic when they differ from the therapist's assessment. Such statements must be taken as the starting point for discussion; they are rarely resolved by tackling them head-on. A more indirect approach is needed that also draws attention to additional issues and seeks to educate the patient, and even relatives or referring sources, about the current state of knowledge in the field.

COMMENT

This overview of treatment planning introduced the idea that treatment may be conveniently divided into five phases—safety, containment, control and regulation, exploration and change, and integration and synthesis—that represent the different issues addressed over time and different interventions that take priority. Underlying these phases is the idea that treatment moves from the use of more structured interventions during the earlier phases to less structured and more exploratory interventions during the latter phases. The therapeutic contract was described in terms of the collaborative goals of treatment, the treatment agreement, and psychoeducation. Establishing a mutually agreed-upon understanding of the framework for treatment begins the process of developing a collaborative relationship with the patient. It also establishes the structure of treatment as an important step toward building a consistent therapeutic process. These developments continue with the use of the general treatment strategies that are discussed in the next chapter.

CHAPTER 7

General Therapeutic Strategies

Earlier discussion of core pathology and the results of psychotherapy outcome studies led to the proposal that treatment should be organized around generic change mechanisms. This chapter extends these ideas by considering the strategies and interventions required to implement this proposal. Four strategies are suggested:

1. Building and maintaining a collaborative relationship.
2. Maintaining a consistent treatment process.
3. Establishing and maintaining a validating treatment process.
4. Building and maintaining motivation for change.

These strategies are independent of the type and duration of treatment, the theoretical orientation of the therapist, and individual differences in patients' personalities and psychopathology.

The consistent use of these strategies brings about changes in core pathology by drawing the patient into a more adaptive relationship. Emphasis on collaboration builds the treatment alliance and addresses problems in working cooperatively with others. A consistent treatment process provides a predictable therapeutic relationship that modifies expectations of inconsistency and unpredictability arising from earlier dysfunctional relationships. Validating interventions convey support and build the alliance. They also help to correct self-invalidating ways of thinking that hinder the formation of a coherent self. Finally, efforts to build motivation create the commitment necessary for change and help to modify beliefs of powerlessness, passivity, and limited self-efficacy that contribute to low self-esteem and perpetuate maladaptive patterns. These strategies also establish the therapeutic relationship and structure required for the effective use of the specific interventions that form the second component of treatment.

The first three strategies largely use interventions that are relationship-based rather than change-focused. Interventions for building motivation, which also incorporate a change-focused element, form a bridge between the general strategies and specific interventions that are more directly concerned with behavioral change.

STRATEGY 1: BUILD AND MAINTAIN A COLLABORATIVE RELATIONSHIP

Priority is given to building and maintaining the alliance because a collaborative therapeutic relationship is inherently supportive and central to managing core pathology. Most treatments emphasize the importance of a collaborative relationship, including psychoanalytic therapy: (Buie & Adler, 1982; Masterson, 1976; Zetzel, 1971), cognitive therapy (Beck et al., 1990), interpersonal therapy (Benjamin, 1993), and dialectical behavior therapy (Linehan, 1987, 1993; Robins et al., 2001). Moreover, a poor alliance early in treatment predicts early termination (Frank, 1992; Hartley, 1985; Horvath & Symonds, 1991; Luborsky et al., 1985; Raue & Goldfried, 1994), and improvement in the alliance during treatment is associated with positive outcomes (Foreman & Marmar, 1985; Luborsky et al., 1993; Westerman, Foote, & Winston, 1995). Although these conclusions are based on the general psychotherapy literature, studies of personality disorder point to similar conclusions (Horwitz, 1974).

Contemporary conceptions emphasize that collaboration is the critical feature of the alliance (Gaston, 1990; Hatcher & Barends, 1996; Horvath & Greenberg, 1994; Luborsky, 1984). Unfortunately, therapists from most schools agree that a collaborative relationship is difficult to achieve with this population. As Benjamin (1993) noted, "The hardest part of treating personality disorder is helping the patient collaborate against 'it,' the long-standing way of being" (p. 240). It takes time for the alliance to emerge and consolidate (Horwitz, 1974). Indeed, an effective alliance is more the *result* of successful treatment than a prerequisite for it (Frank, 1992).

Many factors hinder alliance formation. Many patients lack the relationship skills required for collaborative work. Psychosocial adversity leads to caution about relationships and negative expectations about help and support. Feelings of envy, conflicted attitudes toward authority, and dependency conflicts interfere with the process, as do maladaptive traits. Emotional dysregulation, for example, tends to produce emotionally driven relationships that are unstable. Inhibited individuals, on the other hand, tend to avoid contact with the therapist. Because of these factors, throughout treatment priority is given to building, maintaining, monitoring, and repairing the alliance (Beck, 1995; Beck et al., 1990; Benjamin, 1993; Chessick, 1979; Cottraux & Blackburn, 2001; Meissner, 1984, 1991; Young, 1990, 1994). It may take several months or even years to establish an ef-fective alliance (Masterson, 1976). Empirical studies show that even after 6 months, a good alliance has not been achieved with most borderline pa-tients (Frank, 1992). Subsequently, the alliance is likely to fluctuate: Any deepening of the relationship is likely to evoke feelings of vulnerability, leading to a decrease in the alliance. Work on the alliance typically begins during assessment; patients entering therapy with negative attitudes, hos-tility, and reluctance to engage in the therapeutic process have poor out-comes (Strupp, 1993). An emphasis on the collaborative nature of the alli-ance makes it clear that both partners contribute to the relationship. Descriptions of the working relationship consistently stress (1) the affec-tive bond that the patient establishes with the therapist; (2) the patient's commitment to therapy and capacity for purposeful therapeutic work; (3) the therapist's empathic understanding of the patient and involvement in therapy; and (4) the agreement between the patient and therapist on the goals of therapy (Gaston, 1990). These relationship dimensions remind therapists to separate their contribution to the alliance from that of their patients, and to bear in mind that they, too, may contribute to alliance problems.

Luborsky (1984, 1994; Luborsky, Crits-Christoph, Alexander, Mar-golois, & Cohen, 1983) offered a conceptualization of the alliance that is especially helpful in treating people with personality disorder. For Luborsky (1994), the alliance "is an expression of a patient's positive bond with the therapist who is perceived as a helpful and supportive person" (p. 39). Drawing upon empirical studies, he proposed that the alliance has a *percep-tual component*, in which the patient perceives the therapist and therapy as helpful and supportive and him- or herself as accepting help, and a *rela-tionship component* in which the patient and therapist work together to help the patient.

Strategies for Building and Strengthening the Alliance

The evidence suggests that the alliance is fostered by (1) maintaining a fo-cus on the relationship between patient and therapist, and (2) the thera-pist adopting a collaborative style that focuses on the patient's goals and current concerns (Horvath & Greenberg, 1994; Luborsky, Crits-Christoph, Mintz, & Auerbach, 1988). The evidence also indicates that the patient's perceptions of the alliance, *not* the therapist's, predict outcome (Hartley, 1985; Horvath & Greenberg, 1994).

Luborsky's two-component description offers a systematic strategy for building the alliance. The therapist's task in building the *perceptual and at-titudinal component* is to help the patient understand that his or her condition *can* be treated, that therapy and the therapist are credible, and to en-courage the patient to accept help. With the *relational component*, the task is to establish a collaborative relationship and to help patients recognize and accept this cooperation. Although the perceptual and collaborative components tend to correlate, and many interventions combine both com-ponents, the first component tends to emerge earlier in treatment. Note that it is possible to have high levels of trust and positive attitudes without high levels of collaboration.

Building Credibility: The Perceptual and Attitudinal Component

Before they can form an alliance, patients need to believe that both treat-ment and the therapist are credible and that the therapist is competent and helpful. Therapists can contribute to a *sense of optimism and hope* on which the alliance is built by behaving, from the outset, in a professional manner that conveys respect, understanding, and support, and by educat-ing patients about their problems and the ways that treatment may help them to reach their goals. Even during assessment, the clinician should be mindful of the importance of fostering hope, given that pretherapy expec-tations of success are associated with favorable outcomes (Goldstein, 1962; Strupp, 1993). During these initial contacts, hope is conveyed by questions that indicate understanding, and by the therapist's willingness to work with the patient to establish goals and to work on what may seem to the patient to be intractable problems. During the early stages of treatment, exploration of the patient's doubts or reservations about treatment or the therapist's ability to help may preclude premature termination—a major problem in treating patients with personality disorder (Gunderson et al., 1989; Skodal, Buckley, & Charles, 1983; Waldinger & Gunderson, 1984).

The alliance is also built on the rapport created when *understanding and acceptance* are communicated through careful listening and sensitive responses. Providing regular summaries of the therapist's impressions of the patient's difficulties, beginning with the assessment interviews, also facili-tates rapport. These summaries also address fears that the therapist has pre-conceptions about what is wrong on will not really listen or take the pa-tient's problems seriously.

As noted, realistic goal setting enhances the alliance and the bond be-tween patient and therapist (Borden, 1994) ongoing indications of *support for the goals of therapy* and a consistent focus on these goals are associated with patients' ratings of progress and the quality of the treatment relation-ship (Allen, Tarnoff, & Coyne, 1985). Supporting patients' goals occurs through encouraging patients to talk about the importance of their goals and whether they think they are making progress toward achieving them. Reminding patients of their goals on occasion maintains a focus on change and conveys the idea that the patient's beliefs and wants are important.

Ultimately, it is the patient's experience of change that cements the working relationship. Many patients, however, are reluctant to acknowledge their own progress. For this reason, therapists should *recognize progress* by highlighting even minor changes. Thus, if a goal is to reduce anxiety, occasions when the patient feels that he or she has not overreacted or has managed to contain a sense of panic should be acknowledged and reinforced. The following vignette indicates this process:

A woman in her late 20s, with a long history of psychiatric problems, sought help with relationship difficulties associated with emotional dysregulation (borderline pathology). She was extremely moody, frequently overcome by anxiety and panic, and had uncontrollable angry outbursts. As a result, her relationships were chaotic and volatile. The early treatment sessions were difficult. Extreme affective lability created frequent problems so that treatment was crisis-oriented. It had also been difficult to establish a working relationship. The patient was reluctant to trust the therapist and believe that he was interested in her problems. She constantly accused the therapist of not listening. During the session in question, the patient berated the therapist again for not listening or understanding. She pointed out that it was impossible to work with him when she could not trust him and when she felt that she had to keep him entertained to hold his attention. She maintained that doing so caused an enormous strain for her.

During this barrage, the patient mentioned that she had not consumed any alcohol for a week, and that she had consistently attended AA. The therapist asked her to describe what had happened in the previous week. She said that after the previous session, she had decided not to drink and to attend AA daily. Although the first group that she attended had not been helpful, she had found a second group with which she felt more comfortable. Now she went every evening. The therapist commented that she must be pleased that she had been able to break a habit of 15 years' duration and had been able to go for 7 days without a drink. Somewhat reluctantly, the patient acknowledged that she was pleased. The therapist then went on to note that, although she was describing major problems in therapy, it also appeared that the therapy was helping. Again, the patient reluctantly acknowledged that this was the case, and they began a discussion of the way therapy had been helpful. During the discussion the patient noted that perhaps the therapist was listening, and may even know what he was doing, and that she was benefiting from treatment.

This episode indicates that building the alliance does not require major interpretations. In this case, recognition of progress was sufficient. Explicit acknowledgment of progress need not await major changes. Instead, it is useful to acknowledge small changes early in treatment, as illustrated by the following vignette.

> A fairly withdrawn man with inhibited or schizoid–avoidant traits had attended twice-weekly treatment for about 6 weeks. The early sessions were dominated by his feelings of hopelessness and despondency stemming from negative thoughts about all aspects of his life, and considerable anxiety, uncertainty, and pessimism about the future. His overriding conviction was that that he was a failure. Nothing he tried ever worked out, and he saw few prospects for change.
>
> After being in treatment for about 3 months he took up a sport that had appealed to him for some time, and a few days later he began to pursue an artistic interest. During one session, he commented that things had gone well for him during the previous week, and that he had begun thinking about the future, especially about a career. This had been an unresolved issue for many years, but now several interesting possibilities were raised. Furthermore, these issues were discussed in a more positive and less anxious manner than previously. The therapist noted that he seemed to be feeling a little differently about things. The patient responded by saying that he was now enjoying sports, music, and other activities. The therapist commented that several things appeared to have changed over the last few weeks. The patient was surprised by this comment. After a few moments of reflection, he smiled and said that several simple things were giving him pleasure, but he had not recognized this until the therapist drew it to his attention. The therapist added that it also sounded as if he were feeling a little more optimistic. The patient agreed, adding that he still felt very cautious, because life had been difficult and things had never worked out in the past. The therapist responded that he could understand the caution but that it also sounded as if the patient were pleased with the changes he had made.

This exchange recognized progress to create hope. The collaborative component of the alliance was reinforced, and the interaction moved toward building motivation and instilling a sense of mastery by helping the patient recognize and take credit for the changes he had made.

When acknowledging progress, care needs to be taken to avoid being seen as the source of reinforcement—doing so may foster unhelpful dependency or provoke anger if the patient interprets the therapist's positive feedback as an empty compliment or as minimizing his or her problems. For this reason, it is best to confine positive feedback to comments that the patient seems to have changed, without evaluating or by noting the change, and wondering whether the patient is pleased with it. This stance promotes the patient's capacity to self-reward and self-motivate.

Building Cooperation and Collaboration:
The Relationship Component

The development of collaboration involves translating attitudinal and perceptual changes into behavioral change within treatment. An important
part of collaboration is to *engage in a collaborative search for understanding*,
as captured by the idea of *collaborative description*. In the process, the patient learns skills that can be used outside treatment. *Acknowledging the patient's use of skills and knowledge* acquired in treatment strengthens the
bond by drawing attention to the fact that the patient has learned from
the therapist and now shares certain skills with the therapist.

Most conceptions of the alliance emphasize the patient–therapist
bond and the degree to which the patient feels secure enough to explore
positive and negative feelings (Allen, Newson, Gabbard, & Coyne, 1984;
Luborsky, 1976, 1984; Orlinsky, Grawe, & Parks, 1994; Orlinsky & Howard,
1986). The bond is experienced and expressed as liking, trust, mutual respect, shared commitment to the process, and a shared understanding of
the treatment process and goals (Borden, 1994). It is influenced by a therapeutic style that conveys respect and collaboration and fostered by *language that captures the idea of therapy as a collaborative relationship*. As
Luborsky (1984) noted, comments that include the words *we* and *together*
are a simple way of cementing the relationship. Patients and therapists use
such words more often during successful treatments (Luborsky et al., 1985).
Acknowledging that "we were able to make some progress with that problem" or "in the past we were able to work this out together" promotes cooperation. Used judiciously, such statements move patients away from perceiving the relationship in terms of status or control. The effects of using
the word *we* are often surprising. One patient protested, "I hate it when
you say that . . . it makes me uncomfortable because I don't want to feel
that I'm getting close to you." It is also useful to discuss patients' feelings
about collaborating with the therapist along with their impressions of its
effectiveness. The therapist's feelings about the patient also contribute to
the alliance. Patients who are liked by their therapists tend to do better
than those for whom therapists feel neutrality or dislike (Strupp, 1993). As
Strupp noted, therapists' attitudes function as a self-fulfilling prophecy,
causing therapists to feel more optimistic about outcome and show more
empathy.

An important aspect of close relationships is a shared history that creates the depth and continuity on which trust is built and establishes the
idea that relationships are stable. In therapy, a sense of history is created
by *referring to shared experiences in treatment*. This sharing does not involve
personal disclosure by the therapist or discussion of experiences in common outside treatment. Rather, it involves recalling events when the patient and therapist worked together to solve a problem. Comments such as,

"We spent a lot of time working on those sort of problems in the past, so you must be pleased that the effort is really beginning to pay dividends" serve to deepen the alliance. As therapy progresses, more opportunities arise to refer to past experiences together. As termination approaches, such discussions help to (1) consolidate change, (2) recall how things have changed, and (3) note that the patient and therapist's interaction is different from the way it was in the past.

Monitoring the Alliance and Managing Ruptures

The pivotal role of the alliance in the change process means that the alliance should be monitored carefully and problems addressed immediately, before they escalate. Since ruptures to the alliance are inevitable, an important therapist skill is the ability to deal with these ruptures effectively (Safran & Muran, 2000). When monitoring the alliance, it should be recalled that it is the patient's opinion, not the therapist's, that predicts outcome. Under most circumstances, good indicators of the state of the alliance are rapport, openness (as reflected by the flow of therapeutic material), collaboration, and the patient's commitment to treatment. Periodically it is also useful to evaluate the alliance directly by asking for the patient's impressions about therapy and whether it is helping. Cognitive therapists recommend that this issue be raised in each session (Beck, 1995). Although this practice certainly ensures that the alliance is not neglected, there is the danger that such regular inquiry will be perceived as a stereotyped routine rather than genuine interest.

It is helpful to distinguish between difficulties establishing an alliance and the strains that emerge during treatment (Borden, 1994). Protracted formation of the alliance is common and should not be viewed as "pretherapy" because it provides an opportunity to deal with important interpersonal schemata and model tolerance and empathy. By acknowledging the difficulty, the therapist offers the validation needed to build a relationship. Simply acknowledging that trust must be difficult, given the patient's experience, is often sufficient to move the process along. Difficulty forming an alliance is not always due to patient pathology. It also arises from unclear treatment goals and discrepancies between the patient's and the therapist's understanding of these goals and how they should be attained. Problems may also arise when patients are unsure about the process of therapy and their role in it.

During treatment, disruption of the alliance may occur because of disagreements about the goals or tasks of treatment or due to problems in the bond between therapist and patient (Safran & Muran, 2000). Any deterioration in the alliance should be dealt with promptly and in a supportive and empathic way. This approach usually means dealing with the problem in the here-and-now rather than interpreting it as resistance originating in past relationship problems. Safran and colleagues (Safran, Crocker, McMain, & Murray, 1990; Safran, Muran, & Samstag, 1994) investigated ruptures to the alliance and ways to repair them. Their emphasis on disruptions in the alliance as important opportunities to change dysfunctional interpersonal schemata is particularly relevant to treating patients with personality disorder. They suggest a four-stage process to repair alliance problems. The first stage is for the therapist to notice changes in the alliance—what they refer to as "rupture markers"—such as affect changes, decreased involvement, disagreement with the therapist, and so on, and to focus the patient's attention on his or her immediate experience, including his or her experience of the therapeutic relationship. The second stage is to explore the reasons for the rupture and the patient's thoughts and feelings about the event. If the patient is able to express his or her reactions, including negative reactions, the process moves to the fourth stage, that of resolution of the rupture. Here the patient asserts feelings, fears, and wishes associated with the rupture and the therapist validates these reactions. (Validation is an important part of the process.) If the patient is unable to express his or her reactions in the second stage, a third stage is added: exploration of how and why the patient avoids or blocks recognizing and exploring the rupture.

The value of this approach is that it turns a potentially negative event into an opportunity to apply several change processes. *Recognizing* and *repairing* problems with the alliance are not only necessary components of the change process, they are also important ways to implement change in maladaptive schemata. As Safran and Muran (2000) point out, recognition and repair are the "very essence of change" (p. 13). By recognizing the rupture, the therapist demonstrates empathy; exploring the issue and validating the experience provides a new experience. The process models cooperation and teaches the patient how to solve interpersonal problems. It also communicates the valuable idea that relationships are not fragile and that problems in relationships can be explored, understood, and solved. An important feature is the therapist's acknowledgment of his or her contribution to the rupture. Patients with personality disorder are often excessively critical and readily find fault with their therapists. Usually, however, there is a grain of truth to these criticisms, even if the patient's reaction appears exaggerated (Vaillant, 1992). Therapists should always be scrupulously honest in acknowledging their contribution to alliance ruptures. For patients with severe personality disorder, this acknowledgment can provide the patient with a powerful experience, as illustrated by the following vignette.

A patient with severe emotional dysregulation problems who had been in treatment for several years began one session by saying that she had been very angry after the previous session, and that she was still angry. With a little encouragement, she said that she was angry because the therapist had been late. This was true—a last-minute problem had led to the therapist being about 5 minutes late. The therapist had handled the situation by asking the patient if it would be convenient to extend the session to make up for the lost time. The patient went on to say that she was also angry because, during a previous session, the therapist had discussed an upcoming absence 4 weeks hence. It seemed that she was not important enough for the therapist to be on time, and his absence would be disruptive to her. She had been reluctant to tell the therapist how she felt during the previous session for fear that he would think that she was being unreasonable and that she did not really need treatment. Nevertheless, she was still angry and had to talk about it.

The incident, to this point, had multiple features that warrant exploration. The immediate problem, however, was a significant rupture to the alliance—a rupture to which the therapist had contributed. This contribution needed to be acknowledged before other issues could be addressed. The therapist said that he was sorry that he was late and that he could understand why the patient was angry about it. This made the patient a little defensive. She commented that she did not think it unreasonable to expect him to be on time, given that *she* was always punctual. The therapist agreed, adding that he did not consider it to be unreasonable at all and that what had happened was unfortunate. This comment led to a short, thoughtful silence, after which the patient noted that people did not usually react this way. She had been afraid that he would be angry with her and think her ungrateful. This then led to a useful discussion of the difficulty she had expressing herself because she was afraid others would retaliate, think her silly, or leave her.

The critical feature in this incident was the therapist's acknowledgment that he had contributed to the problem. Usually these steps are all that is required, especially in the early stages of treatment. Later in treatment, it may be useful to help the patient recognize that he or she is hypersensitive to, or hypervigilant for, therapist error. These issues can only be addressed, however, after mistakes are acknowledged. This models openness and interpersonal honesty that makes it easier for patients to reflect on their behavior rather than defend themselves.

Treatment Alliance and Individual Differences

Although only a few empirical studies have explored the effects of personality on the alliance, some patterns that have been identified may alert therapists to potential problems. Gunderson and colleagues (1989), investigating the relationship between the alliance and premature termination, noted that patients with poor motivation and superficial involvement from the outset often remained difficult to engage. A larger group of patients was motivated initially, but patients reacted negatively when confronted with their denial about the severity of their problems and left therapy in anger (see also Allen et al., 1985).

The ability to form an effective alliance is related to the patient's capacity to relate to others (Hoglend, Sortie, Heyerdahl, Sorbye, & Amlo, 1993; Piper et al., 1991). (This observation does not mean, however, that the healthiest patients form the best alliances [Frank, 1992].) A study of hospitalized borderline patients showed that most patients who were distant and uninvolved terminated treatment prematurely and showed little change (Frank, 1992). A useful finding was that patients who formed a negative–oppositional alliance at the beginning but stayed in treatment had a good outcome. These were the typical borderline patients who were chronically self-harming and dysthymic. They became highly involved in treatment but struggled with their therapists over everything, including treatment goals, the contract, and treatment methods. This finding suggests that negative reactions to treatment do not invariably indicate a poor alliance as long they are expressed directly and dealt with early in treatment. Furthermore, overtly angry patients were easier to engage than those who were purely negativistic. Patients in the latter group were more passively resistant, showed more narcissistic features, and denied having problems or needing treatment. Negative feelings about the therapist were difficult to deal with because they were expressed in a covert manner. These patients did not develop a positive bond with the therapist and progressively showed less adherence to the frame.

Finally, Frank described a group of patients who formed a positive and compliant alliance initially, adhering to the frame, but they did not really collaborate with the therapist regarding the treatment plan. They were compliant mainly out of regard for the therapist. To some extent, they were very dependent and behaved in ways that deceived their therapists into believing that they were doing well when they were not. During treatment they regressed and became increasingly disorganized. All did poorly.

These findings point to the complexity of the alliance and the need for careful monitoring. There are also some counterintuitive aspects to the findings: Therapists should be cautious with patients who are compliant in a passive, supplicating manner. Patients who are actively hostile may do well if the problem is addressed promptly. Therapists also should be wary of patients who are distant and noninvolved. In applying these findings, however, it should be noted that treatment was psychoanalytically orientated, and the level of support offered varied across groups, which could account for some of the differences observed among patient groups.

STRATEGY 2: ESTABLISHING AND MAINTAINING
A CONSISTENT TREATMENT PROCESS

Virtually all advocates of intensive psychodynamic treatment of personality disorder emphasize the importance of a consistent frame (Waldinger, 1987; Waldinger & Gunderson, 1989) because of the difficulties patients have with interpersonal boundaries and maintaining stable relationships. In one study, nearly half of the patients with borderline personality violated the frame after 6 months of treatment (Frank, 1992). Consistency starts by defining the frame of therapy and negotiating the therapeutic contract. Consistency, along with therapeutic stance (see Chapter 4) and the situational context of treatment, forms the frame of treatment that creates therapeutic boundaries and a context for therapeutic interactions. When the patient challenges this framework and the therapist's commitment to it, the therapist's responses provide an opportunity for the patient to observe how to maintain boundaries and set limits, and to learn that people can be consistent and predictable.

The frame in conjunction with a supportive relationship helps to contain unstable affects and impulses and regressive tendencies. It is also important in managing unrealistic demands and expectations, and in making patients aware that therapists are not omnipotent and have limited resources (Zetzel, 1971). An explicit frame also helps to ensure a consistent therapeutic process by reducing the danger of the therapist acting out countertransference problems. Furthermore, the frame protects the treatment process from the inconsistency that occurs when treatment is driven by the patient's psychopathology and the therapist's attempts to accommodate the problems and crises that inevitably emerge during treatment.

Strategies for Establishing and Maintaining the Frame

Treatment Context

The office or institutional setting of treatment is an important part of the frame that is easily overlooked. Many patients are acutely sensitive to the context in which treatment is provided and use this context as a source of information about treatment and the therapist. In many settings, patients also interact with other personnel. These multiple interactions create opportunities for inconsistency to creep into treatment. For this reason, it is important that all staff interact with patients in ways that are congruent with treatment. Consider the following incident:

> The therapist was puzzled that a patient, a woman in her early 30s, was not settling into treatment as expected. The patient had presented with multiple problems, including self-harming acts, impulsive

behaviors, alcohol abuse, and associated social and interpersonal difficulties. In the past she had received various treatments, with minimal benefit. Although she had been in treatment for over 6 months,
there was little progress and the crises continued unabated. Rapport
was tenuous and an alliance had hardly developed. Although sessions
were marked by complaints that the therapist did not understand
and that treatment was unhelpful, the patient attended consistently,
something that had been a problem in previous treatments.

The therapist observed that she was usually early for her appointments but did not realize how early until one day when the session prior to hers was canceled. Leaving his office 30 minutes prior
to her appointment, he was surprised to discover the patient in an
intense conversation with his secretary, a warm and sympathetic
woman. Once in session, the patient again complained that the therapist did not understand and that treatment was not helping. Subsequently the therapist learned that the patient always came early and
confided in the secretary, who provided a sympathetic ear, reassurance, and advice. To his dismay, he also learned that these conversa-
tions occurred several times a week, when the patient telephoned for
advice about various matters.

This example illustrates the importance of context and shows how
routine encounters with other staff can influence treatment. In effect, this
patient was in treatment with the secretary, not the therapist. In any treatment setting, staff need to understand how to deal with patients. In private offices, little is required other than advice on nonconfrontational
ways to manage patients and their demands. In hospitals and mental
health centers where contact with other staff is more extensive, attention
needs to be given to organizing the service in ways that are conducive to
treating personality disorder and to developing procedures for dealing with
common problems. These procedures need not be complex. Often all that
is required are simple guidelines, a little education for nonclinical staff
about the nature of personality disorder and the reasons for the policies,
and opportunities for regular staff communication to ensure that problems
are addressed promptly. Such simple steps minimize the possibility of staff
becoming entangled in patient psychopathology and different team members developing conflicting ideas about management.

Regular opportunities for supervision and consultation also help to ensure consistency. Personality disorder is often difficult and stressful to treat.
Therapist stress contributes to inconsistency; hence it is useful to provide
ongoing support or consultation. The proponents of dialectical behavior
therapy even suggest that all therapists engaged in that type of therapy
only work as part of a team (Robins et al., 2001). This is too stringent a
requirement and impractical in many settings. Nevertheless, therapists require regular opportunities to discuss cases, if they are to remain consistent

and effective as practitioners. Ideally, these discussions should occur with a consultant; if this is not available, peer supervision is a useful alternative.

Maintaining Consistency

Consistency may be defined simply as *adherence to the therapeutic frame*. This adherence requires therapists to act consistently in relation to the frame and to intervene when patient behaviors threaten to disrupt it. Explicit agreement about the goals, tasks, and arrangements of therapy are prerequisites. Maintenance of the frame is a major challenge throughout treatment. Unstable self-states, difficulty with cooperation, and habitual distrust prompt ongoing attempts by patients to alter the frame and challenge the therapist's resolve to maintain stability. At the same time, recurrent crises create the practical problem of how to adhere to a treatment plan, in the face of decompensated and unstable behavior, without disrupting the supportive–empathic relationship on which treatment is based. The usual solution is to recognize in a supportive way the pressures that led to challenges to the frame while at the same time confronting the consequences of such violations.

Limit setting is an important and unavoidable part of treatment. The failure to set limits effectively is a common cause of treatment failure. Any behavior that threatens to disrupt treatment needs to be dealt with promptly. Successful limit setting has three components: (1) identification of the frame violation; (2) explicit recognition of the patient's concerns that lead to the violation; and (3) supportive confrontation of the consequences of the violation, which also explains the purpose of the limit.

A common problem is that therapists do not deal with frame violations as they arise but wait until therapy is actively disrupted before taking action. The failure to act promptly often occurs because therapists do not recognize the value of constructive limit setting in blocking self-destructive patterns, or are afraid of damaging the treatment alliance, especially early in treatment. The patient's personality pattern may also contribute to this hesitation. Therapists are often cautious with emotionally dysregulated and dissocial patients who are prone to angry outbursts; typically therapists either fear that the patient will terminate therapy in anger, or the therapists have difficulty dealing with hostility. With inhibited patients, therapists are prone to make a variety of accommodations in an attempt to build a relationship. In both cases, therapists seem to harbor the hope that frame violations will resolve naturally. This stance is almost always a mistake. Failure to act usually causes an escalation of the problem, until the therapist is eventually forced to act, by which time the severity of the violation, along with countertransference reactions often make it difficult to act firmly but supportively. The antidote is to set limits early—and then enforce them.

A second problem is that many therapists find it difficult to confront frame violations in a supportive manner. Part of the difficulty is a misunderstanding of the nature of confrontation, a term that connotes a challenging and coercive approach. Unfortunately, a coercive style often leads to negative outcomes: it increases resistance and activates oppositional behavior and conflicts with authority (Miller, Benefield, & Tonigan, 1993). Nevertheless, confrontation in the sense of *drawing the patient's attention to something that was not recognized* is an important part of therapy. Confrontation in this sense, however, is not a therapeutic style but rather a technique for achieving a particular therapeutic objective. Unfortunately, therapists often only set limits when they feel strongly about the patient's behavior. In such instances, confrontation is the product of countertransference rather than a technique to increase patients' awareness of the consequences of their behavior (Miller & Rollnick, 1991). Confrontations that are loaded with countertransference anger are difficult for the patient to assimilate and tend to lead to deterioration in the alliance (Gabbard et al., 1988).

Successful limit setting usually depends on the therapist's ability to recognize and control countertransference reactions. These reactions are particularly important to monitor in relation to patients with personality disorder, because these reactions tend to be intense. Hence most authorities emphasize the importance of the therapist being able to withstand the patient's verbal attacks without reacting in a retaliatory or withdrawn manner (Gunderson, 1984; Waldinger, 1987). It is not only negative reactions, however, that are important in managing patients with personality disorder; positive countertransference reactions, such as overly protective responses and excessive sympathy (as opposed to empathy), also tend to be intense and may be equally disruptive. Because countertransference is a normal part of treatment, it needs to be managed like any aspect of therapy. This management is best accomplished by monitoring the countertransference and using it as an additional source of information about the patient.

STRATEGY 3: VALIDATION

The importance of validating interventions is recognized by most treatments of personality disorder, ranging from self psychology (Kohut, 1975) to cognitive-behavior therapy (Linehan, 1993). This congruence is not surprising, given the prominent role of invalidating experiences in many etiological theories. Such experiences lead to hypersensitivity to invalidation and the tendency for patients to "test" the therapist to ensure that he or she is not likely to behave as others have done (Weiss, 1993).

For Linehan (1993) the essence of validation is that "the therapist communicates to the patient that her responses make sense and are understandable within her current life context or situation" (p. 223). Kohut, however, seems to refer to something more fundamental: the experience of being understood and affirmed. According to Lang (1987), the goal is "to perceive the ways in which the subjective experience of the patient has a valid psychic reality for him or her" (p. 145). Similarly, Buie and Adler (1982) maintain that patients' capacity to know, value, and love themselves can only develop through experience of being understood, valued, and loved by others. In therapy, the therapist seeks to offer a continual corrective emotional experience by reacting with appropriate expressions of esteem to patients' accounts of their experiences.

Although the therapist's assurance that the patient's experience and behavior is explicable in terms of his or her current situation is important, validation, as used here, more closely resembles Kohut's conception than that of Linehan. Validation is *an active strategy that recognizes and affirms the legitimacy of the patient's experience*. Emphasis is placed on the therapist's nonevaluative acceptance and understanding of the patient's reality. In this sense, validation overlaps with empathy and genuineness—two qualities that Rogers (1951, 1957) considered inherent to a therapeutic relationship. The purpose is to encourage patients to accept the authenticity of their own experience. Providing this encouragement does not mean that the therapist inevitably agrees with the patient's perspective. As Linehan (1993) noted, the therapist should not validate perspectives that are invalid.

Validating interventions are inherently supportive and reduce the need for patients to spend time justifying their feelings and the degree of their distress. In addition to this management function, validating interventions also help to change core pathology. Kohut, and those who adopt the deficit model, emphasized the critical role of therapist empathy in remedying the consequences of empathic failure and defective mirroring. Linehan (1993) also assigns a key role to validating interventions in correcting the effects of invalidating experiences and changing self-invalidating ways of thinking. The combination of therapist empathy and modification of self-invalidating thinking seems to offer an effective way to change core self pathology. Strengthening self-validation also enables patients to trust their intuitive understanding of themselves and others and helps them acknowledge and accept inherent strengths that they may not have recognized. Both processes contribute to self-efficacy and competency. At the same time, the experience of a validating relationship contributes to the establishment of new expectations about relationships that help to correct distorted perceptions.

Strategies to Promote Validation

Recognizing and Accepting Behavior and Experience

Validation is as much an attitude conveyed by tone of voice, listening carefully, and responding with empathy and respect, as it is a set of interventions. Such behavior indicates that the therapist takes seriously what the person says and models acceptance of his or her experiences without questioning or second-guessing them. The expressive component of verbal responses also contributes to validation. Comments that match the patient's tone and rate of speech can contribute to feeling understood, provided that they are not delivered in a stereotyped manner. Empathy alone, however, is not sufficient to promote validation: it is merely a precondition for other interventions that communicate acceptance and understanding.

Validation requires *adequate time to express affects and describe experiences.* Therapists are often tempted to close off expression of painful experiences too quickly, especially early in treatment, by moving to more factual issues or more positive matters, partly out of concern for the patient and partly because they are too distressing to hear. A thoughtful balance needs to be struck between appropriate ventilation and the danger of emotions escalating out of control. This balance is especially important when managing patients with traumatic histories. The task is to support the expression of feelings without promoting unnecessary exploration and additional revelations when these are likely to be counterproductive. It helps if the therapist recalls that the ultimate goal is to help the patient to regulate emotional expression, not simply to ventilate.

Most patients need more than the opportunity to talk about their distress; they also need someone *to recognize the painful and traumatic events that have happened to them.* For example, one patient who had been abused throughout her childhood spent much of one session telling the therapist, with increasing fervor and dyscontrol, about her distress and the basic unfairness of life. She was able to regain control and begin processing the material when her therapist simply commented that, "no one would disagree that what happened to you was absolutely awful."

Faced with a situation in which the patient's beliefs or experiences seem to be invalid, it is often helpful *to accept and acknowledge a belief or feeling but to question its origins and implications.* This two-pronged response requires a distinction between (1) the experience itself, and (2) the *reasons* given for, and (3) the *conclusions* drawn from it. The therapist can validate the experience without validating the causes and consequences of the experience that are considered invalid. This delicate process is illustrated in the following vignette.

A patient with severe personality problems and had been incapacitated for many years held the strong conviction that "I am mentally ill." The patient believed that she had a serious and untreatable psychosis. The belief formed the core of her identity, even though she did not present with any psychotic symptoms. Nevertheless, she offered this belief as an explanation for her inability to manage her life and establish enduring relationships. Previous clinicians had challenged this belief during diagnostic interviews and therapy. Whenever confronted in this way, the patient behaved in a progressively more disturbed way, as if to demonstrate that she was indeed psychotic, and the therapeutic relationship deteriorated. Her life became a quest to find a therapist who agreed with her. Greater progress was made when a therapist accepted that she was convinced that she was psychotic and explored the impact of this belief on her life, especially the way it caused her to adopt a resigned and passive approach to her problems. This acceptance freed her enough to explore the issues, whereas questioning the belief had led to a vigorous defense of her position and ultimately to noncompliance with treatment.

The management of such invalid beliefs begins by accepting the patient's experience of them before exploring the meaning of such beliefs and the way that they influence his or her life.

Facilitating the Search for Meaning

Linehan (1993) suggested that validation is intended to make problematic experiences, responses, and situations understandable. She described three steps leading to validation: (1) listening and observing actively and attentively; (2) accurately reflecting back to the patient his or her feelings, thoughts, and behaviors; and (3) direct validation. The first two steps are part of most forms of therapy. Linehan considers the third step, direct validation, to be specific to her approach. Here the therapist communicates the idea that the patients' responses make sense within the context in which they occur. Linehan recommends that therapists search for the adaptive and coping significance of behavior and communicate this understanding to their patients.

These interventions may be considered part of the more general *search for meaning* that Yalom (1975) considered an important therapeutic factor. This search is especially relevant to treating patients with personality disorder, most of whom find many aspects of their lives and experience inexplicable. For some this bewilderment is a source of considerable distress and a further reason for self-criticism. As one patient noted, "The problem is I don't understand why I am such a mess. I don't seem to be able to do anything right, nothing works out, all my relationships are a mess, and yet there is no reason for it. It is not as if I was abused as a child. My parents really looked after me. I don't know why it is; there must be something really basically wrong with me. I must be flawed in some way." Such instances indicate the value of *providing explanations for psychopathology* that communicate the idea that patients' behavior is explicable in terms of their history and basic physiological and psychological mechanisms. This process begins by incorporating a psychoeducational element to discussions about the treatment contract and continues by weaving brief explanations of psychopathology into the therapeutic dialogue. For example, patients who blame themselves because they dissociate or their thinking becomes confused when distressed are helped by an explanation of the effects of intense affects on cognition. Patients with the emotional dysregulation pattern who are puzzled by their emotional lability and their inability to control their feelings may find it useful to understand the biological and cognitive factors involved in regulating emotions. Many abused patients invalidate themselves by blaming themselves for their current problems and their inability to get their lives in order. Discussion of traumatic events and the way trauma has a lasting influence on behavior helps to validate current feelings and reactions. The purpose of such interventions is to help patients make sense of their problems and symptoms without undermining personal responsibility for change.

The specific component of the search for meaning that Linehan emphasizes is *helping the patient recognize that problem behaviors may be adaptive.* That is, these behaviors may represent the only way to cope with the problem, given the patient's life experiences and situation. Although not all behavior is explicable in this way, it is a useful form of validation for behaviors that can be understood as adaptive. For example, patients who self-mutilate when dysphoric feel validated by the explanation that these acts were the only ways available to the patient at the time to terminate intolerable feelings. It is important, however, to ensure that these explanations do not reinforce the behaviors or prevent the patient from finding alternative ways to handle distress.

Counteracting Self-Invalidation

The tendency to question or second-guess one's experiences is almost ubiquitous in patients with personality disorder. Repetitive invalidation during development establishes a way of thinking that makes it difficult to establish treatment goals and explore problems. Most patients are unaware of the extent to which they question their experiences or how this way of thinking undermines self-esteem and their sense of who they are. Simple comments such as "You seem to confuse yourself" help them to understand how they continually doubt their experience. It takes time, however, for them to recognize the extent and subtlety of the process. The strategy for dealing with enduring behavioral patterns, described in Chapter 4 (identify the broad theme and then focus on specific examples), is a useful way to manage the problem. The incorporation of a psychoeducational component into this process is illustrated by the following vignette.

The patient, a woman in her late 20s, had severe self pathology. She continually questioned and second-guessed her ideas and feelings.

She questioned most statements she made about herself, as to whether or not she really did feel this way, and whether or not her thoughts were real or genuine. The pattern had been acquired from her parents, who regularly told her what she should think and feel, questioned any attempts at self-assertion and self-expression, and criticized her abilities. At the beginning of one session, she proclaimed loudly that she was furious. The therapist asked for details. After a moment's pause, she qualified this by saying that she was angry. Only moments later she said that she thought she was irritated. Each time the therapist tried to explore these feelings, the patient responded by questioning whether she really felt that way. Within a matter of moments, she changed from describing herself as furious to saying that she felt a little annoyed, and she questioned even this. Eventually, she concluded that she was confused.

There are several aspects to this behavior that are important, including the patient's fear of her own anger and of discussing it with the therapist. Although these were themes in other sessions, the therapist used this occasion to comment that she seemed to invalidate her own experience. Although she initially felt furious, she questioned her experience until she ended up feeling confused about what she really felt. He added that she seemed to question and debate everything she felt. Few items were accepted, everything was questioned, and she second-guessed most feelings and thoughts. He added that it was not surprising that she felt confused or that she was unsure of who she was. How could she know herself and know what she wanted if everything was questioned, and not even simple experiences were accepted?

The patient began the next session by saying that she had spent most of the time since the previous session discussing the therapist's comments with a friend via e-mail. Both were interested in constructionist philosophy, and as a result of their deliberations they concluded that she was a "construction of confusion."

This example shows the value of providing explanations of psychopathology that deepen understanding and clarify experiences that were previously inexplicable.

Acknowledging Areas of Competence

A useful form of validation is to recognize and support strengths and areas of competence. It is helpful, for example, to recognize the achievement of a patient who manages to attend therapy regularly, despite a chaotic life circumstance, or the success of a patient who holds down a part-time job despite severe personality problems. This approach seems to be most effective if areas of successful coping are not examined in detail but simply acknowledged as achievements that can be built upon. Acknowledging competence needs to be approached carefully. Patients easily interpret such interventions as an indication that the therapist is insensitive to their pain or is minimizing their distress. Nevertheless, this kind of acknowledgment is beneficial for patients with disorganized lives who feel badly about themselves and their inability to cope. Furthermore, noting assets and achievements often helps them to talk more freely about problems.

Reducing Self-Derogation

Self-blame and self-criticism are common modes of thinking that contribute to dysphoria and self-harm in this population. Given the pervasiveness of these patterns, it is useful for therapists to develop a repertoire of interventions to validate actions that usually evoke a self-critical response. For example:

> "Of course you behaved in that way—what choice did you have? It was the only way you could survive as a child."
> "It is not surprising that you avoid showing your feelings, because you were criticized if you did."
> "It is not surprising that you get angry and full of rage in these situations. They remind you of what happened in the past."
> "It is not surprising that you find these things hard to talk about—no one helped you to talk about your feelings in the past."

Such interventions (1) help the patient to see that the behavior was adaptive in the circumstances in which it developed, and (2) simultaneously hold open the possibility of change.

On other occasions, patients need to recognize that they blame themselves rather than try to understand themselves. Contrasting these responses with those of the therapist, who seeks to understand rather than to blame or criticize, often gives patients sufficient distance to recognize how they maintain a continuous commentary of self-criticism. One patient was helped to recognize the automatic nature of self-critical thoughts when the therapist punctuated one barrage, which seemed unstoppable, with the comment that "There are two people in this room, but only one is on your side—and it's not you." The patient recalled this event long afterward as a point of change that not only helped her to recognize her self-blaming style but also to experience the therapist as supportive and understanding.

Avoiding Invalidating Interventions

An important part of validation is to avoid actions that may be experienced as invalidating, such as minimizing problems by prematurely focusing on the positive; providing inappropriate reassurance that trivializes patients' concerns; interpreting disagreement or refusal to accept an interpretation as resistance; communicating unreasonable expectations of change in self-harming behaviors; and not acknowledging mistakes or lapses of concentration.

In addition to these errors, several other invalidating interventions warrant comment. One is the tendency to *interpret normal experiences and all problems as pathological*. Because clinicians inevitably focus on pathology, it is easy to overlook the fact that frustration, ambivalence, rationalization, and so on, are normal reactions that are not necessarily maladaptive or indicative of personality problems. Interpreting normal reactions as indications of pathology confuses patients who have difficulty distinguishing between what is normal and healthy and what is pathological. A related problem is *to interpret all problems as arising from personality psychopathology or from a single cause*, such as sexual abuse, trauma, or substance abuse. Therapists with strong ideological views or one-dimensional ideas about the origins of personality disorder sometimes fall into this trap. This rigid frame can create the impression that the therapist is not listening and lead to other issues being neglected. Although some patients like the clarity of a one-dimensional perspective, others feel invalidated, especially when they believe that the therapist has preconceived ideas that prevent him or her from treating the patient as an individual. For example, a patient in therapy for self-mutilation also attended an addiction group. He complained bitterly that the group did not take his problems seriously because everything was attributed to alcoholism, and other important issues were ignored. It helps to keep in mind that patients with personality disorder have problems unrelated to their personality pathology. Even when practical problems are due to personality problems, their *practical significance* needs to be recognized.

Managing Validation Ruptures

Invalidating events in treatment are almost inevitable. Patients are hypersensitive to invalidation, so that it is easy for therapists to invalidate inadvertently. As with the therapeutic alliance, it is the patient's view of these events that matters, and therapists always need to be mindful that the communications sent are not necessarily the communications received. If the patient feels invalidated, this response has to be accepted as the starting point for exploration and repair. Modest failures of validation are nodal points that afford the opportunity for useful work, provided that they are handled in ways that do not lead to further invalidation. Such events should be managed similarly to alliance ruptures. The first step is for the therapist to acknowledge the event and his or her contribution. This step in itself is validating and helps to repair the rupture. The therapist's response differs from the patient's expectations and hence offers a new relationship experience that can be used to challenge maladaptive schemata. Indications of the failure of validation vary. With the more emotionally dysregulated or dissocial person, the usual responses are anger, direct criticism, or angry withdrawal. The inhibited individual, in contrast, is more likely to internalize the response so that it is less discernible. The second step is to explore reactions to invalidation, including ideas about its causes and the therapist's perception of the patient. The final step is to validate the patient's responses.

STRATEGY 4: BUILDING AND MAINTAINING MOTIVATION

Motivation to change is essential for patients to seek help and remain in treatment. Unfortunately, motivation fluctuates under the influence of multiple internal and external factors, including core pathology. Motivation, in this sense, is not a prerequisite for change, nor is it a fixed feature that therapists cannot influence (Miller & Rollnick, 1991). Some shorter-term psychodynamic therapies have encouraged a different view by making motivation a criterion for treatment (Malan, 1979; Mann, 1973; Sifneos, 1979). This requirement is understandable with brief therapy, because considerable determination is required to persist with a process that is often painful, and strongly motivated patients have a better outcome (McConnaughty, DiClemente, Prochaska, & Velicer, 1989; Prochaska & DiClemente, 1986). When treating patients with personality disorder, however, the situation is different. The disorder itself limits motivation. Low self-directedness, passivity, demoralization, and difficulty trusting the intentions of others, even those to whom patients turn to for help, reduce motivation. For these reasons, successful outcome depends on the therapist's skills in building motivation. An effective alliance is a prerequisite for sustaining a commitment to change, but additional interventions are often required.

A useful clinical discussion of motivation is found in the volume *Motivational Interviewing*, by Miller and Rollnick (1991). Although written specifically about the treatment of addictive behavior, their ideas have wider currency. Miller and Rollnick characterize motivation as "the probability that a person will enter into, continue, and adhere to a specific change strategy" (p. 19). This probability is not constant—that is, motivation is not a trait—rather, motivation consists of "a state of readiness or eagerness to change, which may fluctuate from one time or situation to another" (p. 14). Although sufficient motivation is required to attend therapy in the first place, subsequent levels of motivation are influenced by therapist behavior, and effective therapists are successful in increasing patient motivation (Meichenbaum & Turk, 1987). Nevertheless, therapists often seem to regard motivation as the patient's responsibility. Statements such as "this patient is not motivated" or "this patient does not want to work on problems" are understandable expressions of frustration in the face of difficult problems, but they overlook the fact that therapists are not powerless in such circumstances. Acknowledging the therapist's role in building motivation does not mean accepting total responsibility for the patient's motivation for change. Assumption of responsibility by the therapist without the expectation that the patient has a complementary responsibility colludes with the patient's psychopathology by reinforcing passivity and promoting unhelpful forms of dependency. It may also cause patients to feel that their autonomy is threatened and evoke reactive and oppositional responses.

Strategies for Building Motivation

Effective alliance building and validation enhance motivation and should be used whenever motivational problems arise. Supporting patients when they feel stuck, recognizing and thereby validating their fears of change, and encouraging a discussion of options are more likely to be effective than confronting "resistance." In addition to these strategies, Miller and Rollnick (1991; Miller, 1985) describe eight interventions for building motivation: giving advice, removing barriers to change, providing choice, decreasing desirability of not changing, providing empathic responses, providing feedback, clarifying goals, and active helping. Although some of these interventions are more relevant to patients with addictions as the primary focus, all are potentially useful.

Using Discontent

Motivation to change is stimulated by discontent with one's behavior or situation. As Baumeister (1991, 1994) noted, discontent is a powerful motivator. As long as personality disordered individuals see their self-harmful behaviors as unavoidable ways of dealing with distress; as long as they believe that their dysfunctional relationships are fun or exciting; and as long as they perceive their maladaptive lifestyles to be normal ways of living, there is little incentive to change.

Discontent is often triggered by a critical incident that leads to a sudden shift in the way individuals see themselves and their lives. Baumeister (1991) refers to this phenomenon as the "crystallization of discontent." The pain associated with this realization seems to mobilize the intention to change. Studies of successful and unsuccessful changes in lifestyles, relationships, and personality among students indicated that those who made major changes reported much stronger negative affects and suffering than those who did not change or changed less (Heatherton & Nichols, 1994b). In treatment, it is sometimes possible to use relatively minor incidents to build motivation by focusing on the discrepancy between the way the person is feeling and living and the way that he or she would like to feel and live. Sufficient discontent is needed to mobilize the commitment to change without increasing demoralization and ruminative guilt. Hope in the form of positive expectations about the usefulness of treatment and the therapist is useful in helping to prevent discontent from spiraling into despair.

The crystallization of discontent usually leads to the commitment to take steps to change. Rarely it may lead to what Miller and C'de Baca (2001) refer to as quantum change. This kind of change was illustrated in Chapter 4 by the vignette of the patient who suddenly decided that she had to change after she had swept everything off the therapist's desk and rushed from the office.

Creating Options

For many patients, motivation is limited by their inability to identify alternative courses of action, and by beliefs that change is not possible, that they are not in control of their lives, and that their options are circumscribed by situational and personal factors. Change is a daunting prospect when alternatives are not apparent. It is important, therefore, to spend time helping patients learn how to be open to other experiences and possibilities, to recognize alternative paths, and to see that choice is possible. Achieving this shift in perspective often involves detailed discussion of problem situations and the way that they and others deal with such situations. Many patients recognize that others react differently from themselves to the same situation, yet they do not feel that the options available to others are open to themselves.

A common reason for an inability to recognize options is that patients often confront themselves with all their problems at once or with problems that are so broad as to be overwhelming. As discussed in Chapter 4, it is often necessary to break down problems into specific components that can be tackled sequentially. At this more specific level, options are more easily identified. This method is similar to the means–end analysis employed in problem solving, in which a problem is divided into concrete components in order to facilitate its solution (Newell & Simon, 1972). Time spent on teaching problem analysis is worthwhile, because this skill will help ensure that changes are retained when treatment ends. Focusing on small steps also increases the probability of success. Motivation is gradually built through a series of modest successes.

Identifying Incentives for Not Changing

Patients rarely examine the costs and benefits of their actions, even when they are obviously harmful or life-threatening. Acts such as self-mutilation and parasuicidal gestures may even be viewed as unavoidable and the costs involved dismissed as inconsequential. As captured by the idea of secondary gain, many maladaptive behaviors benefit the patient in ways that are not always apparent. Thus, as Miller and Rollnick (1991) noted, an important motivational task for therapists is to identify incentives for *not* changing. These incentives may include the experience of relief from emotional distress, as provided by many self-harming behaviors, or gratification of a wide range of interpersonal needs, such as those for receiving care and attention. What matters is the person's *perception* of the costs involved, not the costs in an objective sense. For example, a patient with inhibited traits, a solitary lifestyle, and a long history of self-injury had been in treatment with a community mental health team for more than a decade. The therapist whom he saw weekly was one of the few people in his life. The patient noted that he was afraid to get better because the therapist would stop seeing him and he would have no one with whom to talk. This benefit led him to improve only to a certain level, at which point he would fear the imminent termination and his condition would quickly deteriorate. Cases like this are common in services that offer long-term treatment, and they illustrate the need to identify personal and situational factors that maintain maladaptive patterns and to help patients solve the real-life problems created by change.

Managing Ambivalence

A common obstacle to treatment is the patient's ambivalence about change. Patients recognize that change is desirable and even necessary, but at the same time it often evokes fear and even resentment of the struggle to deal with problems the patient believes are caused by others. Miller and Rollnick (1991) suggested that conflicts between wanting to change and fear of change may be managed by using Lewin's (1935) classic analysis of conflict. Lewin suggested that conflicts fall into three types. *Approach–approach conflict* occurs when the individual is faced with two desirable goals but only one can be achieved (e.g., having two pleasant options for how to spend the weekend). Such conflicts are usually easily resolved. *Avoidance–avoidance conflicts* present a slightly greater problem, in that the individual is faced with two negative goals and is forced to choose between them. *Approach–avoidance conflict* occurs when the goal facing the individual has both positive and negative features. These conflicts are the most difficult to resolve and classically lead to ambivalence.

For many patients with personality disorder, the possibility of change evokes an approach–avoidance sense of conflict. Change is desirable because it reduces distress and opens up new opportunities—but it also has negative aspects: it means adopting unfamiliar behaviors with unknown consequences. As the costs and benefits of changing versus staying the

same are evaluated, patients frequently experience ambivalence about treatment, because of their frustration at feeling stuck and their fear of uncertainty. The danger is that this dilemma will lead to a recurrence of the
maladaptive patterns. Therapists can intervene to change the relative
strengths of the positive and negative aspects of change by increasing the
discrepancy between current experience and the way one would like to experience the self and the world (Miller & Rollnick, 1991). Encouraging individuals to consider the benefits of change and stimulating their desire to
relinquish old patterns can increase the value of the positive side of this
conflict. At the same time, exploring the fear of change and addressing the
concerns raised can reduce the negative aspects of the conflict.

Encouraging Persistence

Maintaining the patient's commitment to change often requires therapists
to encourage patience and persistence. These qualities are needed not because patients give up too easily but because they often believe that progress should be rapid, once a problem is recognized, and berate themselves
for not progressing quickly enough. At this point, it is often useful to introduce information about the way developmental experiences resulted in
habitual ways of thinking and acting that were reinforced repeatedly over
the years. It is also useful to extend the psychoeducational component by
explaining a little about the stability of personality and how the different
components influence each other. For example, a highly submissive person
who recognizes the need for change but finds it difficult to implement may
be less critical and more open to the idea that change takes time if she realizes how this pattern influences the way she thinks and how other people
in her life act in ways that maintain the behavior.

Dealing with Obstacles to Motivation

Obstacles to change can be internal or external to the individual. Many
features of personality disorder, including passivity, feelings of demoralization, expectations that someone or something will provide the solution,
and fantasies of rescue, hinder motivation. Such obstacles can be approached using a stages of change model, in which interventions designed
to change features such as passivity and demoralization are nested within a
broader set of interventions designed to effect change in targeted problems
such as self-harm or maladaptive interpersonal patterns.

External obstacles to motivation arise from person–situation interactions that maintain maladaptive patterns. The tendency to seek out situations and relationships that are compatible with one's personality often
produces formidable obstacles to change. For example, often the patient's
significant others have become familiar with the patient behaving in a par-

ticular way and react adversely to his or her attempts to behave differently. In these cases, significant others may fear change as much as the patient. Their fears may lead them to undermine the patient's initial attempts to behave differently, and the patient may adopt these fears as his or her own. Under these circumstances, patients need help identifying ways to cope with this additional problem; this help may involve conjoint sessions.

COMMENT

The general therapeutic strategies operationalize the nonspecific component of therapy as it applies to the treatment of patients with personality disorder. Applied effectively, these strategies (1) ensure the support required by patients to undergo treatment for severe personality pathology, and (2) create an interactional context for specific interventions. Together the general strategies are likely to account for a substantial proportion of outcome change, and many treatments fail because these strategies are not implemented consistently.

As Linehan (1993) and Clarkin and colleagues (1999) noted, interventions to ensure the safety of the patient and others take priority over all other interventions. Beyond this requirement, *the general strategies have priority over specific strategies.* Therapists faced with a dilemma about which intervention to use in a given situation may find this distinction useful. If the conditions addressed by the general strategies are met—that is, the alliance is satisfactory, the frame is being maintained, adequate validation has been achieved, and the patient is motivated—specific interventions may be used. If not, interventions based on the appropriate general strategy take precedence.

At this point, it is worth reiterating the comment made earlier that an approach using multiple interventions to treat multiple problems runs the risk of becoming unfocused and disorganized, especially when the psychopathology being treated tends to influence, and even control, the conduct of treatment. The general strategies and the above guideline are one of several ideas suggested to resolve this problem (the others are the phases of treatment and the stages of change). Like most clinical maxims, this is not an absolute rule but a guideline that is often useful, especially when problems are encountered and the treatment appears stuck. The following vignette illustrates a situation in which this guideline proved valuable.

> The patient, a woman in her late 20s, had an extensive psychiatric history dating to her early teens. She presented for treatment of problems involving self-destructive behavior, affective lability, and major difficulties with interpersonal relationships, especially difficulty trusting people that resulted by her being socially isolated.

Personality assessment revealed a combination of traits from the inhibited and emotionally dysregulated patterns. At the time of the present event, the patient had been in individual therapy for about 6 months, during which time only modest progress had been made in establishing an effective working relationship. For several months, the patient began each session by telling the therapist that she had nothing to say, that she really did not want to be there, and that she did not know what to say. This pattern proved difficult to change. On this occasion, the patient began the interview immediately by saying that she had been looking forward to the session. While traveling to the hospital, she had felt pleased about the appointment because something important had occurred, about which she wanted to talk. She thought that it would be useful to talk it over with the therapist, whom she thought would understand and have something helpful to say. She then added that, as soon as she entered the room, she realized that the therapist would not understand and would not be helpful. As a result, there was nothing to discuss.

When the therapist attempted to explore these issues, the patient responded, as she had on previous occasions, by saying that she had nothing to add, that nothing seemed worth talking about, and that she could not think of anything to say. The therapist was struck by the two separate images that the patient had formed of him. This seemed like a good opportunity to explore these fragmented person representations with a view to beginning to integrate them. This approach went nowhere. The patient steadfastly maintained that there was nothing to discuss. Eventually, the therapist realized that this approach was not productive and focused on the treatment alliance.

This focus led the therapist to comment that it must be extremely distressing to look forward to seeing him because she thought that he might be understanding and helpful, only to find out that that was not the case. This comment produced a strong reaction. The patient angrily told the therapist that he had no idea of just how terrible it was to come each week, only to find that there was little understanding or help available. A detailed discussion of the patient's disappointment in the therapist and the difficulty she had in trusting anyone followed.

As this discussion proceeded, rapport gradually increased. Eventually, the patient revealed the problem that had concerned her. During the previous week she had learned that her mother, with whom she had had a very poor relationship, was terminally ill and was not expected to live for more than a few months. The information had been devastating. She suddenly realized that it was now too late to resolve problems with her mother and that she would never know what it was like to have a good mother.

This example illustrates the value of the intervention hierarchy. The therapist, struck by the fragmented images that the patient held of him, ignored problems with the alliance and the fact that specific interventions are most effective when the conditions created by the general strategies are met. It was only when the therapist focused on the alliance and the patient began talking about her disappointment that progress occurred.

Although the nonspecific component of treatment is emphasized here, two potential problems should be noted: the failure to progress in therapy, and the development of maladaptive dependency. Both arise when therapists forget that treatment is based on a therapeutic alliance that combines an emphasis on the treatment relationship with the more technical aspects concerned with bringing about change (Borden, 1994; Horvath & Greenberg, 1994). Reliance on generic mechanisms runs the risk of (1) creating a bland form of therapy that makes the patient feel better without effecting change, and (2) establishing a treatment relationship that colludes with, rather than changes, psychopathology. To avoid this eventuality, therapists need to monitor the impact of general interventions and the extent to which they lead to change. Failure to progress, especially in the context of a good rapport, is occasion to review the way general strategies are being applied. It is the balance between the relational and the instrumental in the use of general strategies that prevents the therapeutic process from colluding with patient pathology.

A second potential problem is the development of maladaptive dependency. Dependency in therapeutic relationships is often unavoidable. It is also frequently misunderstood. Dependency is not necessarily negative. For patients with chronic difficulties, dependence on a mental health professional or service is not harmful if it leads to improved quality of life, avoidance of more pathological actions, and prevention of deterioration. Just as one would not consider dependence on a hemodialysis machine to be something to be avoided in patients with chronic renal failure, one should not consider reliance on mental health agencies to be negative for those who are chronically dysfunctional. The real problem with dependency occurs when it perpetuates dysfunctional behavior in patients with the potential for change, or decreases rather than increases coping abilities and efforts.

Deterioration rather than improvement with treatment seems to be common when working with personality disordered patients. Unfortunately, this problem has not received extensive empirical analysis. Clinical impression, however, suggests that it occurs primarily in patients with a history of deprivation, privation, and emotional neglect, and that therapist style is an important factor. Problems occur when the emphasis on general strategies leads to excessive gratification and sympathy, and patients are treated as if they do not have the resources to cope. This style is especially problematic when the therapist also identifies with the patient's trauma. This same problem also seems to occur with intrusive confrontational therapy.

An underlying theme of this chapter is that experiential factors are often more important in creating an effective treatment process than the actual contents of interventions, especially early in treatment (Chessick, 1982), and that a secure working environment is created through a heavy focus on the alliance. In attachment terms, an effective alliance forms a secure base from which problems can be explored. The assumption is that therapeutic progress is attributable to experience of a more adaptive relationship that offers the support and containment that patients have difficulty providing for themselves. The therapeutic stance, the emphasis on a therapeutic process based on collaborative description, and the general therapeutic strategies are designed to offer what Svatberg (cited by McCullough & Vaillant, 1997) has called a "continuous, graded, corrective emotional experience" (p. 17).

CHAPTER 8

Safety and Containment

Treating Symptoms and Crises

The psychopathology of personality disorder is too complex and intertwined to treat in a prescribed sequence. Typically, multiple problems are addressed at each stage of treatment. Nevertheless, the three levels of stability in personality characteristics noted in Chapter 3—crisis behavior and symptoms, trait expressions and non-core aspects of self and interpersonal pathology, and core self and interpersonal problems—form an approximate sequence for tackling problems. They also form a convenient framework for considering how to combine specific interventions with the general strategies discussed previously.

It is convenient to consider crises and symptoms first. Treatment is generally initiated by a symptomatic or crisis state, and containment of affects and impulses is usually an immediate goal. Subsequently, episodes of acute behavioral disorganization often punctuate treatment, at least in the early stages, so that strategies for managing these states are required throughout treatment. Moreover, until a measure of stability is attained, it is difficult to focus effectively on other issues. A final reason for an early focus on symptoms is that improvement is often readily achieved because these features are among the more changeable aspects of personality pathology. Success helps to build the treatment relationship that forms the basis for further work.

Discussion of crises and symptoms is organized around three themes: crises and episodes of acute behavioral disorganization, parasuicidal behavior and associated affective distress, and trauma and dissociation. This chapter deals with the management of crises that either initiate treatment or occur during treatment. It also introduces some general principles that will be used to treat other symptoms. The other topics are covered in subsequent chapters.

CLINICAL FEATURES OF CRISES AND EPISODES OF ACUTE BEHAVIORAL DISORGANIZATION

The clinical features of crisis states (see Table 8.1) vary with severity and personality pattern. The characteristic presentations associated with the emotional dysregulation pattern are considered in detail because these are common.

The core feature is *escalating dysphoria* that typically involves panic-like anxiety, anger, sadness, despondency, despair, and emptiness; this mix-

---

TABLE 8.1. Clinical Features of Crisis States and Episodes of Acute Behavioral Disorganization

Affective dysregulation: intense reactive affects; mixed emotional states that are difficult to label

- Anxiety and panic: generalized anxiety, often associated with panic-like anxiety and usually associated with ruminative thoughts
- Affective lability: rapid mood changes triggered by minimal stimulation
- Generalized dysphoria: escalating state of general dysphoric affects
- Anger and rage: intense irritability
- Low mood: depression and despondency

Behavioral disorganization and dyscontrol: impulsive actions; poor behavioral control

- Suicidal and parasuicidal behavior: deliberate self-harming acts
- Impulsivity: poor behavioral control leading to a variety of impulsive behaviors, with little attention to consequences
- Regression: reduced coping often associated with regressed behavior
- Dissociation: absorption, derealization, depersonalization, amnesic episodes, and unresponsiveness

Cognitive disorganization and dysregulation: confused and disorganized thinking

- Impaired information processing: reduction in coping capacity; logical thinking and rational problem solving reduced
- Transient psychotic features: experiences of illusions and related perceptual phenomena; pseudohallucinations; mild delusions and overvalued ideas

---

ture makes it difficult for patients to label their experiences. This often adds to confusion and inner turmoil leading to the conviction that something fundamental is wrong and prompts desperation that something be done immediately to end the distress. As feelings become intolerable, attempts at amelioration often culminate in an impulsive action such as deliberate self-harm. Although anxiety, depression, and despondency usually predominate, they are rapidly converted into angry, reactive affects if individuals feel too vulnerable. *Behavioral disorganization and dyscontrol*, leading to an increase in impulsive, suicidal, and parasuicidal acts, are characteristic of most crises. In some cases, regression also occurs in which coping sometimes decreases to the point where the individual is unable to manage the tasks of everyday living. *Cognitive disorganization and dysregulation*, involving an array of perceptual and cognitive symptoms, are also prominent features of crises. Thinking becomes disorganized and normal information processing is impaired, so that verbal interventions often have limited effect. As cognitive processes become more fluid, transient psychotic features may emerge. Dissociative behavior is also common and runs the spectrum from mild depersonalization and derealization to episodes of unresponsiveness.

The affective, cognitive, and behavioral components of crises interact to form a positive feedback state in which intense emotions reduce cognitive control, in turn leading to an escalation of affect. When this happens, the main concern is to reduce the dysphoria. At the same time, decreased control increases impulsivity. The resulting parasuicidal and impulsive acts are reinforced because they reduce distress.

Crisis presentations are influenced by personality style. The more florid presentations occur in patients with the emotional dysregulation pattern. Traits such as anxiousness and affective lability reduce the threshold for maladaptive responses to stress and increase reactions to triggering events. The more muted expression of feelings in inhibited or schizoid–avoidant patients leads to a less intense presentation, in which despondency and despair, rather than reactive affects, predominate. Distress is often increased by the exquisite sensitivity and social apprehensiveness experienced by many inhibited individuals. When the anxiousness and affective lability of emotional dysregulation are also present, inhibited patients show some of the classical features of the "borderline crisis," although self-harming acts are usually less dramatic and more secretive. When despondency predominates, the risk of suicide is often greater. The more subdued expression of distress, the tendency to minimize affective expression, and a reluctance to discuss experiences may lead therapists to underestimate the extent to which these patients are at risk. The more dissocial individual tends to react similarly to the emotionally dysregulated patient. Feelings are rapidly externalized and expressed as anger that is likely to be directed at others.

GENERAL PRINCIPLES FOR MANAGING
CRISES AND SYMPTOMS

The key to managing crises is to keep goals and interventions simple. Whether in emergency rooms, crisis clinics, or during ongoing treatment, clinicians often try to achieve too much. Emotional and cognitive dysregulation, however, compromise patients' ability to use anything more than simple interventions. Indeed, more complex interventions may escalate problems. *The primary goal in managing crises is to return the patient to the previous level of functioning as soon as possible.* This goal can be achieved by implementing general treatment strategies, interventions based on an understanding of the chain of events culminating in the crisis behavior, and an optimal sequencing of the different interventions. This approach is combined with medication, as needed, to reduce symptoms and enable patients to make effective use of psychosocial interventions.

Behavioral Sequence

Psychodynamic and cognitive-behavioral theories agree that crisis behavior, including deliberate self-harm, is the endpoint of a sequence of events involving escalating dysphoria, triggering stimuli, and an underlying cognitive–affective structure (Swenson, 1989; see Figure 8.1). The sequence is usually triggered by an interpersonal event that activates maladaptive schemata such as rejection, abandonment, and intrusion. Events in therapy can also function as triggers, such as the sudden frame changes that occur when the therapist cancels an appointment or leaves for vacation without adequate notice. Crises may also be triggered by an early focus on traumat-

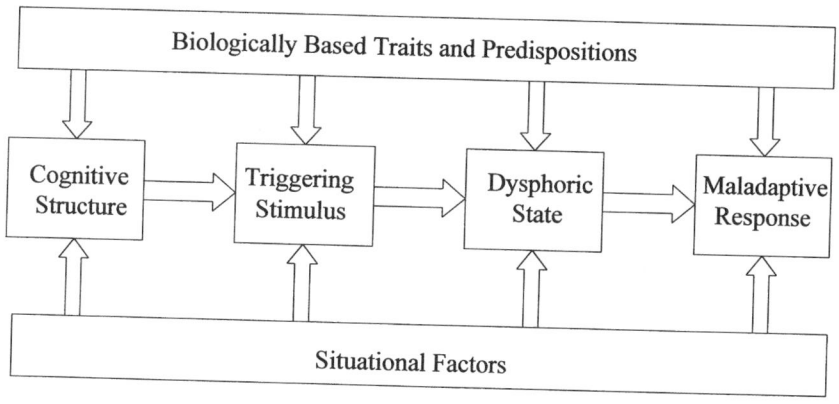

FIGURE 8.1. Behavioral sequence leading to maladaptive behavior.

ic events that arouses overwhelming emotions, or reenactment of earlier, traumatic relationship experiences in the treatment relationship.

Healthy individuals handle everyday interpersonal problems by using an array of coping strategies that includes problem solving, distraction, and self-soothing. Interpersonal problems are more challenging for individuals with personality disorder, because high levels of (1) heritable traits such as anxiousness and affective lability, and (2) defective regulation of emotions and impulses lead to more intense reactions that are amplified by habitual ways of thinking. Many patients ruminate rather than problem solve. At the same time, tendencies to catastrophize and automatic thoughts such as "This should not be happening to me," "I cannot stand these feelings," or "There is nothing that I can do to change the way I feel" increase rather than dampen emotional arousal.

This model of crisis postulates the occurrence of deficits in the mechanisms that regulate emotions and impulses, due to biological predispositions or the effects of environmental adversity or both. This implies a multi-dimensional approach to treatment, in which each component in the sequence—behavior, affective state, triggering situation, and cognitive structure—is a potential target for multiple psychosocial and biological interventions.

Sequence of Interventions

Interventions for treating crises and symptoms are selected on the basis of the following principle:

> Basic Principle: Crises and symptoms are best managed by using a continuum of interventions, beginning with containment strategies, cognitive-behavioral interventions, and medication to control and reduce symptoms and promote affect regulation, followed by less structured interventions that address the cognitive, affective, and interpersonal processes leading to symptoms and maladaptive behavior.

This principle is based on evidence that cognitive-behavioral interventions and medication are effective in treating impulsivity and affective instability. This evidence, as it relates to the treatment patients engaging in self-harm, is reviewed in the next chapter.

The five-phase sequence of interventions (safety, containment, control and regulation, exploration and change, and integration and synthesis) discussed in Chapter 6 constitute different steps along this continuum. The first step in crisis management is to ensure safety, followed by interventions of support, structure, and medication to contain unstable behaviors and affects. As containment is achieved and reactivity settles, behavioral, cognitive, and pharmacological interventions are used to control and regulate impulsive and parasuicidal behavior and manage emotional instability.

Once affect management skills are acquired, attention is given to more exploratory work, often requiring less structured interventions, designed to help patients understand the interpersonal context of symptoms, the cognitive and emotional processes underlying these behaviors, and the factors involved in symptom formation and maintenance. This process inevitably produces some degree of affect arousal. For this reason, these interventions are best left until the patient has learned to tolerate and regulate emotions.

This sequence essentially describes the overall treatment of personality disorder, because the fourth phase of exploration and change begins to address (1) interpersonal and self problems, (2) the developmental experiences that underlie these acts, and (3) the traits that contribute to their occurrence and persistence. This phase leads gradually to the final stage of developing more adaptive self and interpersonal systems. The sequence involves a gradual transition from more relationship-based and structured interventions to more change-focused and less structured interventions.

SAFETY

The challenge in managing crises is to ensure patients' safety without acting in ways that are experienced as invalidating. Nevertheless, interventions needed to ensure safety take priority over other interventions, regardless of their effects on the alliance. However, awareness of the problem often makes it possible intervene in ways that do not damage the treatment relationship.

Crisis management begins by evaluating the patient's mental state and level of coping, including assessment of potential dangerousness and his or her ability to manage self-harming impulses without external interventions (Kjelsberg, Eikeseth, & Dahl, 1991). Making this determination requires evaluation of suicidal and parasuicidal risk, as discussed in Chapter 5 (see Table 8.2). Evaluation of suicidal intent is difficult in patients with chronic suicidal ideation, for whom contemplation of suicide is "a way of life." Hence it is important to distinguish between chronic ideation and immediate intent and risk. Key considerations in evaluating the degree of risk are *level of intent* and whether intent has changed, as indicated by the formulation of a more detailed plan in patients with chronic suicidal ideation, and *level of impulse control*. Risk is increased when (1) cognitive control is reduced by intense affects and impulses or alcohol and drugs; (2) consciousness is impaired due to dissociative reactions, alcohol, or drugs; and (3) transient psychotic episode and quasipsychotic symptoms are present. Risk factors associated with borderline personality disorder, however, have limited predictive value (Paris et al., 1989); indeed, accurate prediction of risk is not possible with any psychiatric disorder (Hirschfeld & Russell, 1997; Mann, Waternaux, Haas, & Malone, 1999).

TABLE 8.2. Managing Crises: Ensuring Safety

General goal: Enable the patient to return to previous level of functioning as soon as possible.

Specific goals

- Ensure the safety of the patient and others.
- Contain affects, impulses, and behavioral disorganization.
- Prevent an escalation of psychopathology.
- Establish or maintain the basis for ongoing treatment.

Evaluate suicide risk

- Change in suicide intent
  - Change in intensity
  - Formulation of detailed plan
- Level of impulsivity
  - Intensity of affect arousal
- Level of control
  - Changes in consciousness due to
    - Alcohol, drugs
    - Dissociative behavior

Take appropriate action

- Admit to inpatient facility
- Arrange additional structure and support
  - Admit to day treatment program
  - Family and social support system
  - Additional appointments

When assessing risk, it is useful to note how personality influences presentation. As noted earlier, the intense reactive affects of emotionally dysregulated individuals may mask severe depressive features, leading to an underestimation of suicidal risk (Kernberg, 2001). Similarly, the more muted expression of distress and depression in the inhibited individual may lead to an underestimation of risk. On the basis of this evaluation, one of the following decisions is made: admit to an inpatient facility, arrange partial hospitalization or day treatment, treat as an outpatient, arrange additional structure and support for patients in treatment, or continue with scheduled treatment.

Indications for Inpatient Treatment

Inpatient treatment should only be used when there is no other way to ensure safety. Patients with borderline personality disorder in particular make extensive use of inpatient treatment (Kent, Fogarty, & Yellowlees,

1995; Williams, Weiss, Edens, Johnson, & Thornby, 1998). Common features leading to multiple admissions are anorexia, psychotic symptoms, and suicidality (Hull, Yeomans, Clarkin, Li, & Goodman, 1996). Surprisingly, depression did not predict frequent admissions. Despite high utilization, there is little evidence that inpatient treatment has lasting effects or that it is useful in managing parasuicidal behavior or threats (Paris, 2002). Moreover, many patients appear to regress in inpatient settings, and there are serious risks associated with inpatient treatment (Miller, 1989). For this reason, admissions should be brief.

The indications for inpatient treatment include:

1. Danger to others
2. High risk of suicide or other serious high-risk behavior that cannot be managed in any other way
3. Transient psychotic episode that cannot be managed in ambulatory care or is considered to increase risk
4. Severe dissociative reaction involving either an amnesic or a non-responsive state.

None of these indications is absolute. Posing a serious threat to others is an uncommon reason for admission. Suicidal and parasuicidal ideation is not an indication for admission unless the risk is high, as revealed by levels of intent and impulse control, and other ways to manage this risk are not available. The exception would be a patient in treatment who is out of control and who requires a brief admission of a day or so to allow things to settle down. Chronic suicidal ideation alone is not an indication for admission: there is no evidence that inpatient treatment changes this behavior. Indeed, clinical observation suggests that thoughts of self-harm often continue long after self-harming acts have ceased. Similarly, transient psychotic episodes are not, in themselves, an indication for admission, unless the patient is unable to comply with treatment. The management of patients in hospital settings is discussed later.

There is also no evidence that long-term admission is useful in treating patients with personality disorder. Even with chronically self-harming individuals who inflict serious injuries on themselves, by penetrating or opening a body cavity, and who cannot be treated in the community, it is doubtful whether lasting change occurs; often the self-harm continues even after years in hospital care. However, there may be occasions when a longer admission of a month or more is indicated to disrupt a repetitive cycle of self-harm that cannot be terminated in other ways. In some situations, repetitive self-harm elicits a strong reaction from the community, including responses from social and health care service personnel. The ensuing turmoil makes treatment difficult, so that a respite sometimes gives an opportunity to organize a coherent management plan without always having to respond to another crisis. Instances such as these are relatively infrequent. In both examples, a more extended admission is used not because it is needed to manage personality disorder but because treatment has failed and the health care system is unable to manage the serious condition.

This conservative use of hospital treatment is not recommended by some authorities, nor is it adopted in some settings. The Practice Guidelines for treating borderline personality disorder (American Psychiatric Association, 2001), for example, appear to advocate greater use of hospital admission and suggest indications for extended inpatient treatment. However, there is little evidence to support these recommendations (Paris, 2002). Even after extended admission to a facility designed to manage these problems, patients still show serious pathology (McGlashan, 1986). In most situations, however, extended admission is usually made to a general long-stay psychiatric service rather than a specialized facility. Not only is there no evidence that this course of action is valuable, but clinical experience suggests that the outcome is often poor. The unfortunate reality is that many patients do badly in hospital environments. Many find the experience distressing and humiliating. And, all too often, hospital treatment appears to lead to reduced capacity to manage problems and initiates an escalating cycle of crises and repeated admissions that is difficult to break.

Other Treatment Options

The preferred option is to manage crises without an inpatient admission, or if admission is unavoidable, to keep the patient in the hospital for a brief time, preferably no more than 48 hours. Partial hospitalization or day treatment programs are an effective way to provide short-term treatment for people with personality disorder (Bateman & Fonagy, 1999, 2001; Piper et al., 1993, 1996). When available, they are preferable to inpatient treatment. Patients can either be admitted directly or following a very brief inpatient admission of a day or so. The indications for partial hospitalization include:

1. Ongoing crisis behavior, with acute behavioral disorganization that cannot be managed in outpatient or office treatment
2. Failure of outpatient or office treatment to contain affects and impulses effectively
3. Serious regressive behavior or other symptoms, including a comorbid disorder, that severely interfere with the routine activities of daily living and self-care.

Often sufficient support and structure can be provided to ensure safety without inpatient treatment by mobilizing family and social support systems and offering frequent appointments for patients not currently in treatment or extra appointments and telephone contact between sessions for those with a regular therapist. When patients are not admitted, clinicians often use a verbal or written no-suicide contract in which patients agree to inform a relative or health-care professional if they are suicidal, rather than acting on the intent. However, there is no evidence that these contracts are effective (Stanford, Goetz, & Bloom, 1994). Indeed a survey of clinicians indicated that although 57% used no-suicide contracts, 41% of those using them reported that they had patients who completed suicide or made serious attempts (Kroll, 2000). Interestingly, the use of no-suicide contracts decreased with number of years in practice. Although this study did not compare the use of contracts in different diagnostic groups, it raises serious doubts about the value of this approach. Clinicians may be lulled into a false sense of security by the patient agreeing to a contract and fail to take appropriate steps to ensure safety. As Kroll noted, the limited value of a contract does not mean that the clinician should not try to get a commitment from the patient to use resources available, if needed. However, the contract itself seems to have little efficacy.

CONTAINMENT

Following practical steps to ensure safety, the next task is to provide the support and structure required to contain behavioral disorganization and emotional instability, by using interventions based on the general treatment strategies (see Table 8.3).

Interventions

General Interventions

Interventions are based on the assumption that patients in a crisis want relief from emotional pain and to feel understood, rather than help in understanding their problems (Joseph, 1983; Steiner, 1994). Relief comes from feeling a connection with someone who understands. This occurs when the therapist is able to align with the patient's distress in a way that conveys *support and understanding*. Support helps to contain behavioral and emotional turmoil by reducing fear, suspicion, and mistrust. As captured by the idea of collaborative description, the therapist seeks to see the world as the patient sees it and convey an understanding of this perspective without necessarily agreeing with it. Minimal exploration occurs: one only explores sufficiently to understand the patient's feelings and make informed decisions.

Containment is weakened by (1) failures to acknowledge the patient's distress, (2) lengthy attempts to clarify feelings, and (3) interpretations of

TABLE 8.3. Managing Crises: Providing Containment

Goals

- Prevent the escalation of psychopathology.
- Return the patient to the previous level of functioning as quickly as possible.

Therapeutic stance

- Align with the patient's distress.

Interventions

- Convey support and understanding.
- Establish a connection with the patient.
- Focus on affect rather than content.
- Use straightforward, concrete statements that reflect an understanding of the current situation and the patients' experience.
- Reframe only to reduce intense self-derogation.
- Stabilize the environment.
- Set limits supportively.

---

the origins of thoughts, feelings, or impulses (Steiner, 1994). Thus a *focus on affect rather than content* (Linehan, 1993) and *the immediate present rather than the past* is indicated. However, the task is not to promote ventilation but rather to achieve affect regulation by acknowledging feelings without attributing motives. This acknowledgment is best made in the form of *straightforward, concrete statements that reflect an understanding of the current situation and the patient's experience.* Anything more risks (1) overwhelming the patient's capacity to process information, and (2) being experienced as invalidating or interpreted as evidence that the therapist does not understand or care. Statements that incorporate the patient's own words reduce the chance of misunderstanding. In highly reactive states, patients are remarkably intolerant of therapist error. Hence it is better to reflect what the patient says than to attempt even a modest reframing of problems. When reframing is used, it is best confined to attempts to reduce any self-criticism that is exacerbating the situation.

The therapist's presence as a stable, consistent, caring, nonpunitive person who is able to survive the patient's distress and anger and continue providing support and understanding is often more effective in achieving containment than the actual content of the therapist's comments (Buie & Adler, 1982). Similarly, the way understanding is communicated is often more important than the actual words. In highly reactive states, it is important to "get the music right" because patients often interpret language differently. When the patient is extremely distressed and unable to function, it may also be important for the therapist to talk to establish contact and avoid anxiety-inducing silences (Ryle, 1997). Words convey a bond and a connection while creating structure that can be reassuring. Therapist talk needs to be monitored carefully, however, to avoid creating the impression that the clinician is not interested in what the patient has to say or has prematurely decided what is wrong.

In crises, therapists should not be misled by the intensity of the distress into assuming that the patient is not attending closely to what the therapist says. Most patients are hypervigilant on these occasions, even when in a dissociated state. They worry about not being understood and whether the clinician is angry or judging them unfavorably. The therapist's reactions are examined carefully not because patients hope to gain insight but because the reactions may reveal something about the therapist's attitude toward them (Steiner, 1994).

When dealing with these states, therapists are often tempted to address intense affects directed to the therapist with transference interpretations. As Steiner (1994) pointed out, interpretations that take the form "You are afraid that I will . . . *because* . . . " often fail to contain distress because they do not match patients' ideas about what they need. The inclusion of an explanation may also be perceived as critical or as evidence that the therapist does not understand. These interpretations also tend to overwhelm the patient's capacity to process information. Simpler statements such as "You see me as . . . " or "It seemed to help when you felt that I understood" are more effective (Steiner, 1994). Interpretations also can create a sense of intrusion and increase mistrust. Even questions that are designed to clarify the patient's feelings may be experienced as an attack, and felt to be intrusive and challenging, when what the patient wants is understanding and acceptance.

These ideas about containment as the basic approach to crises differ from the emphasis that Kernberg (1984; Clarkin et al., 1999) places on interpreting the patient's rage or hostility toward the therapist as contributing to "acting-out" behavior and attempts to control the therapist. The current approach acknowledges that it is easy to construe behavior in this way and that these behaviors may serve such a function. However, the assumption is that crisis behavior arises primarily from an underlying biological predisposition to emotional dysregulation and impaired self-regulation, which suggests the need for a more supportive approach.

Stabilizing the Environment

Most crises are triggered by interpersonal situations involving either temporary or more enduring instability in the immediate environment. In these circumstances, it is helpful to make the social environment more predictable and supportive (Vaillant, 1992). Achieving this stability is one of the functions of inpatient treatment—it creates a respite for all involved. Other ways to stabilize the environment include (1) providing other kinds of respite, (2) temporary avoidance of the social situation or relationship that contributed to the crisis, and (3) working with the patient and their significant others to defuse the situation. Significant others who are involved can often modify their behavior in the relationship and avoid being reactive or doing things that exacerbate the problem, once they understand the nature of the patient's difficulties and are informed about ways in which they can help.

Preventing an Escalation of Psychopathology

An important objective of crisis management is to prevent an escalation of psychopathology and reduce the risk of future crises. Short-term escalation is minimized by effective containment and intervening to dampen feelings. It is also minimized by avoiding (1) challenges to coping mechanisms, (2) interventions that increase impulsivity and dysphoria, and (3) extensive use of interpretations, excessive control, criticism, or a confrontational stance. Successful crisis management reduces the risk of future crisis presentations. As several authors have noted, many patients do not appear to be helped by the health-care system and some may even deteriorate (Frances, 1992; Rockland, 1992). Indeed, Kroll (1988) maintained that patients with severe borderline personality disorder are made, not born. Maladaptive behavior is often unintentionally, and sometimes unavoidably, reinforced. Parasuicidal acts, for example, force gratification of needs for care and attention simply because self-injuries have to be treated. Although it is not helpful to view these behaviors simply as care or attention seeking, they can produce considerable secondary gain. In other patients, the reinforcements may be very different. The excitement and drama associated with crises are reinforcing for patients who are highly sensation seeking. Even the harsh and unsympathetical stance shown by some health-care professionals toward deliberate self-harm, in the mistaken belief that this response will minimize gratification of assumed needs for dependency or attention seeking and reduce the chances of recurrence, can serve as reinforcement. Such reactions invariably fail because they overlook the fact that victims of abuse often unwittingly seek out abusive situations. Far from reducing the probability of future episodes, these responses increase the risk because they either provide the punishment that some patients think they deserve, or patients feel the need to convince all concerned that they really need help.

Therapist Reactions

Effective containment depends on clinicians managing their reactions to their patients. These reactions take many forms. Perhaps the most benign are attempts to do too much to alleviate distress; these attempts risk overwhelming the patient's ability to manage information. Some therapists also try to reduce intense distress by focusing on the positive aspects of the individual's life or minimizing problems. Such interventions rarely work; indeed, they encourage escalation to make the clinician understand. It is usually better to acknowledge the distress without minimizing it. Statements such as "Most people would find it difficult to cope with these problems" or "Given the problems that you have described, it is not surprising that you are feeling overwhelmed" are more likely to reduce distress because they convey understanding rather than attempt to change the way the patient feels.

More troublesome reactions occur when therapists attribute motives to patients' behavior. Tendencies to see these acts only in terms of the transference leads to assumptions that they are motivated by hostility or attempts to control, manipulate, or gain attention. Such attributions are rarely helpful and foster unhelpful confrontation and nonsupportive limit setting. Yet these behaviors are, indeed, a "test" of the therapist: They test the therapist's ability to survive these episodes with support and empathy intact.

Containment Interventions throughout Treatment

Containment interventions are useful throughout treatment to manage episodes of behavioral disorganization. In the early stages of treatment, in particular, these interventions should be used whenever the patient is emotionally overwhelmed or has difficulty processing information. Over time, fewer containment interventions are required as increased ability to regulate affects permits greater affect arousal and more active exploration of psychopathology. This use of containment is illustrated by the following incident that occurred in the treatment of Natasha, a patient discussed in Chapter 6:

> Natasha began one session by saying that she was having difficulty coping and felt overwhelmed. These problems began the previous day. While walking through a car park, she suddenly felt overwhelmed, confused, and trapped. This progressed to feelings of helplessness and passivity, and she decided that she might as well give up. Since the incident, she had been so depressed she had not eaten. She was not sure what triggered these feelings, but she thought it was the memory of an abusive experience. The incident clearly contained important material that needed to be addressed at some point. However, the patient had difficulty describing events; she felt confused and her thoughts were disorganized. These reactions had occurred frequently in the past and often heralded dissociative behavior and deliberate self-harm. Given difficulties processing information, there was little value in exploring the incident. Indeed, attempts to do so were likely to cause further problems. Instead, containment interventions,

focusing on the distress and the feeling of being overwhelmed, were used. When the immediate emotional reaction was contained and thoughts became more organized, the episode was examined in terms of the connection between feelings of passivity and abusive experience.

MEDICATION

Although the current state of knowledge suggests that the treatment of personality disorder is largely psychotherapeutic, medication is an important part of a comprehensive treatment plan. The evidence suggests that medication is useful in managing cognitive disorganization, impulsivity and aggression, and depressed, anxious, and labile mood (Soloff, 1998, 2000). A focused approach, in which medication is used to treat specific symptom clusters rather than global personality disorder, is recommended. There is little evidence that core interpersonal and self pathology respond directly to currently available agents. However, symptomatic improvement has a synergic effect on treatment, making the patient more amenable to psychotherapeutic interventions.

Although numerous medications have been used to treat patients with personality disorder, only a few have been shown to be effective in controlled trials. It should also be noted that most studies have involved patients with borderline personality disorder. The evidence particularly supports the use of neuroleptics and selective serotonergic reuptake inhibitors (SSRIs) as first-line agents (Markovitz, 2001; Soloff, 1998, 2000).

Perceptual and Cognitive Symptoms

The major medication to consider in the immediate management of crises is a neuroleptic. Low doses of these agents are useful in managing perceptual–cognitive symptoms, such as confused and disorganized thinking, transient psychotic episodes, and quasipsychotic features (e.g., paranoid ideation and pseudohallucinations). This approach is supported by several controlled trials and many open trials on adults and adolescents (Cowdry & Gardner, 1988; Goldberg et al., 1986; Kutcher, Papatheodorou, Reiter, & Gardner, 1995; Leone, 1982; Schulz, Camlin, Berry, & Jesberger, 1999; Serban & Siegal, 1984; Soloff et al., 1986; Soloff et al., 1993; Zanarini & Frankenberg, 2001). The original study using typical neuroleptics (Goldberg et al., 1986) reported that beneficial effects were confined to reducing quasipsychotic features and hence there was little reason to continue with medication once symptoms had settled. Currently, atypical neuroleptics are preferred because of a more favorable side-effect profile. These medications also appear to have broader effects, and hence there is reason to continue with them once the crisis is mitigated. For example, olanzapine led to improvement in psychotic features, depressed mood, interpersonal sensitivity, and anger in a small sample of patients with borderline personality disorder in an 8-week open label trial (Schulz et al., 1999). A randomized control trial of the same drug reported changes in anxiety, depression, paranoia, anger and hostility, and interpersonal sensitivity (Zanarini & Frankenberg, 2001).

Low doses of atypical neuroleptics are also useful in managing hypersensitivity, a trait that has not received the attention warranted. Many patients, regardless of their personality pattern, feel overwhelmed by any form of stimulation, including experiences, feelings, and everyday events. This low threshold increases reactivity that leads to further distress. For example, one patient noted that "everything seemed to have the volume turned up"—sounds were too loud, colors too bright, and feelings too intense. In this hypersensitive state, he was exquisitely "touchy," a quality that caused strong reactions to events that others considered trivial. As the Schulz (Schulz et al., 1999) and Zanarini and Frankenberg (2001) studies showed, low doses of atypical neuroleptics reduce interpersonal sensitivity, which is probably a facet of the broader trait. This dampening of hypersensitivity allows patients to reflect on their experiences rather than struggle to contain them.

Beneficial effects of neuroleptics are usually apparent within a few days but may take several weeks. Prolonged occurrence of psychotic-like symptoms, despite medication, is reason to review the diagnosis (with the exception of those with schizotypal personality disorder). Currently there is little empirical evidence to indicate the optimal duration of medication use or to support long-term usage. A reasonable trial of neuroleptics is about 12 weeks (American Psychiatric Association, 2001). If a response has not been obtained, it is appropriate to consider another agent. It has been suggested that if the perceptual–cognitive symptoms do not improve, the dose be increased into the range used to treat Axis I disorders (American Psychiatric Association, 2001). There is, however, limited evidence to support this proposal. To avoid the problems of overmedication, higher doses are best confined to patients with severe quasipsychotic symptoms who do not respond to lower doses. Higher doses do not seem indicated for those being treated only for hypersensitivity. The problem with higher dosages in patients with personality disorder is that coping may be adversely affected.

If a good response to medication used in a crisis situation is obtained, it is appropriate to continue it for some weeks after the crisis has resolved. If used to manage more persistent perceptual and cognitive symptoms or hypersensitivity, longer-term use may be appropriate. Longer-term use would also be indicated if low-dose neuroleptics lead to improvement in impulsivity and anger–hostility. A problem with longer-term or chronic use, however, apart from unwanted side effects, is that compliance progressively decreases (Cornelius, Soloff, Perel, & Ulrich, 1993; Kelly, Soloff, Cornelius, George, & Lis, 1992).

Patients who experience recurrent transient psychotic episodes can sometimes be taught to self-monitor their mental state and use neuroleptics immediately, when symptoms first appear. In this way, some episodes may be aborted. In some cases, it is useful to involve relatives or significant others in monitoring symptoms.

Affective Symptoms and Instability

Patients with depressed, angry, anxious, and labile mood should be treated initially with a selective serotonin reuptake inhibitor (SSRI) or related agent (Soloff, 2000). There is consistent evidence that SSRIs are valuable in treating depressed mood, anxiety, and impulsive aggression (Cornelius, Soloff, Perel, & Ulrich, 1990; Kavoussi, Liu, & Coccaro, 1994; Markovitz, 1995, 2001; Markovitz, Calabrese, Charles, & Meltzer, 1991; Norden, 1989; Salzman et al., 1995; Soloff, 1998, 2000). Although mood symptoms do respond to SSRIs, it is less clear if these agents are effective in treating the trait of affective instability that is a central feature of the emotionally dysregulated or borderline pattern and present in most forms of personality disorder.

The advantage of these agents is that they are relatively safe if an overdose is taken. They also have fairly broad effects, leading to improvements in depressed mood, anxiety, and impulsivity, including self-harming behaviors. In some studies they also reduce anger and hostility and psychotic-like symptoms (Markovitz, 2001). The beneficial effects on anger and hostility appear to be independent of effects on other affective features (Salzman et al., 1995).

Clinical opinion suggests that a reasonable trial of an SSRI is at least 12 weeks (American Psychiatric Association, 2001). Most controlled studies have investigated fluoxetine. However, open trials suggest that sertraline has similar effects (Kavoussi et al., 1994; Markovitz, 1995, 2001), as does venlafaxine, which works as both a serotonin and noradrenaline reuptake inhibitor (Markovitz & Wagner, 1995). Most patients with personality disorder appear to tolerate SSRIs reasonably well, although compliance is always a problem. Effect on sexual functioning is a common problem affecting compliance in women, although the occasional patient who has problems controlling sexual urges and boundary difficulties finds this unwanted effect beneficial.

If a poor response is obtained with the first agent, consideration should be given to changing to a second SSRI or related antidepressant. Soloff (2000) advocates caution about using tricyclic antidepressants in patients with borderline personality disorder. If a poor response occurs with the second agent, it is suggested that consideration be given to augmenting with a neuroleptic (Soloff, 1998, 2000). Although there is little empirical evidence to support this strategy, it is worth considering, given the beneficial effects of low-dose neuroleptics on mood and hostility. This combination should also be considered for patients with prominent mood symptoms and hypersensitivity. It is suggested that patients with affective instability who are also anxious may benefit from a benzodiazepine in addition to an SSRI (American Psychiatric Association, 2001). There is, however, very limited empirical support, at present, for the use of benzodiazepines in treating patients with personality disorder. Given problems with abuse, dependency, and reports of serious behavioral dyscontrol with a short-acting agent (Cowdry & Gardner, 1988; Gardner & Cowdry, 1985), it is not clear that these agents have a role in treatment. If it is considered necessary to use benzodiazepines to treat anxiety, clonazepam is preferred because it has a long half-life (Soloff, 2000).

Second-line agents for treating affective instability are the monoamine oxidase inhibitors (MAOIs) and mood stabilizers. Although there is reasonable evidence of the efficacy of MAOIs (Cowdry & Gardner, 1988; Soloff et al., 1993), their side-effect profile and need for dietary restrictions in patients with low compliance suggest that they have a limited role in treating patients with serious personality disorder. A variety of mood stabilizers has used to treat personality disorder, including lithium carbonate, valproate, and carbamazepine. However, there are few controlled studies to support their use. The use of lithium is supported by a few studies showing that it is useful in reducing impulsivity (Links, Steiner, Boiago, & Irwin, 1990), with modest effects on day-to-day mood variation (Rifkin, Quirkin, Carrillo, Blumberg, & Klein, 1972). After reviewing the literature on the benefits of lithium in treating borderline personality disorder, Markovitz (2001) concluded that it should be regarded as a second-line treatment, given its limited effects on affective instability (which continues following treatment, although at a reduced level) and its potential lethality in overdose. Lithium also produces such severe side effects that compliance is a problem with most patients (Rifkin, Levitan, Glaewski, & Klein, 1972). There is a lack of evidence to support the use of carbamazepine and valproate; some open trials report benefits but not others (American Psychiatric Association, 2001). Carbamazepine also has been reported to lead to melancholic depression in some patients with borderline personality disorder.

Impulsivity and Aggression

Besides effects on depressed and anxious mood, the SSRIs have also been shown to improve impulsivity, including self-harm and aggression. These effects are independent of the effects on depression and anxiety (Coccaro

& Kavoussi, 1997). For these reasons, an SSRI should be considered for patients who engage in impulsive acts. The effects of these agents on impulsivity and anger are often observed before antidepressant effects, sometimes within a few days.

Lithium has been shown to reduce impulsive–aggressive symptoms in adults and adolescents (Sheard, 1975; Sheard, Marini, Bridges, & Wagner, 1976; Tupin et al., 1973), and controlled trials have shown that MAOIs can be used to reduce impulsivity (Cornelius et al., 1993; Soloff et al., 1993). Safety considerations, however, suggest that lithium and MAOIs should be used cautiously, as second-line agents. Low doses of neuroleptics also have a beneficial effect on impulsivity.

A practical approach to medication is to consider initially the indications for low-dose neuroleptics and SSRIs. Low-dose neuroleptics should be considered when managing crises in patients with perceptual–cognitive symptoms. They are also indicated for patients in whom hypersensitivity is a problem. An SSRI is indicated for patients who engage in deliberate self-harm and those with significant mood symptoms. Low-dose neuroleptics also have a beneficial effect on mood symptoms and impulsivity. Hence many patients benefit from a combination of these agents. However, every effort should be made to avoid polypharmacy. Most patients are usually on a mixture of medications, with unclear benefits. Soloff (2000) provides algorithms for treating cognitive–perceptual, affective dysregulatory, and impulsive–behavioral symptoms, as well as suggestions for strategies to use for nonresponsiveness.

Principles Underlying the Use of Medication

The demonstrated value of medication raises questions about how to incorporate medication into the treatment framework. Within the current treatment model, medication is considered a specific intervention that should be used with the same attention to the general therapeutic strategies as other specific interventions. For this reason, there does not appear to be any significant reason why the therapist should not also prescribe appropriate medication, when this is possible. Objections that this arrangement complicates the treatment relationship and the transference are not pertinent to the present approach. Indeed, there are major advantages to the therapist prescribing. Doing so avoids involving others in the patient's care—a situation that is always a potential source of problems. When the therapist does not manage medication, it is important that both professionals have an explicit understanding of their respective roles and that they maintain good collaboration and frequent communication.

Several other factors about the use of medication need to be considered (see Table 8.4). Medication is used to treat specific symptoms rather than personality disorder per se (Soloff, 1998, 2000); medication should

TABLE 8.4. Medication Management

- Within the framework of general and specific interventions, medication is merely another form of specific intervention.
- Medication should be used in the context of the general therapeutic strategies, especially the treatment relationship.
- Medication is used to target specific symptom clusters rather than disorders per se.
- Effects of medication on core pathology are likely to be limited to "ripple effects."
- Education is important to ensure that patients and significant others do not develop unrealistic expectations about the likely effects and benefits of medication.

not be expected to have a major effect on all domains of personality pathology. It is important to ensure that the patient (and, if necessary, significant others), clearly understands what the medication is being used to treat, what changes may be expected—and, equally importantly, what the medication is *not* likely to change. Receiving this information reduces (1) unrealistic expectations about the likely benefits, and (2) the pressure to change medication frequently in search of a "cure." It also reduces unnecessary polypharmacy. It is important to remind patients of the importance of psychological work and that medication is not a panacea. The decision to use medication should be made collaboratively with the patient, following discussion of the likely benefits and possible side effects. To avoid medication being viewed as something imposed by the therapist, the final decision should be the patient's. In crisis situations, however, such a perogative may not always be possible. Nevertheless, the patient should be involved as much as possible in the decision-making process and the issue reviewed when the acute state begins to diminish. Compliance is typically a major problem and needs to be approached collaboratively to avoid polarization of patient and clinician.

INPATIENT TREATMENT

Earlier it was suggested that inpatient treatment should be used to ensure safety when there is serious risk of suicide or serious self-harm, as indicated by levels of intent and impulse control. Admissions are usually to general units that manage a wide variety of disorders, including psychotic conditions. Unfortunately, the milieu of many general facilities is not conducive to managing patients with personality disorder. As noted, admission should only be used when alternatives are not available, and then the admission should be brief. Problems often arise if patients remain in hospital beyond the short time required for crises to recede, because the patient's psychopathology begins to interact with unit dynamics.

Treatment Goals

The goals of inpatient treatment, like those of crisis management generally, should be modest and appropriate to the changes that can be achieved during a brief admission (see Table 8.5). Usually these goals are to (1) ensure safety, (2) return the patient to the previous level of functioning as soon as possible, (3) establish or maintain the basis for ongoing outpatient treatment, and (4) initiate treatment of any comorbid mental disorder.

The primary focus is on reducing the symptoms related to the current crisis (Williams, 1998). However, patients and therapists frequently collude in setting goals that are unrealistic, given the time and resources available (see Chapter 6). Unrealistic goals cause staff frustration because planned outcomes are not achieved, and patients are disappointed with their progress—both scenarios readily lead to further problems. Prolonged admissions in an attempt to achieve more extensive changes are another side effect of unrealistic goals. Such hopes for extensive changes are rarely met. Instead, longer admissions create opportunities for the enactment of maladaptive patterns on the unit, in interaction with ongoing staff dynamics, leading to increased impulsivity and new management problems. Sometimes longer admissions are suggested to encourage patients to accept outpatient treatment; however, this is rarely a valid reason—even after

TABLE 8.5. Inpatient Treatment

Goals

- Ensure safety.
- Return the patient to the previous level of functioning as soon as possible.
- Establish or maintain the basis for ongoing outpatient treatment.
- Initiate treatment of any comorbid mental disorder.

Therapeutic processes and interventions

- *Respite*: the provision of a safe haven and removal from an unstable environment
- *Structure*: the provision of a holding environment through the routines and schedules of the unit
- *Containment*: emotional holding through the consistent use of containment interventions
- *Reintegration*: the promotion of reintegration and interpersonal involvement
- *Medication*: to treat specific symptoms and any comorbid disorder

long admissions, good alliances with a staff therapist are rare and collaboration limited (Allen et al., 1985).

A therapeutic contract covering the goals and duration of inpatient treatment should be developed before admission. Some centers require no-suicide and no-parasuicide contracts that include the consequences of such actions, such as discharge if the patient engages in a suicidal or parasuicidal act. As noted earlier, there is no evidence that these contracts are effective, nor do they help to build the alliance. Challenge to the contract is almost inevitable, and contract violations create a management dilemma. If the contract is followed and the patient is discharged, even if in a suicidal or parasuicidal state (the state that led to admission), the admission was probably pointless. On the other hand, failure to follow through on the contract undermines the frame and leads to inconsistency that complicates future management and limit setting. It is best to avoid such contracts and to avoid establishing conditions for treatment that have a high probability of failure or are likely to cause additional management problems.

Treatment goals can usually be achieved fairly quickly: in most cases, behavioral disorganization recedes in 24–72 hours. This time frame provides a window for discharging into outpatient or office treatment. For patients who are already in treatment, the admission may be even shorter. For example, it may be sufficient to keep the patient in the emergency room overnight, or even for a few hours, until the dyscontrol or dissociation has diminished sufficiently for the patient to manage until the next scheduled treatment session or until an extra session can be arranged.

Therapeutic Processes and Interventions

As with crisis management generally, less active intervention is often better than intense treatment. Consequently, to contain impulsivity, limit regression, and promote coping, inpatient management relies primarily on the provision of a structured, containing, and supportive environment rather than on specific interventions. Important elements of treatment include: respite, structure, containment, reintegration, and medication (see Table 8.5).

Respite

Although the primary purpose of hospital treatment is to ensure safety, it also provides a retreat from an unstable and destabilizing environment (Swenson, 1992). Invariably crises are triggered by interpersonal problems—an intense, engulfing relationship, rejection or abandonment, overwhelming intrusiveness, or isolation. In many cases, these interpersonal situations become self-perpetuating. Admission removes the person from the pressures of the situation and provides the opportunity for things to settle down and for the individuals involved to reintegrate. In many cases, respite is all that is needed.

Structure

In addition to offering a retreat, hospital treatment provides a structured and stable environment with a fixed routine, clear expectations, and firm schedule that disrupts chaotic and self-perpetuating crisis behavior. Routine activities of the inpatient unit provide boundaries and structure that help to anchor the person in reality. This structure also helps to limit regression and render maladaptive behaviors ungratifying. The value of this component of care is that it is does not depend on the activities or interventions of any given member of staff. Instead, structure is built into the way the unit functions. This system reduces the conflicts and struggles that readily emerge when structure and limit setting are dependent on the actions of a given person.

Fixed schedules of activities and expectations applicable to all patients are the inpatient unit's equivalent to the therapeutic frame. The effectiveness of this structure is strengthened by the explicit understanding reached with the patient prior to admission concerning the goals and duration of the admission. These decisions reinforce the frame provided by the unit and establish boundaries around the process. This frame is an essential part of treatment; hence it is important that staff members are consistent and objective in the way that they maintain the frame. As with frame violations discussed in Chapter 7, problems need to be addressed promptly and firmly in a way that conveys commitment to the frame and support and understanding of the patient's reactions and concerns. This supportive firmness has a settling effect on patients.

Containment

Containment interventions provide an emotional and interpersonal dimension that complements and reinforces the restraint and holding provided by the structure and routine of the unit. As with containment generally, the goal is to convey understanding of the patient's feelings and problems. This aspect requires more active interventions by staff and interaction between the patient and specific members of the unit. This contact provides an opportunity to convey support and to build hope to counteract demoralization and low self-esteem. These objectives are achieved most readily when staff members have an explicit understanding of what should be achieved and the interventions that are most useful. Consistency is a critical part of the process.

Containment also involves the promotion of coping skills and the use of affect-regulating interventions. Given the intensity of inpatient settings, it is useful to recall that effective containment requires the avoidance of interventions that are likely to increase emotional expression and impulsivity or foster regression and dependency. Containment is hindered by a number of factors, including a confrontational stance, failure to convey understanding, critical responses, invalidation, interpretations, active exploration of trauma, inappropriate ventilation of affect, and attempts to minimize distress. Regression and dependency are fostered by excessive sympathy as opposed to empathy and persistent advice giving as opposed to encouraging problem solving. These kinds of intervention are destabilizing; they undermine coping skills and generate affects that are difficult to contain. As result, a considerable amount of time may be spent managing the consequences of regression induced by the way the patient is treated. For this reason, active exploration of trauma and abuse should be minimized. These themes should be acknowledged and validated, if raised, but not actively explored.

Reintegration and Interpersonal Involvement

Inpatient treatment provides the opportunity to interact with other patients who are also in crisis, something that is not readily available with community treatment. Although most patients are absorbed with their own issues, unavoidable contact with others with similar or even worse problems helps to counter alienation and isolation. Inpatient milieu provides many formal and informal opportunities to reinvest in the world and to take an interest in others. As Vaillant (1992) noted, an effective way to help patients with strong dependency needs and regressed behavior is to encourage an interest in others. This strategy is often more effective than addressing these needs directly. Altruism is a powerful antidote to regression. Every opportunity should be taken to foster is this kind of reintegration, and staff need to be alert to the benefits that can accrue from helping patients interact with one another and take an interest in each other's well-being.

Establishing and Maintaining the Basis for Ongoing Treatment

One function of inpatient treatment is to establish the conditions for subsequent ambulatory care (unless a crisis management approach is used, in which crises are treated as they arise, without ongoing therapy). Successful resolution of the crisis and the development of good relationships with staff form the foundation for future work. As the crisis settles, treatment goals may be extended slightly to include a discussion of the interpersonal situations that trigger these problems. This shift begins to focus patients' attention on the causes of their difficulties and establishes a focus for future therapeutic work. Most patients are amenable to this idea. Others, however, are only interested in getting help for immediate distress and are not interested in continuing treatment. Sometimes supportive confrontation helps them to recognize the need for further treatment, but for some patients several admissions are needed before this is recognized.

Medication

Medications are usually part of inpatient treatment of the symptoms contributing to admission. As noted, the most immediate benefits are likely to be derived from the use of neuroleptics to treat cognitive dysregulation and transient psychotic symptoms; in most cases these recede quickly. In patients with impulsive behavior and affective lability, an SSRI will usually be prescribed during the admission, but improvement will probably not be observed during the few days that the patient is in the hospital. A further indication for medication is the presence of any comorbid syndrome. When medication is used, the guidelines discussed earlier (see Table 8.4) should be followed to avoid creating the impression that medication will improve all problems, thereby undermining the patient's responsibility to manage symptoms and impulses.

Common Pitfalls and Problems

All too often inpatient treatment of people with personality disorder is frustrating for patients and staff alike. Although some problems are inherent to treating personality pathology, many are due to unclear and unrealistic treatment plans and the lack of explicit treatment guidelines. Common problems include continuation of suicidal and parasuicidal acts, or a recurrence of these acts, leading to difficulty discharging patients and to conflict between the patient and staff and within the treatment team.

Since crisis behavior usually recedes quickly following admission, continued impulsivity should lead to a review of the treatment plan to determine whether treatment strategies are exacerbating problems. Unclear plans promote inconsistent management; treatment objectives may differ across the treatment team, and patient and staff may have radically different expectations of treatment outcome. It is sometimes difficult to formulate a collaborative plan when the admission is compulsory or when the patient was too disturbed to participate. When this happens, a collaborative plan should be established at the first opportunity.

Continued difficulties are a reason to review unit policies and dynamics. The lack of clearly stated policies and guidelines and the presence of different ideas about effective interventions create inconsistency in the way patients are managed. Differences in staff attitudes about personality disorder is another fertile breeding ground for problems. Many inpatient services are also ambivalent about treating personality disorder. Some staff are unsympathetic to patients who engage in deliberate self-harm, and others are frustrated by the repetitive nature of these acts.

Some degree of inconsistency is inevitable in inpatient treatment. The decision to admit implies that the patient is unable to manage impulses and feelings, yet an important part of treatment is to encourage the patient to assume responsibility for doing just that. Hence, despite behavioral instability, it is important to avoid responding as if the patient were out of control because this invariably leads to the patient behaving as if this were the case. Likewise, hospital admission and the care provided in a crisis are dependency inducing—and dependency promotes regression, decreased coping, and interpersonal demands that are difficult to meet.

The seeds for problems during inpatient treatment may be sown before admission by the way the admission was handled. Polarization between staff and patient occurs all too easily in crisis situations, such as emergency rooms, when assessing clinicians are frustrated at having to deal with another case of deliberate self-harm, another angry patient. These attitudes inevitably evoke further hostility and color patients' interactions with inpatient staff. This problem is often exacerbated for those who have been abused, whose behavior unwittingly evokes further abuse and victimization. Under the pressure of emergency situations, it is easy for health-care personnel to act out the patient's anger and guilt. Even if the more overt responses are controlled, patients are very attuned to negative reactions and anything that hints of criticism and invalidation.

The recurrence of suicidal or parasuicidal behavior following a period of remission can also be reduced by a well-defined treatment contract and guidelines. The problem often occurs when patients are kept in the hospital too long after the crisis has settled, leading to conflicts with unit personnel and stresses within the treatment team. A typical scenario occurs when a patient establishes a close relationship with one or more staff members and becomes increasingly open about problems and feelings. If this interpersonal dynamic is managed in ways that increase emotional expression rather than emotional regulation, increased demands for staff time to deal with the ensuing feelings will be the result. At some point, the patient becomes disappointed when the staff member "fails" the patient in some way. This perceived failure provokes anger and impulsivity, and the cycle that initiated admission begins again.

This situation is often further complicated by divisions within the treatment team about the way the patient should be treated. Although these divisions are often attributed to "splitting" by the patient, the situation is usually more complex. Patients rarely create these problems; rather they home in on sensitive issues, and their psychopathology begins to interact with preexisting staff problems. Disagreements among staff inevitably get communicated to the patient, leading to further problems. Although these issues can usually be managed on units designed to manage patients with personality disorder, it is difficult to establish the appropriate milieu on general inpatient services that are primarily designed to manage acute psychoses and related disorders. Awareness of the problem and good staff communication and morale often mitigate these effects in the short term, but in the longer term these problems are unavoidable.

Longer admissions often lead to unrealistic goals and to pressure from the patient to deal with major problems and pathology. In the process, expectations are built that set the stage for disappointment and frustration, and destabilizing affects are mobilized. The convergence of dashed expectations and destabilizing affects leads to a recurrence of suicidal and parasuicidal behavior, making it difficult to discharge the patient, leading to prolonged admission—and so on. In most circumstances the best solution is to use short admissions in combination with good outpatient support.

COMMENT

Crisis management is a crucial component of treatment. It is all too easy for patients to get caught up in an endless series of crises and short-term hospital admissions that have a minimal or even negative impact on the course of the disorder and serve only to reinforce maladaptive ways of coping. An understanding of the nature of crisis behavior suggests a conservative approach that relies heavily on general strategies implemented through interventions designed to effect containment. Inpatient treatment is considered to have a limited and circumscribed role in patient treatment. Emphasis is placed on settling crisis behavior as soon as possible and the use of management strategies that minimize the probability of adverse consequences arising from the way problems are handled.

CHAPTER 9

Regulation and Control

Treating Affects and Impulses

Once acute behavioral disorganization has settled, albeit temporarily, attention can be given to the third phase of intervention, *regulation and control*. The general goal of this phase of treatment is to improve self-management of impulsivity, self-harming behavior, and emotions. The specific goals include:

1. Facilitate recognition of the behavioral sequence leading to self-harm, with a view to initiating early identification and self-management of reactions to triggering stimuli.
2. Reduce and eventually cease self-harming behavior.
3. Increase control over affects and impulses.

FOUNDATIONS FOR AN APPROACH
TO THE TREATMENT OF SELF-HARM

The general approach to treating self-harming behaviors and associated dysphoria is based on (1) an understanding of the behavioral sequence leading to crisis behavior, and (2) the principle that symptoms are best managed using a continuum of interventions beginning with safety and containment and followed by cognitive-behavioral interventions and medication, as discussed in the previous chapter. The behavioral sequence of a triggering event that activates maladaptive schema and an escalating dysphoric state that leads to maladaptive behavior provides a useful way to conceptualize treatment. Each step in the sequence is the target for multiple interventions (see Figure 9.1). The more fully the links in the chain are understood, the more opportunities there are to identify links that can be changed. Treatment is also based on assumptions about the causes and functions of self-harm and the stages of change model.

Rationale for Intervention Strategy

The rationale for using cognitive-behavioral interventions and medication is based on: (1) evidence of the efficacy of cognitive-behavioral interventions in reducing symptoms, including parasuicidal behavior (Davidson & Tyrer, 1996; Evans et al., 1999; Koons et al., 2001; Linehan et al., 1991, 1999; Perris, 1994; Piper & Joyce, 2001); (2) clinical observation that strong emotions are destabilizing for many patients, so that exploration of adversity is best deferred until the self-management of affects and impulses improves; and (3) evidence that medication modulates impulsivity and affective symptoms.

The efficacy of cognitive-behavioral interventions has been demonstrated in several studies. Linehan and colleagues (1991) reported the results of a randomized clinical trial of dialectical behavior therapy versus treatment as usual, usually individual therapy, for borderline personality disorder. Cognitive-behavioral treatment consisted of 1 hour of individual therapy and 2½ hours of group therapy for 1 year, incorporating skills training, problem solving, contingency management, and cognitive restruc-

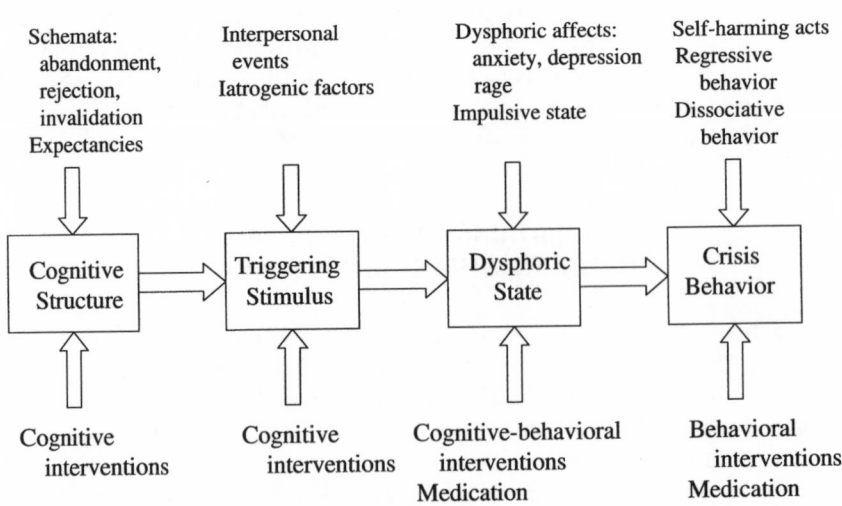

FIGURE 9.1. Behavioral sequence leading to self-harm and targets for change.

turing. Cognitive interventions led to greater improvement in parasuicidal behavior, experience and expression of anger, social role functioning, and greater retention in treatment, fewer and shorter inpatient admissions, and improved employment status. Differences were not found for levels of depression, hopelessness, or suicidal ideation. Unfortunately, not all members of the control group received treatment, a situation that substantially favors dialectical behavior therapy (Piper & Joyce, 2001). Follow-up 6 months later showed that patients who received dialectical behavior therapy were significantly better than controls on anger, anxiety, social adjustment, and work performance, although these effects were less marked after 1 year (Linehan, Heard, & Armstrong, 1993). Linehan and colleagues (Linehan, Tutek, Heard, & Armstrong, 1994) concluded that 1 year of dialectical behavior therapy achieves some symptomatic improvement, but it is not sufficient—patients are still miserable and core self and interpersonal problems remain.

The treatment looks promising, however, and the results have been replicated (Koons et al., 2001; Linehan et al., 1999), although the total number of patients treated is still small. It is not clear, however, that dialectical behavior therapy is a comprehensive treatment for borderline personality disorder. Limited attention is paid to interpersonal pathology and to the integration required to promote more adaptive interpersonal and self systems. The method is also labor-intensive; patients received 3½ hours of therapy each week for 1 year and thus may not be suitable for routine clinical practice (Davidson & Tyrer, 1996). Nevertheless, studies of dialectic behavior therapy point to the value of cognitive-behavioral interventions in promoting behavioral stability and reducing parasuicidal behavior.

This conclusion is supported by other studies. A case study evaluation of a 10-session treatment of borderline personality disorder showed that all three patients improved in target problems (Davidson & Tyrer, 1996). Perris (1994) reported on a similar approach that sought to address dysfunctional self and interpersonal cognitions in 13 patients. Treatment was tailored to the individual and lasted approximately 2 years. As with the Linehan and colleagues study, premature termination was low, and parasuicidal behavior and hospital admissions decreased. Increased social functioning observed at termination showed further improvement at a 2-year follow-up.

One interesting application of a cognitive approach provided patients with a manual covering problem-solving strategies, basic cognitive techniques to manage emotions and negative thinking, and relapse prevention strategies (Evans et al., 1999). Compared with treatment as usual, the treated group reported fewer suicidal acts and lower self-rated depression. Given that the intervention only took an average of 2.7 treatment sessions, the results are promising. Other studies also point to the value of a skill-building approach in treating social skills deficits, communication problems, social anxiety (Piper & Joyce, 2001), and improving parasuicidal behavior and depression in patients hospitalized for suicide attempts (Lieberman & Eckman, 1981).

These studies suggest that cognitive-behavioral interventions are useful in achieving behavioral stability, reducing parasuicidal and impulsive behavior, and improving affect regulation and impulse control. The destabilizing effects of emotional arousal suggest that exploration of issues that evoke intense feelings such as trauma, abandonment, and deprivation in patients with (1) histories of extreme adversity, (2) limited capacity to relate to others, (3) difficulty using therapist support, and (4) limited ability to regulate and contain affects or "self-soothe" should be deferred until stability has been achieved and affect tolerance and regulation improves. It is also important to manage emotional arousal because intense emotions, especially anxiety, can adversely affect the treatment alliance. These considerations apply to all personality patterns. The destabilizing aspects of emotional arousal are most apparent in patients with emotional dysregulation and dissocial traits. With the inhibited pattern, however, early exploration of trauma and neglect can similarly exacerbate problems by intensifying despondency and despair.

Functions of Self-Harm

The management of deliberate self-harm is shaped by assumptions about its functions and causes. A crucial issue is whether these acts are primarily motivated by the need to achieve interpersonal goals or attempts to change intolerable dysphoric states. This distinction colors attitudes toward self-harm and determines treatment strategies. The assumption that self-harm is motivated by hostility, attention seeking, or the need to control and manipulate others is likely to lead to an early focus on motives and the interpersonal aspects of these behaviors. It is also likely to encourage a more confrontational stance. The assumption of interpersonal motivation also encourages a focus on the overall disorder and underlying dynamics rather than on the behaviors themselves. On the other hand, the assumption that these behaviors are primarily attempts to terminate intolerable feelings is more likely to evoke a supportive response and a specific focus on these behaviors and on finding alternative ways to handle feelings.

Given these different assumptions, it is not surprising that there is disagreement over whether it is best to adopt a general focus on the disorder or a specific focus on self-harming behavior. Psychodynamic approaches often focus more generally on the overall disorder and the motives, processes, and structures that are assumed to underlie these acts (Clarkin et al., 1999; Kernberg, 2001). Similarly, the interpersonal approach of Benjamin (1996) considers these behaviors to be manifestations of underlying dynamics—the recreation of a particular version of incest that involved pleasure and pain, helplessness and love, loneliness and intimacy. In contrast, cognitive-behavioral treatments tend to focus on specific self-harming behavior and the factors that initiate and reinforce these acts (Evans et al., 1999; Linehan, 1993; Linehan et al., 1991).

Given the considerable differences between these approaches, it is important to be explicit about the model of self-harming behavior that guides treatment. Unfortunately, there is limited empirical evidence on whether a specific or general focus is most effective. Clinical observation, however, suggests that acts of deliberate self-harm are primarily attempts to change feeling states, although they may also serve other functions. Many patients who cut themselves, for example, report feeling better once the blood begins to flow. Linehan (1993) expressed this view clearly by stating that deliberate self-harm is adaptive—that is, it is the best way that the patient has identified to reduce distress. The approach proposed here adopts this position: it assumes that the immediate purpose of deliberate self-harm is *to regulate affects and alleviate anger, anxiety, guilt, or emotional pain* (Suyemoto, 1998; see also Kemperman, Russ, & Shearin, 1997).

Self-harm reduces dysphoria in several ways. For some patients, self-inflicted injury produces relief and an emotional high. As one patient noted, "Cutting is like taking a good dose of sublingual Ativan." Such actions are not usually painful, although for a few patients the physical pain they do experience may be useful in blocking emotional pain. The relief produced has promoted suggestions that the opiate antagonist naltrexone may be successful in blocking these effects. Unfortunately, this possibility has not been evaluated in controlled trials, although two reports suggest that it may be useful (McGee, 1997; Sonne, Rubey, Brady, Malcolm, & Morris, 1996). Self-harming acts also create a sense of being in control of intense feelings and situations. One patient stated: "Everything is about control of feelings—of not feeling anything. Cutting, overdosing, blacking things out, trying to keep things in boxes, street drugs—they are all about *not* feeling." These acts also help to organize chaotic and disorganized thoughts and alleviate feelings of emptiness and despondency. For some individuals, dysphoria is reduced because self-mutilation is a form of self-punishment that lessens guilt or self-directed anger. In these cases, guilt increases to the point that it is intolerable, and self-harm then produces relief. At the same time, these acts are often a source of considerable conflict—they are deeply satisfying and, at the same time, a source of shame. The self-punishing aspect of self-mutilation reflects the tendency of most personality disordered patients (except those with dissocial traits) to turn anger against the self. This self-punishing tendency may be due to conflicts about expressing anger, fears of retribution, or fears of the anger getting out of control. The self-sacrificial aspect of this tendency may create countertransference problems for clinicians who get drawn into acting out the patient's anger.

Although emphasis is placed on the adaptive, affect-regulating functions of deliberate self-harm, other factors may also contribute to these actions. As Kernberg (1984; Clarkin et al., 1999) noted, anger and aggression may play a role. However, it is useful to focus initially on the affect-regulating function. The therapist's acknowledgment that self-harm has a purpose is, in itself, reassuring and validating (Linehan, 1993), for it offers a different explanation from the ones that patients offer to themselves or are offered by other mental health professionals. The acknowledgment reduces the self-criticism and self-loathing that increases dysphoria, and enhances the alliance by aligning the therapist with the patient, avoiding the polarization that readily occurs when self-harm is attributed to such motives as control and attention seeking. Once the patient is freed from the need to justify such actions, change becomes a possibility. Deferring the exploration of interpersonal factors contributing to self-harm until an effective alliance has been established also reduces the risk of the therapist being seen as critical. This strategy is particularly important in the early stages of treatment when the alliance is being used to achieve containment and stability. However, patients *are* confronted with the consequences of their actions, but the discussion occurs in the context of support and validation.

Stages of Change

The final component of this approach to the treatment of deliberate self-harm is the *stages of change model*, used to (1) identify problem behaviors and establish a commitment to change, (2) explore the behavioral sequence leading to self-harm, (3) develop alternatives to self-harm and more effective ways to manage dysphoria, and (4) generalize and maintain the new learning. However, to deal with the immediate problems created by self-harm, the stage model is modified by limiting the initial exploration to the identification of immediate triggers of dysphoria and self-harm, followed by an active focus on reducing the self-harming behavior and the dysphoria. Direct attention is paid to these acts whenever they occur because they are distressing, have serious consequences for the individual, and disrupt treatment. Once a measure of control is achieved, attention moves to exploring and changing (1) the maladaptive schemata activated by triggering events that initiate and maintain these behaviors, and (2) any cognitive styles that contribute to the process. Subsequently, attention moves to dealing with the sequelae of psychosocial adversity.

REDUCING AND CONTROLLING PARASUICIDAL BEHAVIOR

Problem Identification

Problem identification and the establishment of a commitment to change may seem unnecessary with obviously maladaptive behaviors such as cutting or overdosing. Denial, however, is a major problem: Many patients do not fully acknowledge, even to themselves, that such acts are harmful. Instead, the acts are often considered natural and effective ways to cope with distress. For example, one patient argued that it was all right to cut because it did not hurt and she felt better afterwards. She saw no reason to stop because it did not cause lasting harm. She maintained this position, despite the limited movement in her arms due to scarring and tendon damage. Hence it cannot be assumed that patients want to relinquish these behaviors without first exploring their perceptions of these acts and their commitment to change. Patients are sometimes reluctant to commit to change because of the relief and feeling of control that comes from deliberate self-harm. This reluctance should be acknowledged and discussed. When the negative consequences of self-harm are denied, a cost–benefit analysis of the behavior as discussed in Chapter 4, may help to change perceptions by gently highlighting discrepancies in the patient's account.

Exploration: Defining the Behavioral Sequence

Once a commitment to change is established, no matter how tenuous, the next step is to begin delineating the sequence of events leading to self-harm, giving particular attention to triggering stimuli (see Figure 9.1). This exploration is usually combined with behavioral interventions. The immediate goal is not to terminate these acts but to delay their onset and reduce their frequency.

Triggering events usually activate maladaptive schemata such as rejection, "badness," and abandonment that originated in adversity. Patients do not often fully recognize triggering events, so it is usually necessary to examine specific acts of self-harm in detail to identify triggers, as illustrated by the following vignette:

> The patient with inhibited traits (DSM-IV diagnosis: avoidant personality disorder) had a history of frequent overdoses associated with intense, overwhelming dysphoria. Attempts to uncover factors that triggered these states were unsuccessful. The patient consistently maintained that the distress "just happened," and he was irritated by the therapist's attempts to understand the underlying details.
>
> He began one session by revealing that he had nearly taken an overdose the previous day because one of these episodes had occurred again. When asked when the event started and where he was at the time, the patient said that he had felt fine until he attended a discussion group at a local community center. During the discussion he suddenly felt overwhelmed. He had no idea why. Initially the therapist's attempts to explore the event were rejected. Gradually, the patient recalled that the group leader had suggested that everyone identify a positive feature about him- or herself. The patient suddenly felt anxious because he could not think of anything. Fur-

ther discussion revealed that he also felt that other members of the group would find it easy to identify good qualities about themselves and that they would know that he must be struggling because there was nothing positive about him. He felt criticized and rejected.

It was only by focusing on the details of this event that the trigger became apparent. Further exploration led the patient to recall that the leader's comment triggered an overwhelming sense that he was bad. He went on to add that he had thought of himself in this way throughout his life. As a child, he had decided that he must be bad for his mother to treat him so abusively.

This vignette illustrates the value of a detailed analysis of specific events—something that many patients try to avoid. Patients who have difficulty identifying triggers may find it useful to keep a log recording self-harming acts and accompanying thoughts and feelings. Sometimes a stepwise approach is useful; the patient begins by keeping a record of self-harming behaviors, which is extended to include thoughts and feelings only when he or she has become more comfortable with the process.

A preliminary understanding that self-harm is a response to a dysphoric state that is triggered by specific interpersonal events begins to impose meaning on events that may have seemed unrelated and inexplicable previously. This new sense of meaning helps to consolidate the commitment to change because it implies that these behaviors can be identified, controlled, and changed. Identification of triggers may also provide information about factors that reinforce self-harm and suggest alternative ways to react to the triggering events themselves. As the sequence leading to self-harm becomes clearer, it is useful to work with the patient to construct a simple diagram showing the links between triggering events, dysphoria, and self-harm. This diagram helps the patient examine the sequence more objectively and reinforces the point that the sequence can be modified by aborting some link in it before emotions get out of control (e.g., use of distracting behaviors).

These discussions of the sequence provide an opportunity to integrate a psychoeducational component into treatment by introducing the idea that self-harming behavior (including bingeing or alcohol abuse) may occur because patients need to be soothed and cannot identify any other way to end their pain or distress. Presenting this idea builds the alliance, validates, reduces self-derogation, and improves self-esteem. At some point, it is also useful to explain how the emotional, cognitive, and behavioral components of crises interact to produce an escalating state. This information, along with an understanding of the behavioral sequence, helps patients understand the reasons behind specific interventions. It is also useful to distinguish between *ideas* of self-harm and self-harming *acts*, because ideas of self-harm usually continue long after the behavior has ceased.

There is some suggestion that self-harming ideation has a heritable component, whereas self-harming behavior is largely learned (Jang, Livesley, Vernon, & Jackson, 1996). Hence patients need to learn to tolerate thoughts of self-harm and accept that they do not need to act on them.

Preliminary Interventions to Reduce Self-Harming Behavior

Achieving lasting change in self-harming behavior depends on finding alternative ways to handle affects and impulses and changing the cognitive and affective structures that contribute to these acts. It is rarely sufficient merely to block such actions without finding alternatives, or to deal only with the behavior without addressing contributing factors. Nevertheless, early in treatment, simple behavioral interventions such as *distraction, substitution, avoidance, reducing ego-syntonicity of self-harming acts,* and *promoting adaptive help-seeking behavior* may reduce the frequency of such actions, thereby providing an opportunity to focus on the cognitive and emotional processes underlying self-harming behavior and on developing more effective coping strategies. Although each intervention may be comparatively ineffectual, a combination of interventions, often in conjunction with medication, may produce modest changes.

The success of behavioral interventions depends on the quality of the therapeutic relationship; in each session time should be spent on general interventions. Success also depends on being clear with the patient that the goal is not to eliminate these behaviors immediately but to delay their onset and reduce their frequency as a step toward replacing them with more effective and less harmful actions. It is unreasonable to expect longstanding self-harming habits to stop abruptly. (The exception, of course, is with life-threatening acts.) These modest goals are readily attainable at a time when therapeutic successes are needed to consolidate the alliance and build motivation.

Distraction

With some patients, a distracting activity reduces the probability of enacting deliberate self-harm. Various types of activities can be used for this purpose, such as engaging in pleasant or absorbing activities, changing sensory input (e.g., listening to soothing music), or refocusing attention to more pleasant images or thoughts. Once the therapist has introduced the idea of distracting attention from the self-harming pattern, it becomes a creative exercise to identify activities that are congenial to the patient. This focus provides an opportunity for collaborative work early in treatment and introduces the idea of problem solving. For some patients, exercise reduces tension and eases the urge to harm themselves. With others, the distractions may range from listening to music to watching romantic movies. Any occasion when an episode of self-harm was delayed or aborted should be considered a success and used to reinforce the idea that these feelings and acts can be controlled.

Distracting activities are also useful in dealing with other forms of self-harm, such as eating problems or drug misuse and to control rage or violent behavior. For example, a patient with an eating disorder and personality disorder may have the urge to vomit for about 30 minutes after eating. Engaging in distracting activities during this time diverts attention from feelings of fullness. One patient found that playing computer games was a useful distraction; another did crossword puzzles.

Substitution

With self-harming behaviors such as cutting, burning, or hitting, substitute actions can sometimes be identified that also reduce tension (Rosen & Thomas, 1984). Often, a certain amount of ingenuity is required in working with the patient to identify possible alternatives. Many of these alternatives involve inflicting pain that is less damaging than burning or cutting. One simple method that occasionally reduces the urge to cut is to hold ice cubes in both hands until they melt. Some patients note that the method is more effective if the ice cubes are dyed red with food coloring, because this gives the impression of blood, which reduces tension even more effectively. Presumably the red coloration is a conditioned stimulus that is associated with tension reduction.

Avoidance

With a few compliant patients it may be possible to reduce self-inflicted injuries by taking simple steps to ensure that instruments that could be used for this purpose are not readily available. For example, many patients carry knives, razor blades, or can tops so that they always have something available with which to cut themselves, should the need arise. As the therapeutic relationship improves, it is sometimes possible to encourage these patients to give these articles to the therapist for safekeeping or to stop the habit altogether.

The strategy of avoidance may also help when self-harm is triggered by a specific situation or event that the patient can avoid. For example, one patient could not pass a store that sold knives without going inside and taking a knife from a display to cut herself. For a while, she reduced the frequency of cutting simply by avoiding these stores. This reduction in the target behavior afforded the opportunity to work on ways to reduce the dysphoria; previously, these events had disrupted treatment and prevented this focus. Similarly, individuals who get the urge to commit suicide by jumping off balconies in shopping centers or off bridges may be encouraged to avoid these situations. For example, if they have to cross a bridge, they should do so using public transport. Again, the objective is not to terminate these behaviors but rather to reduce their frequency so that treatment is not always focused on crisis resolution.

Reducing Ego-Syntonicity

As noted earlier, acts of deliberate self-harm are often ego-syntonic: They are felt to be natural ways to reduce distress, a belief that is supported by the fact that many self-injuries are painless at the time. Change depends on making these acts ego-dystonic. Exploration of these behaviors and discussion of the way the patient thinks other people perceive them and the way that they would react to someone who hurt themselves in this way help the patient to view these acts more objectively. This process can be assisted by wondering why minor accidental injuries hurt, whereas self-inflicted injuries do not. One patient, for example, noted that when she tried to take the blade out of a disposable razor, she accidentally cut herself on the plastic—and the cut hurt. She then cut herself deliberately without feeling any pain. Questioning these experiences helps to make these behaviors slightly more ego-dystonic. This dissonance is increased by encouraging patients to ask themselves, the next time they cut themselves, why it does not hurt—something that is often difficult to do without feeling pain. The first inkling that an action is no longer ego-syntonic should be highlighted. For one patient who had cut herself for many years, this moment occurred when she briefly "felt sick at the idea" of cutting herself. The therapist noted that this seemed to be a new feeling and wondered what the patient thought about it.

Adaptive Help-Seeking Behavior

Early in treatment it is often helpful to encourage patients to seek help at the beginning of a crisis, before feelings become uncontrollable. Various alternatives should be explored, such as contacting a relative or friend for support, contacting the therapist, attending an emergency room or crisis clinic, or seeking support from community groups. As with other interventions a graded approach can be adopted, in which patients are encouraged to seek help the moment they feel that their emotions are getting out of control and that they are likely to harm themselves. Over time, the interval between the onset of the dysphoria and the help seeking can be increased until the patient is able to wait until the next scheduled appointment.

   Interventions to promote more adaptive ways to seek help include providing education about how to act in a crisis. Many patients cannot communicate distress or ask for help in ways that elicit positive responses from others. Information on more effective help-seeking behavior is often useful (Layden et al., 1993). Emotionally dysregulated or borderline patients, for example, tend to act in a demanding way that others find aversive. They are also inconsistent: They demand help while, at the same time, protesting that it is not likely to be forthcoming or rejecting help that is offered. The inhibited person often reacts by withdrawal and fails to communicate distress effectively; the more dissocial individual reacts angrily, causing others to withdraw. In many cases, patients try to control others or manipulate them into providing help, because they believe that they cannot trust others to help without using coercion. They are also unaware that they repel others by the way they elicit support. Rather than demanding help, they need to learn to *ask* for it; rather than angrily accusing others of never helping, they need to learn to express their needs more openly and less insistently; and rather than withdrawing, they need to learn to reveal a little about themselves. Essentially these changes involve learning how to communicate effectively and relinquishing the assumption that others know what is needed without being told.

In the long run, the effects of behavioral interventions are limited. Early in treatment, however, they are useful in helping to contain self-harm, and later they form a small but valuable component of self-management skills. Initially, they are most likely to be effective if simple, small steps are taken to achieve control. Complex behaviors involving multiple steps overwhelm highly aroused and regressed patients and also evoke underlying passivity—patients may not use them because they are "too much trouble" or seem unlikely to work. Smaller steps seem less effort-intensive and help to ensure experiences of success. For example, one patient with emotional dysregulation (i.e., borderline pathology) and major eating problems was unable to maintain adequate food intake. Suggestions about diet were not effective—the patient did not feel sufficiently hopeful even to try them. Progress was made only when small steps were taken to improve food intake. Initially these steps included using an alarm clock to remind her to eat. When a routine of six small meals had been established, attention was paid to diet—to ensuring that different food groups were included in the diet. Later the focus expanded to planning balanced meals. This incremental strategy worked, whereas other interventions had failed.

CONTROLLING AND REGULATING DYSPHORIA

A second approach to treating self-harming behavior is to promote more adaptive ways of managing dysphoria by increasing affect tolerance and affect regulation capacities. The assumption that deficits in emotional control arise from genetic predisposition and psychosocial adversity implies a combination of psychosocial interventions, including skill training (see Linehan, 1993) and medication.

Identifying Emotions

It is difficult to learn to tolerate and regulate emotions unless they can be recognized and labeled. Many patients find this task difficult; many emotional states are complex mixtures of feelings that are difficult to tease apart, and these patients have a tendency to move rapidly from impulse to action without noticing or thinking about the feelings involved. More fundamentally, this inability may be part of a more general failure to develop an intuitive understanding of human nature.

The skill of identifying and labeling emotions is often taught as a separate exercise, with the aid of handouts. Although this method is useful, it is often not sufficient. It is more effective to clarify and label feelings, as they emerge in treatment, by slowing down the therapeutic interaction and encouraging patients to reflect on their experiences. In this way they learn to recognize the many ways that they avoid, suppress, or block feelings. This approach also allows the therapist to regulate emotional expression. By taking the time to inquire about feelings, the therapist models tolerance of both positive and negative feelings. This tolerance often contrasts with previous experiences, in which patients' feelings were criticized or dismissed, and validates and strengthens patients' confidence in the authenticity of their experience. The process of clarifying and differentiating emotions also promotes a more global differentiation of self-experience—an important contributor to the long-term objective of developing a more adaptive self system.

Psychoeducation about Emotions

The process of identifying and labeling emotions and discussing how the individual handles feelings is an opportunity to discuss their value and adaptive significance. Many individuals with personality problems believe that feelings, especially negative feelings, are bad. This impression can be partly corrected by providing information on the benefits of both positive and negative feelings—how feelings enrich experience and contribute to interpersonal relationships and the attainment of personal goals. The idea that emotions may be useful is a new idea for many patients and sheds light on the maladaptive relationships that led to dysfunctional ideas about emotions. Information about the genetic basis of emotions, and that emotions play an important role in communication and social interaction, also helps to build tolerance.

Affect and Distress Tolerance

Most individuals with personality disorder have difficulty tolerating feelings. In individuals with the emotional dysregulation pattern, this intolerance largely involves negative feelings. In some cases, individuals are almost phobic about negative affects. In those with the inhibited or schizoid–avoidant traits, intolerance extends to all kinds of affects. Lasting change depends on building affect tolerance and altering the cognitions associated with affect arousal as part of a broader strategy of promoting self-acceptance. Acquisition of affect tolerance begins by encouraging the patient to examine feelings as they occur in treatment. Attention is drawn to positive and negative changes in emotional state, and the therapeutic relationship is used to help the individual "hold" and tolerate the feelings involved.

The cognitions associated with emotional arousal often contribute to intolerance by amplifying distress. Patients frequently tell themselves that they cannot stand their feelings any longer, they will never go away, anything would be better than what is happening, and they could not stand feeling this way again. Many patients also catastrophize about the situation and their reactions, whereas others ruminate over problems and experiences as if a tape describing painful or embarrassing events were continually playing. These thinking habits become so familiar that they are barely recognized or taken as normal. Change requires increased awareness of how such self-talk increases distress. Patients need to understand that anyone who talked to themselves in these ways would feel upset, and that such thoughts undermine self-esteem and any sense of mastery and control.

Increased tolerance depends on challenging such maladaptive thoughts as "I cannot tolerate feeling this way, and these feelings are never going to go away" or "These feelings are going to get worse and something terrible is going to happen" and replacing them with more adaptive versions such as, "These feelings are terrible, but they have occurred many times before, they do not last long, and I have always survived them" or "I feel bad but the chances of a disaster occurring are not very high, and if a disaster does occur, I will cope." Cognitive restructuring may be hindered by the difficulty some patients have in recalling times when they were not dysphoric, or occasions in which they coped with these feelings successfully. To challenge these beliefs, the therapist often has to act as the memory for the patient by recalling how he or she coped with similar experiences in the past.

Affect Regulation

The second set of interventions for improving self-management involves developing skills to regulate emotions that compensate for the regulatory deficits. Many of the behavioral interventions used to manage self-harm are also useful in modulating emotions. Individuals with anger problems as part of either the emotional dysregulation or dissocial pattern may also find these techniques helpful when anger is the major cause of dyscontrol.

The key to successful application of these techniques is for patients to use them as soon as problematic emotions are aroused, before they become so preoccupied with the intensity of their feelings that they cannot use the interventions. Therefore, patients need to identify the situations that are likely to evoke intense reactions and employ these techniques before feelings escalate. Initially, many patients have difficulty applying this strategy, because they cannot spot problems early enough or they deny that the cycle is starting again.

Promoting Self-Soothing Skills

One of the primary ways that people regulate feelings is by doing pleasurable things. Simple things such as giving oneself a treat or listening to a favorite piece of music can settle and soothe the self because they are pleasurable and familiar. Individuals with personality disorder have usually failed to learn how to take self-soothing actions; indeed they often feel guilty or undeserving if they do something enjoyable for themselves, and they typically resist the idea of managing feelings in this way. Considerable encouragement is needed to help them accept the idea that it is permissible to do enjoyable things for themselves. It is also helpful for such patients to recognize the lack of compassion that they show toward themselves and to contrast this lacuna with their concern for others. As with other interventions, self-soothing measures are more effective if used before feelings get too strong.

Grounding Techniques

Patients who experience intense panic-like anxiety and dissociative reactions, such as loss of contact with immediate reality, depersonalization, or derealization, can learn to thwart these responses by using grounding techniques (Baum, 1997). In these states, the panic creates a positive feedback loop in which intense anxiety leads to loss of contact with surroundings and a preoccupation with inner experience leading to further panic. It is often possible to settle the panic and the tendency to dissociate with a simple exercise that involves placing one's feet firmly on the ground, feeling a solid object, such as the arms of the chair, and concentrating on the texture and solidity of them, looking around and focusing on specific objects in the environment, and increasing abdominal breathing by placing one's arms around the back of the chair. These steps shift the patient's attention toward external stimuli and away from chaotic inner experience.

Grounding techniques are best introduced early in therapy and on an occasion when the patient begins to show dissociative behavior or describes a recent incident when he or she lost control and dissociated. The method is best explained by taking the patient through the different steps. Success depends on the quality of the treatment alliance, so that it is not helpful to introduce the technique when the alliance is impaired. The exercise is a useful way to initiate active collaborative work, and any success can be used to enhance the alliance and the patient's commitment to change.

In some cases it is constructive to involve significant others or friends who can take the patient through the different steps when he or she feels overwhelmed. Arranging for such support helps to ensure that the patient applies the technique in everyday situations. In the process, the patient is encouraged to collaborate with others. Incorporating significant others into treatment enables them to understand why crises occur and helps them to act supportively. The task also gives both parties something to do when problems arise, which counters the helplessness that they often feel in these situations—a helplessness that only increases the patient's distress. This use of grounding exercises is illustrated by the following case:

> Sheila, who had been severely abused in childhood, became intensely distressed and dissociated whenever she saw someone with a specific facial characteristic that reminded her of her abuser. In this state, she often engaged in serious self-harm. These episodes commonly occurred in public situations, such as busy streets and shopping malls, and they usually resulted in the patient being taken by ambulance to the nearest emergency room. These reactions even occurred when her partner or a friend was with her; the other person usually became alarmed about what was happening and enmeshed in the panic.
>
> In therapy, Sheila was taught grounding exercises. These were effective in containing distress and dissociative behavior in treatment, but Sheila could not use them elsewhere due to the intensity and speed of emotional arousal. Sheila thought that if her partner understood what happened to her at these times and was aware of the exercise, he would be able to coach her. This idea was implemented. Whenever Sheila encountered a trigger, she told him, and he would promptly encourage her to ground herself by placing her feet firmly on the ground, holding onto something solid, such as a handle or rail, and focusing on events around her. On many occasions, he was able to talk her through these episodes and abort negative outcomes. They continued this practice until eventually the patient was able to use the method without help. The transition occurred when Sheila was in an elevator alone and the lights went out and the elevator stopped. This reminded her of childhood events when she was locked in a dark closet and abused. She began to panic, but then she recalled her partner's voice and was able to grasp a cold metal rail in the elevator and use this to ground herself. She told herself that the situation was different from the past and that she was alone and there was no one there to harm her.

Skill Development

Improvement in self-regulatory skills may be achieved using specific training modules or by integrating skill development into the treatment process. When the patient is attending a day treatment or partial hospitalization program, it is convenient to use skill-training groups, provided steps are taken to ensure integration with other components of treatment. In individual treatment, skill development is seamlessly incorporated into the overall treatment process.

A brief consideration of common skill deficits suggests the need for affect management, including stress and anger management, and interpersonal skills development, including communication training, social skills training, and assertiveness training. Here the main concern is the management of emotions. A common component of many methods used to develop these skills is relaxation training, which provides a useful introduction to other interventions.

Relaxation Exercises. Most patients benefit from relaxation training. However, many of the techniques used in cognitive and behavioral therapy, such as progressive relaxation (a systematic tensing and relaxing of muscle groups), are too involved for use with patients with severe personality disorder, especially early in treatment. Such exercises require considerable practice at home with the aid of audiotapes. Most patients are not sufficiently motivated or convinced of the exercise's value to practice regularly; moreover, progressive relaxation often evokes the paradoxical fear of losing control. A simpler technique that is easily incorporated into a treatment session is breath training: slow abdominal breathing, with attention focused on exhalation. As patients breathe out, they are instructed to say a single word, such as *calm* or *relax*, and to let themselves go loose. Care is necessary in choosing this word, because many patients heard words such as *relax* when being abused.

This exercise works well because it produces almost immediate benefits while evoking minimal fears of losing control. Any difficulties that are experienced can be discussed, and the therapist and patient can collaborate in identifying solutions. Later in treatment, following the establishment of a more collaborative working relationship and stronger motivation, more systematic exercises can be introduced, if needed. One advantage of the technique is that it is easy to use in everyday situations. It can also be used to manage other feelings. Patients who get into rages with others because of assumed slights, jealousy, or rejection can learn to control these feelings using this approach. The intent is to demonstrate that feelings *can* be controlled as a preliminary step toward building a greater sense of self-efficacy.

Attention Control Skills. Affect regulation requires the ability to shift attention away from unpleasant thoughts rather than ruminating on them. Control can be improved by learning to shift attention away from a painful, triggering stimulus and toward a more pleasant, relaxing stimulus. The exercise is a version of systematic desensitization (Wolpe, 1958) that builds on the relaxation exercise discussed previously. Systematic desensitization uses short exposure to minimal amounts of an anxiety-evoking stimulus, followed by relaxation to control anxiety. The purpose is to extinguish fear or other distressing responses. Here the technique is used to show that emotions can be controlled and to build affect tolerance and affect regulation. Later the technique will be used to desensitize fear reactions to traumatic stimuli.

The first step is to identify the stimulus that triggers an escalating emotional state or dissociative reaction. Typical stimuli are memories of traumatic incidents, words or phrases used by an abuser, interpersonal events that activate maladaptive schemata, and losses. When memories evoke uncontrollable emotions, it is helpful to identify components of the stimulus that evoke less intense reactions, rather like the hierarchy used to desensitize phobias. Next, the patient is asked to identify a pleasant scene or memory that is easily visualized and recalled. This image is used to help the patient relax. While relaxed, the patient is asked to shift attention to the triggering stimulus. As affect begins to rise, the patient is asked to shift attention back to the pleasant stimuli and helped to focus on it and relax until the affect settles. Initially, attention is diverted to the pleasant stimulus as soon as distressing emotions are aroused. This may only be a matter of seconds. Over time, this interval is increased, while keeping affect arousal within tolerable limits. When relaxation occurs, the cycle is repeated. On the first occasion it is useful to complete three or four shifts in attention (this takes about 10 minutes). Over time, more traumatic stimuli are introduced.

Although the intervention can be practiced at home, it is helpful to introduce it during a treatment session. Once the patient understands the exercise and has experienced several successful shifting sequences, practice between sessions can be encouraged and the method taught to significant others. The value of this technique is that it is gradual and patients are exposed to minimal anxiety. For this reason, the exercise should not be introduced when the patient is in a highly aroused state. It also helps if the exercise is introduced when the patient has described an incident wherein he or she was distressed by a flashback or other triggering stimulus. The technique is then introduced as a way to control these feelings.

The exercise is interactive and involves the patient working collaboratively with the therapist. For this reason, the exercise should only be introduced when the alliance is positive. Reviewing the experience immediately afterward provides an opportunity to use a successful outcome to strengthen the alliance and the patient's motivation for change, as illustrated by the following vignette:

> The patient, an unemployed woman in her early 30s, living alone, presented with acute distress and dysphoria that had been especially intense during the previous 6 months, although she had longstanding dysthymic tendencies. She had a long history of deliberate self-harm, labile moods, chronic thoughts of suicide, inability to maintain relationships, and a chaotic employment history. She showed features of emotional dysregulation and inhibitedness. The DSM-IV diagnoses were dependent and borderline personality disorders. She said that she became more depressed after an incident that had occurred 8 months earlier, in which someone who lived nearby deliberately killed her dog. Whenever the patient thought about her dog or passed the place where the dog was killed, she became acutely distressed. Assessment was spread over two sessions and a treatment plan developed. The patient placed high priority on learning to cope with her feelings about the incident. Over the subsequent few weeks, the immediate distress settled and the patient began to form a satisfactory treatment alliance.
>
> In one session she presented in a relatively calm state but noted that the event continued to bother her. Indeed earlier in the day she had thought about it and became very distressed. She said that she could not continue in this way. This seemed an opportune moment to introduce the attention control exercise. The procedure was explained and the patient asked if she would like to try this approach. She was encouraged to imagine a pleasant scene and taught simple relaxation measures. When she said that she was feeling relaxed, the therapist suggested that she shift her attention to her dog. Almost immediately she felt intense distress and was asked to shift back to the pleasant scene. The therapist had to talk about the pleasant scene and ask the patient to concentrate on it and describe the image for a few minutes before the patient could focus on it. When she felt relaxed again, she was asked to imagine the incident. Again affect arousal was intense and rapid, whereupon she was asked to shift to the pleasant image. This procedure was repeated several times, until she could shift attention more readily and tolerate thinking about the incident for a few seconds longer. Subsequently the dialogue between patient and therapist went as follows:

THERAPIST: What was that like?

PATIENT: I really enjoyed relaxing. I didn't think I could do it.

THERAPIST: You had not tried relaxing in this way before?

PATIENT: No. I didn't think I could do it. I was surprised ... I relaxed.

THERAPIST: So we have just done something that you hadn't thought possible?

PATIENT: Yes ... it was good ... I think I'm going to try this at home.

THERAPIST: If you do, you will probably find that you will be able to do it more easily with practice.

PATIENT: That would really help.

THERAPIST: It also seemed that you were able to shift your mind away from your dog.

PATIENT: I was really surprised about that. I never thought it possible (*surprised tone to voice*).

THERAPIST: And you were able to control your feelings about your dog.

PATIENT: I was, wasn't I? I didn't think that I would ever be able to think about my dog without bursting into tears. I can't even say *dog* without breaking down. I never thought that I would be able to say *dog* without getting upset ... Oh! I've just said dog three times and I'm not upset ... and I have just said *dog* again.

THERAPIST: So this is a change for you.

PATIENT: Mmm-mmm! A big change! It can't be possible.

THERAPIST: It seems that we have been able to work together on this just now, and we were able to find a way that helped you to learn to control your feelings—something that you didn't think possible before.

PATIENT: I didn't think it was possible. I think that I am going to try this at home.

THERAPIST: That would help you get better at controlling your feelings, but you may want to concentrate on imagining the pleasant scene and learning to relax before thinking about your dog and the way he died.

This incident illustrates the implementation of some of the basic ideas of this approach to treating personality disorder. The vignette demonstrates the therapist's careful attention to the general therapeutic strategies as well as the application of a specific intervention. The intervention was only used when the alliance was satisfactory. Subsequently, the therapist used the modest change experienced by the patient to comment on the way the patient and therapist had worked together to bring about the change to foster hope and motivation. Within the framework being discussed, this aspect of therapeutic interaction is as important as the specific benefits derived from the intervention. The example also illustrates how an affect-regulating strategy is applied: minimal affect arousal was allowed to occur before the patient was encouraged to shift attention. This aspect is important (1) because patients are afraid of these feelings, which easily spiral out of control, and (2) to ensure a successful outcome for these early interventions. This success was achieved by focusing on small steps and modest change.

MORE DETAILED EXPLORATION

As crises and incidents of self-harm decrease and emotional control increases it becomes possible to use the A-B-C model (see Chapter 4) to explore, in more detail, the behavioral sequence that leads to dysphoric states and self-harming acts. This more precise focus requires a detailed evaluation of current environmental factors that initiate and maintain maladaptive behavior and the maladaptive schemata contributing to these problems.

Focusing on Consequences

Relatively early in treatment, it is useful to explore the way self-harm affects the person and his or her relationship with others. Most patients are oblivious to these issues; the self-harming acts are reinforced regularly by tension reduction, and the negative consequences are ignored or dismissed because they occur later. Change involves *reducing the positive reinforcement of self-harming acts and accentuating awareness of negative consequences*. This goal is achieved by examining the personal and interpersonal costs and benefits of these behaviors, as discussed in Chapter 4. Despite relief from distress, most patients feel embarrassed or guilty about these acts and berate themselves afterward. However, these distressing reactions have little impact because they occur too long after the self-harm has occurred, and they may not be fully acknowledged. Nevertheless, discrepancies between initial relief and future consequences can be highlighted to increase awareness of longer-term effects on self-esteem and other feelings about the self.

Similarly, the impact of self-harming behavior on relationships with others is only partially acknowledged. Negative reactions are usually taken as further evidence that people do not care or understand. Once the reactions of others are understood and accepted, however, they become a further incentive to change. The issue can often be addressed when the patient mentions the reactions of family, friends, and emergency room staff to these acts. Patients are often puzzled and angry about the critical, and even hostile, reactions of others, including health-care professionals. This provides an opportunity to discuss the way patients' behavior affects others and influences the way others treat them. Comments such as the following extend the focus of therapy: "You are talking about how distressing it is when other people criticize and blame you for cutting yourself, and how they get angry with you rather than trying to understand and help. But if you hurt yourself, you make it easier for other people to hurt you. If you abuse yourself, you make it easier for others to abuse you." Discussing this topic begins to make patients aware of how they create the situations to which they react and lays the basis for exploring maladaptive interpersonal patterns (see Chapter 11).

An important part of focusing on consequences concerns the effects of self-harm on the treatment process. In Chapter 7 a hierarchy of interventions was proposed, in which safety issues take priority, followed by general treatment strategies and specific interventions. Suicidal threats and acts and deliberate self-harm often threaten the continuity of treatment. It is essential that the patient be made aware of these implications. An active focus on this issue is an important part of limit setting, which protects the treatment process and helps to strengthen the patient's ability to control deliberate self-harming acts.

Additional Contributing Factors

Exploration of the behavioral sequence underlying self-harm should include an evaluation of the role of current circumstances in initiating and maintaining maladaptive behavior. Identifying this component extends the analysis of the functions of self-harming behavior beyond the initial focus on affect regulation. Most self-harming actions are influenced by multiple factors that have a variety of reinforcing consequences. For many cases, increased attention and care from family, friends, and professionals satisfy dependency needs and create a sense of being cared for and even loved. These acts may also provide a vehicle for expressing underlying traits such as dependency and sensation seeking. The case discussed in Chapter 1 illustrated the multiple sources of reinforcement that maintain these acts. The immediate reinforcement for cutting was reduction of dysphoria—the patient felt better when the blood began to flow. She usually cut in a public place that brought a rapid response from security personnel, paramedics, and the police. This scenario satisfied dependency needs, and the ensuing chaos satisfied her need for excitement. The excitement was so important an element that the profound boredom she experienced following the cessation of these acts threatened treatment. Being strapped to a gurney by the paramedics and the attention she received in the emergency room produced a sense of containment that also reduced the dysphoria. Subsequent treatment further satisfied needs for care and attention.

For other patients, these acts are also vehicles for expressing anger and rage. The act becomes a way of punishing themselves or significant others for perceived failures, rejection, or harm. Thus *exploration of the functions of deliberate self-harm is a two-stage process.* The initial focus is on the affect-regulating function—improving regulation and control and building the alliance. Once progress has occurred in this area, attention can shift to other factors. This principle should not be followed slavishly, however, especially when there is considerable secondary gain involved in the self-harm. This point is illustrated by the following case.

The patient, a woman in her late 20s, who had attended several mental health programs for the treatment of borderline personality disorder for about 5 years, had been in treatment with her current therapist for about 9 months. In addition to emotional dysregulation, she also had anorexia nervosa. When assessed, she was in a decompensated and regressed state and found it difficult to organize her life on a day-to-day basis. She engaged in multiple high-risk activities, such as taking serious overdoses and walking on the tracks of a busy commuter line and on ledges of high buildings. The eating problems were serious, although the other forms of self-harm were more immediately life threatening.

Early interventions were largely cognitive-behavioral in nature, designed to reduce regression and introduce structure into daily activities, including regular mealtimes. Multiple methods were used to instill regular eating habits, such as working out meal plans in advance, setting an alarm clock to remind her of the next meal, and so on. Distraction techniques were used to control parasuicidal actions and to reduce the self-induced vomiting immediately after eating. Avoidance strategies were used to minimize her exposure to situations that evoked self-harm.

These strategies worked for a while. Her eating became more regular, her weight improved, body fat became more normal, and parasuicidal behavior decreased. Yet there was always an occasional problem, so that the therapist found it difficult to address additional issues. A meal would be "forgotten," and the patient would "collapse," as a result, usually in a public place, whereupon she would be taken to an emergency room. Frequent hospital admissions disrupted treatment, which was always dealing with the latest life-threatening crisis. These crises occurred, however, against a background of modest improvement. Every few months a relapse also occurred, and problems returned with their original ferocity. Limit setting that focused on the potentially serious consequences of these acts and their effects on treatment did not produce lasting change.

The patient began one session by saying that she was not eating and had lost several pounds and that her daily routine no longer existed. After discussing the problem and expressing concerns about the threats this situation posed for her health and treatment, the therapist focused on the treatment alliance and motivation for change. The therapist noted that the patient seemed very disappointed that so little lasting progress was being achieved and that everything was so difficult. This led the patient to comment that she was looking to her physicians for help and was prepared to do anything they recommended. The therapist noted that although the patient said that she was prepared to follow the recommendations of physicians responsible for her physical care, she was rarely able to follow their advice. The patient agreed but added that she would like to do so. When discussing this point, the therapist commented that although the patient said that she wanted to get well, there seemed to be another part of her that was not so sure.

This comment led the patient to reveal that she was afraid of getting better. Whenever her weight increased, she immediately thought that she would have to get a job. This was a great worry because she did not know what she wanted to do. A job would also bring her into contact with other people. Her previous experiences in employment had been painful, and she did not think that she could go through a similar experience again. Putting on weight also reminded her that her partner wanted a child. She was afraid of pregnancy, and she was worried that if she got better, her partner would make sexual demands that he did not make when she was underweight. The self-inflicted cuts also "put him off." Further discussion led her to recall that family and friends told her how much they loved her and cared about her when she was ill—something that they did not normally do. This made her feel special. For the first time in her life, she felt that other people really cared. A bit of her still longed for those expressions of love, and she wondered if she would receive them if she got well.

An understanding of the factors that reinforce self-harm is important in identifying the maladaptive schemata and interpersonal patterns that contribute to these acts. One goal, as already noted, is to increase the perceived costs and decrease the benefits of these acts and increase choice by identifying less maladaptive ways of satisfying needs and expressing traits. The elaboration of these factors begins to move therapy into the next phase of exploring and changing maladaptive interpersonal patterns and cognitive styles.

Reframing Triggering Situations

Many of the interventions discussed earlier were concerned with changing reactions to stimuli by regulating affects and impulses. An additional perspective on change is to modify the way triggering events are perceived and understood. Patients tend to assume that triggering situations are separate from the self, and that the ways in which they interpret these situations are natural responses that cannot be changed. Most resist the basic idea of cognitive therapy that the *interpretation* of an event, rather than the event itself, determines one's reactions to it. Over time, however, as reactivity recedes and trust in the therapist and treatment increases, the idea that events can be interpreted in different ways becomes more acceptable.

Opportunities to reframe the triggering situation depend on the nature of the trigger. When it is a stimulus associated with traumatic or abusive events, restructuring is less important than desensitization, an issue that is discussed in the next chapter. When the trigger is an interpersonal event, however, such as a perceived rejection, slight, humiliation, or abandonment, it may be possible not only to modify responses to the event but also to reframe the way the event is perceived. Change largely involves slowing down reactions and encouraging a Socratic approach whereby the patient questions whether he or she is seeing this situation appropriately and whether there is another explanation for what has happened. Implementing this new perspective involves changing core schemata that contribute to crises, self-harming behavior, and associated affects (see Chapter 11).

COMMENT

This chapter and the previous one describe a general framework for treating crises and symptoms and demonstrate how specific interventions may be combined with the general treatment strategies. The specific interventions suggested are intended to be illustrative rather than definitive. They are not intended to be used in a fixed order, nor will all be necessary in every case. Over time better interventions will be developed. The framework offered should be able to accommodate these developments. The creative challenge for therapists is to find or develop specific interventions that are tailored to the patient's needs and problems and are congenial with his or her style.

Early sessions are likely to be dominated by immediate problems and the need to build the relationship. As the alliance emerges, specific interventions are introduced to address specific problems or symptoms, beginning with the regulation and control of affects and impulses. During this work, it is important not to lose sight of the alliance and the value of a consistent therapeutic process and hence the need to deal promptly with therapy-disrupting behavior. It is also important not to become so preoccupied with control and regulation that other aspects of self-harm, especially its underlying causes, are neglected.

Throughout the process, the intent is to reduce self-harm, recognize the steps leading to maladaptive behavior, improve self-management of emotions, modify reactions to triggers, and acquire more effective self-monitoring. The development of these skills and consequent reduction in self-harm involve a gradual process. Although the frequency of these acts should gradually decrease, frequent relapses are likely. When they happen it is important that they are taken seriously but without overreacting. As with addiction-related relapses, it is best to focus on the positive: those occasions when self-harm was delayed or aborted, and the days in which it did not occur. Relapses are best viewed in this context rather than as incidents of failure.

CHAPTER 10

Regulation and Control

Treating Trauma and Dissociative Behavior

This chapter deals with two additional symptom clusters that are common: the sequelae of developmental trauma and dissociative behavior. Many of the methods used to treat these problems are extensions of methods discussed in the previous chapter. Successful treatment of trauma often involves greater levels of exploration than has been discussed so far and hence combines the regulation and control and exploration and change phases of treatment. Dissociation and trauma are discussed here because they follow naturally from a consideration of the treatment of affective and impulsive symptoms; however, this is not necessarily the sequence in which they are tackled. Dissociative behavior often has to be addressed early in treatment because it is disruptive. The treatment of trauma is a different story; it requires a more cautious and graded approach. Although the sequelae of trauma surface regularly during treatment, many of the more definitive interventions are used later in treatment because they require a stable therapeutic relationship and patient skills in tolerating and regulating the emotions that are inevitably aroused.

TREATING THE CONSEQUENCES OF EARLY TRAUMA

It was noted in Chapter 3 that psychosocial adversity can lead to traumatic memories and associated symptoms that have enduring effects on personality. Three clusters of symptoms were described that are similar to those observed in posttraumatic stress disorder (PTSD): (1) reexperiencing or intrusive symptoms (e.g., flashbacks, unwanted thoughts, intrusive images), (2) hyperarousal symptoms (e.g., hypervigilance, anger, sleep disturbance, and impaired concentration), and (3) avoidance symptoms (e.g., decreased interest, emotional numbness, restricted affect, emotional detachment, and avoidance of thoughts, feelings, and experiences associated with the event). Although personality disorder is more than chronic PTSD (Kroll, 1988), cognitive and information-processing models of PTSD help to explain reactions to trauma in personality disorder, and interventions based on these models are useful in treatment.

Cognitive-Behavioral Models

Behavioral explanations of the sequelae of trauma incorporate two models based on learning theory (Mowrer, 1960). First, it is assumed that fear is acquired through a process of classical conditioning. Just as Pavlov's dogs learned to salivate to a bell that rang just before feeding, so fear responses evoked during the traumatic event may become associated with other stimuli present at the time. This mechanism explains the emotional and autonomic reactions to any sight, sound, or smell associated with the trauma. For example, a woman who was abused in childhood by a male relative with a facial mole may develop a fear of men with facial moles; furthermore, the fear may generalize to men with any skin lesion, or even all men. The second mechanism explains avoidance behavior. Escaping from stimuli associated with trauma is reinforced by a reduction in fear and distress. Consequently, avoidance becomes a learned way to reduce distress. Avoidance, in turn, prevents the fear response from being extinguished by learning, through exposure, that the evocative stimulus is not harmful. Thus treatment should involve exposure to evocative stimuli under conditions that lead to extinction of the fear response.

Cognitive models extend these ideas by explaining how the experience of trauma leads to dysfunctional thinking patterns (Follette, Ruzek, & Abueg, 1998). Traditional cognitive therapy assumes that emotional reactions are influenced by the way traumatic events are interpreted. Trauma is assumed to modify or shatter basic beliefs about the self and the world (Janoff-Bulman, 1992). The unpredictable and uncontrollable nature of the trauma—in particular, the loss of control occurring during the event—affect beliefs about personal safety and vulnerability, trust in others, personal efficacy, self-worth, and intimacy (Basŏglu & Mineka, 1992; McCann & Pearlman, 1990; McCann, Sakheim, & Abrahamson, 1988). Thus it is important to challenge and restructure maladaptive beliefs, reestablish beliefs that some things are predictable, and promote a sense of mastery and control.

A second cognitive perspective extends these ideas by showing how fear responses become elaborated in memory into "fear structures" that consist of information about feared stimuli, fear responses, and interpretations of the meaning of the feared stimuli and responses (Foa & Rothbaum, 1998; Foa, Steketee, & Rothbaum, 1989; Meadows & Foa, 1998). Change in these structures (schemata) is assumed to require (1) the activation (through exposure) and extinction of the fear response, and (2) restructuring of the fearful beliefs through acquisition of new information.

A third perspective examines the way traumatized individuals struggle to develop narratives that give meaning to their experiences (Meichenbaum & Fong, 1993). Change is assumed to involve altering both these narratives and the meaning assigned to the traumatic events. Finally, trauma also influences basic cognitive processes, such as attention, memory, and information processing, which mediate the way in which the individual responds to environmental events.

Treatment based on these ideas has two components: (1) reexperiencing, to reduce the anxiety and fear; and (2) cognitive interventions, to modify maladaptive beliefs, fear structures, and meaning structures. Most therapies for trauma involve reexperiencing the event with an accompanying emotional arousal and working through the experience to attenuate its effects. Indeed most cognitive-based treatments for anxiety disorders involve exposure to anxiety-provoking stimuli, whether internal or external (Brown & Barlow, 1992). In the case of PTSD, the evidence indicates that exposure, particularly prolonged exposure, is effective for the reexperiencing and hyperarousal symptoms but not so effective for the avoidance symptoms. These may respond better to dynamic psychotherapy and skills training (Blake & Sonnenberg, 1998).

Application to Trauma Associated with Personality Disorder

Studies of PTSD suggest a multidimensional approach that is consistent with the proposed approach to treating personality disorder. The general interventions provide the interpersonal dimension recommended for treating avoidance symptoms; specific interventions are added to (1) provide exposure to, and subsequent extinction of, the fear response, and (2) restructure maladaptive beliefs. Prolonged exposure to evocative stimuli that allows anxiety to rise and then habituate is more effective than brief exposure. In vivo exposure (i.e., experience with the actual stimulus) also appears to be more effective than images of the stimuli or descriptions of events (Goldfried, 1985). The exposure component leads to intense emotions. This intense arousal presents a problem when treating patients with personality disorder. Although overwhelming anxiety is detrimental in treating any patient with PTSD (Jaycox & Foa, 1996), the problem is more serious with personality disorder. Imaginative or in vivo exposure may be overwhelming and trigger dissociative episodes or self-harming behavior (Feeny, Zoeller, & Foa, 2002). Moreover, many patients actively avoid dealing with these problems, so that attempts to address them are resisted and may even threaten therapy.

Clinical investigators who advocate prolonged exposure to treat the sequelae of sexual trauma suggest that the approach can be used without modification to treat trauma associated with personality disorder (Feeny et al., 2002; Meadows & Foa, 1998). This recommendation is based on the fact that investigations of prolonged exposure did not exclude individuals with a history of childhood sexual abuse and incest. Individuals with borderline features (some of whom may have had borderline personality disorder) did not have difficulty with either imaginal or *in vivo* exposure (Feeny et al., 2002). However, individuals with acute suicidal behavior were excluded, so that individuals with moderate to severe personality disorder were probably not treated. Moreover, the outcome of cognitive-behavioral treatments of patients with a primary diagnosis of PTSD with and without borderline personality characteristics (not disorder) indicates that patients with borderline characteristics benefit from treatment, but the outcome is poorer than for patients without these characteristics.

These findings suggest caution in applying these methods to treat the sequelae of childhood sexual abuse in patients with severe personality disorder. A prudent change would be to *explore trauma and abuse and to use exposure only after an effective therapeutic relationship has been established and affect tolerance and regulation skills have been acquired.* This approach could be considered a "Catch-22" situation, in which the treatment of trauma is delayed until stability is achieved—whereas stability depends on changing reactions to trauma. However, stability is also promoted by an effective relationship and the acquisition of affect-regulation skills.

Interventions

A graded approach is used in which less evocative material is explored and worked through before the more distressing events. Careful attention is paid to the quality of the alliance and the level of emotional arousal. Whenever emotions threaten to become overwhelming, cognitive functioning deteriorates, as evidenced by feelings of confusion or indications of dissociative behavior, supportive and validating interventions, containment strategies, and affect-regulation interventions are implemented to keep arousal within tolerable limits. A common problem encountered in following this approach comes from the fact that information about trauma is often revealed early in treatment. If such revelations occur during episodes of behavioral disorganization or before the development of a satisfactory relationship and effective affect-regulating skills, the therapist's task is to validate feelings and concerns while containing the affects aroused. Emphasis is placed on validation and on dealing with the impact of the trauma on current functioning rather than exploring past events. Exploration is limited to eliciting sufficient information to permit effective validation and containment. When the individual is insistent on dealing with these issues, the therapist validates this desire while maintaining containment. If necessary, the therapist can recognize that "these are important issues that we need to deal with when you are feeling a little more settled and you think that you can handle it. Until you feel more settled and less distressed, it would be best if we concentrated on how these thoughts and memories affect you when they happen now and what we can do to reduce their impact."

Education about the Effects of Trauma

Patients who are not aware of the many consequences of trauma blame themselves for having symptoms or feel guilty about the symptoms. Many also worry that these problems mean that they are "losing their minds." Information about trauma can often be introduced early in treatment to correct these beliefs. Initially it is useful to describe intrusive, hyperarousal, and avoidance symptoms so that the patient realizes that these experiences are typical reactions to trauma. The explanation can also include an account of the mechanisms involved in symptom development, including an explanation of autonomic responses. It is also helpful to point out that memories are difficult to control voluntarily, and that one cannot control the thoughts that come to mind—only what one does with those memories and thoughts subsequently. Later, explanation can be extended to cover the effects of traumatic experiences on beliefs, thinking styles, relationships with others, and ideas about the self. The goal is to make the patient's experiences explicable and normalize reactions, as far as possible, by showing that they are typical responses to trauma.

Description and Exposure

Many patients have not had an opportunity to describe traumatic experiences in detail. Moreover, victims of childhood abuse were often told that the event did not occur, that they were lying, and some were even punished for suggesting such a thing. Even when events were acknowledged, the patient may have been forbidden to talk about them. As a result, considerable effort is put into avoiding thinking about these events, even when memories are intrusive. A detailed description can begin the process of change by serving as a critical incident stress debriefing (Kubany & Manke, 1995). While retelling experiences, opportunities occur to (1) examine maladaptive beliefs about the event and reactions to it, and (2) address feelings of guilt and anger. Retelling is also a form of exposure that

can gradually be extended to more evocative material, as control over anxiety and fear is achieved. An informal approach often works best: The
therapist deals with traumatic material when it is raised by the patient,
rather than adhering to a prescribed procedure and timetable. Issues can be
selected over time as a way to deal with the trauma in increasing depth
and detail. Such a sequence may involve:

- Descriptions of (1) stimuli or situations that evoke symptoms in
  the present, and (2) intrusive material such as nightmares or flashbacks occurring in the present, with a gradual increase in detailing
  the emotions aroused.
- Broad and relatively superficial description of the original traumatic
  events, with minimal emotional content; exploration of the way
  these events affect current relationships and feelings about the self.
- Detailed description of the original events, including feelings, thoughts,
  and other reactions at the time; description of current reactions to
  the recalled information.
- Imaginative exposure, with detailed description of these events in
  the present tense—that is, as if they were actually occurring now.
- *In vivo* exposure to actual avoided situations and stimuli, if possible
  or relevant.

Working through trauma in this way may take many months or longer.
Typically issues are dealt with for a while and then put aside, to return
later for work at greater depth.

Traumatic material is best approached during a period of stability and
when the alliance is strong enough to provide the support needed to contain fear and deal with avoidance. It is convenient to begin with descriptions of current intrusive symptoms, such as nightmares or flashbacks, or
current abusive relationships, when these are mentioned in treatment. Initial inquiry often yields superficial responses, such as, "It was just a night-
mare," so that it is usually necessary to press for elaboration. The affect-
regulating exercises and attention-shifting technique discussed in the previous chapter can be used to manage emotional arousal, including fear reactions, in response to specific images and stimuli. Overwhelming reactions to a specific event are dealt with by constructing a hierarchy of
stimuli associated with the event, from the least fear-evoking to the most.
In the early stages of treating the consequences of trauma, priority is given
to building confidence that these events can be discussed without catastrophic consequences and that the fear and anxiety can be controlled.
Later more prolonged exposure is used to extinguish the fear.

Detailed description of symptoms usually evokes memories of early
trauma. Initially these events can be talked about in broad terms, with an
emphasis on the impact of these events on current relationships and feel-

ings about the self, and minimal exploration of feelings. As avoidance decreases and comfort in disclosure increases, it becomes possible to elicit
more detailed description of actual events, including the feelings, thoughts,
and other reactions that occurred at the time. Description of current reactions to retelling these experiences both deepens the experience of retelling and provides opportunities for affect regulation.

The important step is to prolong exposure until the anxiety begins to
settle. In the treatment of PTSD this step is usually achieved through
imaginal exposure, in which patients are encouraged to describe events in
the present tense, while in a relaxed state with their eyes closed (Foa &
Jaycock, 1999; Meadows & Foa, 1998). This step needs to be approached
slowly and with adequate preparation. In some cases prolonging exposure is
only possible after extensive treatment; in others, it may not be necessary.

Cognitive interventions for PTSD usually incorporate various kinds of
"homework" that the patient does between sessions. Homework assign-
ments are not always effective with patients who have severe personality
disorder. When intense affect and dissociative behaviors are likely to occur, exposure should be limited to the treatment sessions and the patient
encouraged to use grounding exercises, relaxation, and attention shifting
to deal with problems experienced in everyday situations. This process is
illustrated by the following vignette:

> Sandra was a single woman in her late 20s who lived alone. She had
> an extensive psychiatric history, with frequent hospital admissions for
> self-harm and intense affective lability. There was also a history of
> drug and alcohol abuse. During crises she became severely regressed
> and found it difficult to manage even everyday chores. She had dis-
> sociative episodes lasting anywhere from a few minutes to several
> hours, when she was unresponsive as if catatonic. She had a history
> of severe, repetitive sexual and physical abuse by multiple perpetra-
> tors that stretched from mid-childhood to late teens. These events
> had a profound impact on her day-to-day functioning and on her
> personality structure. Particularly problematic were frequent flash-
> backs and intrusive memories that appeared to occur with minimal
> warning and which led to intense anxiety, dysphoria, dissociative
> behavior, and often self-harm. She followed a limited lifestyle in that
> she avoided going to places where she might encounter stimuli evo-
> cative of memories of the trauma. She had difficulty going out after
> dark, because one particularly traumatic event had occurred in the
> early evening one dark winter night, when the patient was about 13
> years old. The memories of this incident were so intrusive that she
> avoided opening the door of her home after dark.
>   Over the course of about 2 years of treatment, progress was
> made in dealing with the self-harming behavior and in reducing the
> affective lability. Severe regressive behavior had virtually ceased, dis-
> sociative reactions had decreased, but trauma remained a problem

and became the focus of attention. There were many aspects to the trauma and a wide variety of traumatic events and multiple perpetrators. An approximate hierarchy was established, according to degree of distress evoked. Over time, events were dealt with sequentially, beginning with the least traumatic. These achievements did not have much impact on the event that had occurred at the age of 13, but they did provide the basis for beginning to deal with the problem. As her affect-regulation skills increased and her mood and behavior stabilized, attention was focused on this event. Over a period of several months, the patient acquired relaxation skills, using the focus on breath approach, and was introduced to the attention-shifting exercise that she used successfully to desensitize several evocative stimuli.

The patient gradually described the event in increasing detail. It began when she was in the house alone in the early evening, when it was dark, and someone knocked at the door. When she looked outside she recognized the person, so she opened the door and spoke to him on the doorstep. She soon became concerned about his intentions and tried to close the door. He blocked this attempt; she recalled his arm extending around the door, reaching her. Subsequently, he managed to gain entry and assault her. She found it impossible to disclose this event to anyone, although it rapidly became known among her peers, and she was taunted about it at school for many years. Over time, the fears generalized to the current point where she could not open the door in the evening. When she was alone and there was a noise outside, she would experience flashbacks and intrusive images of the man's arm coming around the door.

Recalling this information caused considerable distress. At times she was overwhelmed by emotions; transient episodes of behavioral disorganization occurred that included cognitive confusion and dissociative reactions. These were managed with containment interventions and medication. The gradual approach described earlier was used, so it took many weeks to elicit all the details. As the fear settled a little, it was possible to begin desensitization within sessions. The patient was encouraged to imagine the door at her home and to discuss her reactions to it. The attention-control exercise was used to help control the fear. The patient also described how, when she was at home alone, she would imagine the arm coming around the door as it did when she was a child. This memory was gradually incorporated into the sessions. Over time, her fears receded, and the patient was able to describe experiences in detail without fear. Unfortunately, she could not apply these techniques when she was actually alone at home. The fear continued, and she continued to be distressed by vivid images of the hand coming around the door. Her nights remained filled with anxiety.

The desensitization process was then continued at home. A hierarchy was constructed. The first step was sitting alone at home in the middle of the day, looking at the door and using that as a stimulus for the attention-shifting exercise. Control over fear responses to looking at the door was achieved fairly rapidly. The exercise was extended to images of the hand coming around the door during daylight hours. The next step was for the patient to open the door for a short period of time and close it. Again, progress was fairly rapid in extinguishing the fear. Gradually, the time of day in which the exercise was conducted was changed to late afternoon, to dusk, then finally evening. The nighttime situation was the most problematic, but the patient was able to tolerate looking at the door, imagining opening it, and then closing it without too much difficulty. The next step of actually opening the door and slowly closing it was much more difficult. Once this was resolved, the door was opened for increasingly long periods, until the patient could step out into her front yard.

Reframing

The second component of treatment is to restructure or reframe maladaptive schemata that are triggered by evocative situations. Self-blame and guilt are common; most individuals who have experienced abuse blame themselves for what happened; indeed many feel that they "did something" to provoke the abuse. As result they believe that they are "bad" or that something is fundamentally wrong with them, not only as a result of the abuse but also because they caused it. Hindsight is used to blame themselves—they feel that they "should have known what would happen" or did nothing to stop repeated abuse. These reactions form a background of constant negative self-talk that is so familiar, it is not always recognized as a problem that contributes to distress and mood symptoms. Interventions focus on restructuring these beliefs and helping patients to view events in terms of the understanding and resources available at the time, rather than with the hindsight of adult understanding.

Managing Anger

Anger is a common but neglected reaction to trauma in patients with a history of childhood sexual abuse. Although it is not usually as apparent as fear, depression, and distress, it is part of the hyperarousal symptoms and activated by the same stimuli that evoke other symptoms in the cluster. When present, anger impedes the treatment of PTSD (Novaco & Chemtob, 1998) and creates problems when treating trauma associated with personality disorder. When anger is the primary response to trauma, it is often difficult to modulate it sufficiently to address the problem. Rapid arousal and the speed with which anger leads to action makes it difficult for patients to reflect on what happened long enough to construct an understanding of events. The problem is exacerbated when associated with dissocial or psychopathic traits; these patients become preoccupied with retaliation rather resolving the problem, as illustrated by the following vignette.

> Jill was a single woman in her mid-30s who presented for treatment with a longstanding history of labile moods, impulsive self-harming behavior, severe interpersonal problems, and labile anger. She gave a history of severe childhood sexual abuse and further abusive episodes in adolescence and early adulthood. During assessment she expressed intense anger toward the men who had abused her and talked about her desire to hurt them for what they had done to her. She was diagnosed initially as having DSM-IV borderline personality disorder. She was referred for long-term group psychotherapy. In the group, it soon became apparent that her anger toward her abusers had generalized toward all men. In one early group, she was very critical of another member who described difficulties relating to women. The man in question was a slightly inhibited individual with considerable fears of interpersonal hurt and rejection. Jill played on his sensitivity and vulnerability and openly denigrated him. When other members intervened, she was contemptuous of their concerns. In ensuing weeks, she successively attacked each man in the group and made it almost impossible for them to be open about their problems. The attacks were vindictive in that her primary concern seemed to be to hurt. When the therapists and other group members tried to draw Jill's attention to this pattern, their feedback was rejected. Jill adamantly insisted that everything she said was deserved and she felt no concern about hurting men because of what they had done to her. It was this remorseless quality, rather than the anger, that hindered the development of any kind of self-understanding. It became apparent that Jill saw the group not as an opportunity to develop understanding of her maladaptive patterns and dysfunctional traits but rather as an opportunity for revenge.

With the emotionally dysregulated or borderline patient, anger is often masked by fearfulness and general distress. It is only when traumatic events are explored that it emerges as a major factor. The addition of anger often produces a sharp increase in distress that poses a further obstacle to treatment, especially when the anger is used to reduce feelings of vulnerability. When anger is recognized, it is often experienced as intense unfocused rage that is readily turned against the self, leading to a recurrence of deliberate self-harm, even late in treatment. One patient with emotional dysregulation traits, who experienced overwhelming distress that lead to serious self-harming acts, described the fear and panic-like feelings evoked by events that reminded her of serious childhood abuse, commenting: "I don't know that I am really afraid. I thought that I was terrified, but I think I'm really angry. It's the anger that I'm afraid of. I think I'm going crazy. I can't stand it. I don't want to think about it. I think that's why I do these things [acts of deliberate self-harm]. It's the anger that makes me do it. I'm afraid of what I might do, so I take it out on myself." Although anger has adaptive features and may give a sense of power and control, it did not have this effect on this patient; indeed it added to her reluctance to deal with her problems, because it intensified the distress and made her feel that she was "losing her mind." In this case, it was necessary to focus on the anger by identifying triggers and using behavioral and affect-regulating interventions, similar to those discussed earlier, until she could modulate the anger. This example also illustrates the progression in treating self-harm, discussed in the previous chapter. The initial focus was on self-harm as a way to regulate feelings, which, in this case, included anger. When a moderate level of control was achieved, attention was focused on the anger more directly.

The Problem of Acceptance

Radical change ultimately involves accepting that the traumatic events happened and cannot be changed. This is a new form of acceptance that does not include condoning or minimizing the events or engaging in ruminative self-blame. Although patients recognize, on a rational level, that nothing can be done to change events that are part of their history, they act as if this were not the case. Much time and energy is spent denying that events occurred and wishing that things had been different. Patients fantasize, at length, about how their lives would have been if these things had not happened. Intense anger over "why me" perpetuates these reactions and the distress. Change requires that patients direct these energies toward changing what can be changed—the ways in which they continue to react to trauma, the extent to which it still evokes distress, and the way it affects their current lives. This degree of acceptance is difficult to achieve and usually only emerges during the later stages of longer-term treatment. In earlier stages, patients often feel that to change in this way would devalue the devastating significance of these events.

Common Problems

It is may be useful at this point to consider some problems that are commonly encountered when treating the consequences of trauma. The commonest problem is reluctance or outright refusal to deal with traumatic material, even when it is intrusive. Manifestations of this reluctance range from simple refusal to talk about events in the detail needed for effective intervention, to overwhelming affective responses or dissociative reactions that prevent descriptive exploration of traumatic material. Moderate reactions may be managed with support, containment, and affect regulation. More severe dissociative behaviors, especially those in which the patient is unresponsive, as if catatonic, are more difficult because verbal interventions do not work. Initially, all that can be done is to keep that patient safe until the episode subsides. Achieving this safety may require a brief admission or at least a few hours in an emergency room. In these cases, a more supportive approach is required and definitive treatment of trauma should be left until dissociative behaviors are controlled. With some highly vulnerable patients, the use of exposure may not be appropriate.

One serious consequence of exploring trauma occurs when the patient is left in an irresolvable distressed state that often includes severe regression. Affects flood experience uncontrollably and coping deteriorates. This usually occurs in severely traumatized and deprived individuals who have minimal capacity to manage affects and self-soothe and who are exposed to the trauma prematurely, with minimal attention given to affect-regulation strategies and insufficient attention given to building a therapeutic relationship that can support the stress of dealing with traumatic material. Problems also arise when catharsis is stressed rather than affect regulation. The need for a cautious approach to exploration is in order, especially with patients who have a history of extensive early abuse and deprivation. In some cases, this problem of overwhelming affect is linked to severe guilt and self-hatred, which is common in people who have experienced severe trauma and, as a result, failed to develop effective ways of managing their emotions.

Shame and Self-Hatred

One of more intractable problems is intense shame about abusive experiences. Shame forms a major obstacle to treatment because patients go to great lengths to avoid discussing both what happened to them and, more importantly, current reactions to the abuse. The intense shame affects self-worth, influences most forms of interpersonal behavior, and leads to highly submissive behavior that leaves the patient open to further abuse. In some cases, the shame can be dealt with directly, by exploring its origins and restructuring the cognitions involved. Greater problems are encountered when the shame is associated with intense self-hatred. Often in these cases, modest improvement and greater behavioral stability are followed by suddenly erupting crises, and the self-punishing aspects of the deliberate self-harm become more apparent. It is as if self-hatred suddenly hypertrophies. In retrospect, the self-hatred was always there but was not so apparent because other issues took center stage, and affect and impulse regulation were the main focus of therapeutic endeavor. As self-harming acts decrease in response to treatment, the self-hatred becomes more apparent. This is often a testing time for treatment, because progress seems to halt. Guilt and shame are often increased by the fact that many patients think that they should be better by this point, and the presence of new problems leads to further denial.

These reactions—shame, guilt, and self-hatred—become intertwined and self-perpetuating, forming a closed system in which patients blame themselves, feel guilty, and then punish themselves by deliberate acts of self-harm, which only lead to further self-blame and guilt. These reactions are closely connected to family-of-origin pathology especially when the perpetrator of the abuse was/is a family member or someone close to the family. In these situations, a combination of familial denial and the tendency to hold the patient responsible for what happened forms a further obstacle to treatment. Patients feel that they are betraying the family by revealing secrets, and doubts instilled by family denial increase the sense of shame and contribute to a reluctance to discuss these matters. Patients also feel shame because they accept the attributions of responsibility placed on them by family members and believe that what happened was their fault— that they are weak because they let it happen and are unable to handle the consequences. Others people's critical reactions to self-harming behavior confirm and intensify guilt and self-blame. At this point improvement seems to reach a plateau, as illustrated by the following vignette:

One patient who had made good progress in reducing self-harming behavior and self-managing feelings and impulses, to the point where she could hold down a part-time job—something that she had not been able to do previously—continued to self-mutilate every few months. This pattern continued for about 1 year. Significant issues had been discussed, but progress had slowed down or even stopped. The self-harming episodes had decreased in frequency but not in immediate intensity; however, the crises were shorter and, as the patient noted, "I bounce back faster." The episodes then increased in frequency. Although the patient was reluctant to discuss the triggers, it was apparent that they were memories of severe childhood sexual and physical abuse that evoked terrifying feelings of depersonalization and derealization. Being unable to tolerate these feelings, she cut herself severely or hit herself with a hammer.

The sexual and physical abuse had occurred throughout childhood and continued into early adulthood. She was part of a large family, and the perpetrators were family members. They and other members of the family blamed her for what had happened. From an early age she was told that she was being punished severely, for her own good, because she was bad. She was told that the sexual abuse was her fault because she was seductive and provocative, although she was only about 6 years old when the abuse started, and the perpetrators were adults. When the abuse continued into early adulthood in other relationships, the incidents were interpreted as further evidence of her inherent "badness." The patient accepted her family's interpretations. She blamed herself for past and present problems. "I am a bad person" was a core schema. She felt that she deserved to be punished for what had happened and what was happening in her life. The self-mutilation reduced the guilt and changed intolerable feelings of depersonalization. She was not sure that she deserved help and thought that she deserved to suffer for what had happened. This system of ideas and actions became even more self-contained because her family blamed her for harming herself and verbally abused her for being ill. She, in turn, interpreted the self-mutilation and depression as further evidence that she was indeed bad.

The events and beliefs described in this vignette are shown in Figure 10.1. Intrusive memories of childhood abuse triggered the depersonalization and dysphoria that led to self-mutilation. The abuse and the family's responses caused shame, guilt, and self-hatred that contributed to self-mutilation, which was also a form of self-punishment. In the current situation, self-mutilation was a further reason for the family to blame her, which, in turn, only increased the self-hatred. A closed system that resisted change was firmly established. Achieving change was difficult because it depended on changing the way she thought about herself and the family's behavior. She needed to accept that the family was abusive and punitive rather than benignly concerned about doing what was best for her, as they maintained and she struggled to believe. She could not accept these ideas about her family because she was closely enmeshed and feared

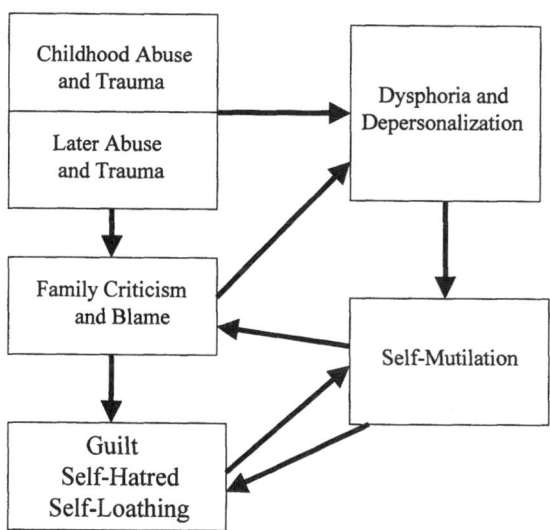

FIGURE 10.1. The closed cycle of trauma, self-hatred, and self-harm.

that she could not cope without them. As Fairbairn (1952) pointed out, even a bad relationship is better than no relationship.

The treatment situation becomes even more complicated when patients feel that they do not deserve to receive help or to get better because they are so bad. The situation is akin to Freud's (1923) description of the negative therapeutic reaction: a situation in which patients act in ways that oppose recovery because they think that they deserve to suffer. This response makes for an even more closed and enmeshed system, because the guilt and the need to suffer block progress. In the most severe forms, the guilt is about actually existing at all, given what has happened and what they allowed to happen. In these situations changing guilt and self-hatred is difficult. Suggestions are made in the literature on trauma for cognitive restructuring of the guilt and self-hatred. It is difficult to fault such recommendations, but they do not seem to capture the intensity of the reaction or the way attempts to generate new understanding or to reframe fixed ways of perceiving the situation are used as a further reason to persecute the self.

At these times, the treatment alliance comes into focus again. Issues of trust and cooperation emerge in more intense form. Earlier in treatment, patients learn to trust the therapist enough to develop some confidence that the therapist knows what he or she is doing and can be relied upon to provide help and understanding. The question of trustworthiness now moves to a deeper level of whether the therapist can be trusted *as a person* (as opposed to a professional). As one patient put it, "Of course I trust you, you have helped me a lot. I just don't know that you will like me if I talk about the things that I am ashamed of."

Little is gained from challenging these closed systems of reactions and self-hatred directly. Such actions simply consolidate the self-hatred and reinforce the status quo. It seems best to maintain a supportive stance and offer an understanding of what is happening: the dilemma that the patient faces and the reasons why he or she feels so stuck. Sometimes therapists are tempted to take a different tack—that of taking sides in this struggle—but this strategy also is fraught with problems. Siding with the patient as he or she struggles with memories of past abusive relationships may lead to further self-persecution if the patient feels undeserving of support. Sometimes however, taking sides in the struggle helps to resolve the impasse. One patient, trapped in the closed system of shame, self-hatred, self-mutilation, traumatic memories of abuse, and current criticism and blame within her family, asked her therapist: "Do you think I am a bad person? Everyone in the family tells me it's my fault and that I am only getting what I deserve. Do you think they are right? You have to tell me." The therapist replied, "You have told me about the many bad things that happened to you, and the bad things people have done to you, but that doesn't mean that you are a bad person. Bad things happen to good people." The patient replied, "Thank you. . . . Now I can tell you about the shame I feel, which I have hidden from you and avoided all this time."

Change to these closed and self-perpetuating structures of patients who have histories of severe deprivation and abuse, and few supports and inner resources, is primarily achieved through a supportive, empathic, and validating therapeutic relationship. What seems to matter is the experience of a relationship in which the therapist is simply present and where hatred and blame are not experienced. Confrontational stances are usually ineffective because it is so easy for these patients to misconstrue even moderate confrontation as critical and abusive.

DISSOCIATION

Dissociative reactions are prevalent in patients with personality disorder. Environmental and genetic factors contribute to this response. Dissociative behaviors are common sequelae of sexual, emotional, and physical abuse. However, dissociative behaviors are not an inevitable consequence of abuse and do not necessarily indicate a history of sexual trauma (a common assumption). Nor are dissociative behaviors influenced only by experience. Twin studies show that dissociative behavior, as assessed by the Dissociative Experiences Scale (Bernstein & Putnam, 1986), is heritable (Jang, Paris, Zweig-Frank, & Livesley, 1998). Dissociative behavior may also be due to drugs (Good, 1989; Krystal, Bennett, Bremner, Southwick, & Charney, 1995). Although many agents have these effects, those commonly used by patients are alcohol, benzodiazepines, and cannabinoids. Hence the occurrence of dissociative behavior should not lead the clinician to assume specific causes. Instead, it is reason for a careful review of possible contributing factors. In many cases, a combination of factors is involved, including genetic predisposition, trauma, and current drug misuse.

Various explanations of dissociative behaviors have been advanced, and most suggest that dissociation is linked, in some way, to affect regulation. Ludwig (1983), for example, suggested that dissociation serves adaptive and defensive functions that include automatization of responses, efficiency and economy of effort, conflict resolution, escape from reality, isolation of catastrophic experiences, catharsis, and the enhancement of the herd sense. Putnam (1991) suggested that it also creates a state of analgesia and detachment. Wagner and Linehan (1998) expressed these ideas in behavioral terms: the "primary function of dissociative phenomena is the regulation of exposure to cues related to trauma experiences" (p. 203). These ideas suggest that dissociative behavior serves a similar function to that of deliberate self-harm—both are affect-regulating responses used to reduce fear, anxiety, rage or distress.

Interventions

Given the assumed affect-regulating function of dissociative behavior, any intervention that reduces the overall level of emotional arousal, especially fear and anxiety, is likely to reduce the frequency of dissociative phenomena. Consequently, the frequency of these behaviors is likely to decrease, without specific interventions, simply with improvements in the capacity of the therapeutic relationship to support and contain affects, and foster the patient's ability to self-manage emotions. The value of these indirect measures should not be minimized. In many cases, they are sufficient to produce a significant improvement. When specific interventions are needed to supplement these effects, they may be approached through the stages of change model used to treat parasuicidal behavior.

Problem Identification

As with any undesirable behavior, changing it begins by identifying the problem and establishing a commitment to change. In most instances dissociative behaviors are readily apparent. Some patients, however, do not fully understand these behaviors, and an explanation of dissociative reactions aids the recognition process. Although most patients are motivated to change and willing to acknowledge that these behaviors cause difficulty, a few patients are reluctant to relinquish them because they are effective in reducing distress. One patient noted that, "I can't not do this [dissociate]. It's the only way that I can tolerate what happens." In these cases a commitment to change may develop out of a discussion of the consequences of these acts and their impact on lifestyle and relationships with others. It may also develop as measures that foster tolerance of distress take effect. Somewhat more difficulty is usually experienced when drug misuse contributes to affective lability and dissociative reactions. Many patients who use drugs to enhance mood are reluctant to discontinue. It usually takes considerable time and frequent supportive confrontation to build a commitment to change.

Exploration: Analysis of the Behavioral Sequence

The first step in mapping out the chain of events leading to a dissociative response is to identify triggering stimuli. This is often complicated by the reluctance of many patients to discuss these episodes because they are afraid of provoking further incidents. Descriptions of the sequence are most readily constructed when dissociative responses are relatively mild, such as with states of slight depersonalization and derealization. Patients are also usually able to identify triggers when the stimuli are relatively specific, such as seeing someone with the same physical characteristic as an abuser. With more severe reactions, such as unresponsive states, the onset is often so rapid that patients are not aware afterward of what triggered their reaction. In these cases considerable persistence and support is required to identify precipitants by examining specific instances. Success often depends on detailed analysis of an episode that occurs during a treatment session.

When such an episode occurs, little can be done at the time other than wait until it settles—which may mean waiting until the next session. Then the event can be reconstructed in detail. For example, one patient who suddenly became unresponsive in a session could not recall much of what happened prior to the event when it was discussed in the next session. Careful review of the event eventually revealed that she initially noticed an intense feeling of vulnerability and the need to protect herself. The immediate effect of this feeling was to evoke a "freeze" response in her. Further discussion led to the realization that she felt vulnerable when she thought that someone was saying something that could be interpreted in several ways. This ambiguity made her confused about the person's intention and evoked memories of similar feelings about a parent who was physically abusive.

Developing Alternative Responses

Many of the techniques used to self-manage dysphoria and self-harm reduce dissociative responses. Once triggers have been identified, it is often possible to reduce the frequency of these reactions by *avoiding* contact with the stimuli that evoke them. This gives a respite that makes it possible to learn other methods. Similarly, *control* of dissociative responses can be increased using the grounding exercise discussed earlier. Again, it may be helpful to enroll the assistance of significant others in implementing this exercise. The attention-control exercise used to build feelings of mastery and affect regulation is a useful way to *reduce the emotional significance of triggers*. Here it is used to desensitize the evocative stimulus in much the same way as it is used to treat phobias. This exercise works well with specific stimuli, such as seeing a man with a limp that was similar to that of an abuser. However, these kinds of interventions are not usually sufficient. They also need to be supplemented with interventions that address maladaptive cognitions. In the case of the patient who dissociated when she saw a man with a limp, it was also necessary to (1) address the tendency to confuse past and present, and (2) reduce the intense long-held guilt that was based on unreasonable expectations of what a child could do. She believed that, even though she was a young child at the time, she should have been able to resist someone with a handicap. Control was only fully established when these beliefs were reframed.

COMMENT

This chapter concludes our discussion of specific strategies for treating symptoms and affect and impulse problems. Most common symptom clusters have been considered. Other symptoms, such as the "pseudoseizures" that occur in some severely personality disordered individuals, can be dealt with using the same basic stages of change approach. It seems appropriate at this point to reiterate two points. First, the techniques and interventions discussed are most effective when the general conditions of therapy are given careful attention. Second, exploration of the consequences of trauma is approached cautiously and gradually, as the therapeutic relationship develops and the patient acquires skills in managing affects. In highly vulnerable patients who have a history of deprivation and a limited ability to tolerate anxiety and fear, exploration may be minimal and the more modest goals of gaining control over current sequelae of trauma are adopted. Premature exploration can cause considerable harm by arousing memories and feelings in patients who lack the resources to tolerate, contain, and resolve the issues raised.

In this connection, it is also important to consider the controversial issue of how to distinguish true from "false" memories of trauma. Most patients with personality disorder who have histories of traumatic experiences are usually aware of those experiences; they are rarely repressed, although they may be suppressed. Nevertheless, the experiences are usually on the fringes of awareness, even if patients deny that these things happened and actively avoid thinking about them. Most patients disclose these traumatic experiences early in treatment, once the alliance has developed and trust emerged. Problems arise when therapists are convinced abuse must have happened, given the patient's history and presentation, and convey this assumption to the patient. Many vulnerable individuals readily accept this idea because they are compliant and suggestible and are searching desperately for explanations of their pain and the chaos in their lives. Considerable harm may be done to these patients and their families when therapists search for traumatic memories that are not there. The evidence does not provide a rationale for this approach: No symptom or set of symptoms or behaviors is an infallible indicator of trauma.

CHAPTER 11

Exploration and Change

Treating Self and Interpersonal Problems

The strategies for treating symptoms and crises discussed in previous chapters eventually lead to a consideration of underlying mechanisms and processes. As symptoms settle and affect tolerance and regulation improve, it becomes possible to focus on the more stable aspects of personality disorder—self and interpersonal problems, and the maladaptive trait expressions that contribute to these problems. This is the fourth phase in the intervention sequence of safety, containment, regulation and control, exploration and change, and integration and synthesis. It should be recalled, however, that these phases merely represent differences in emphasis and overlap substantially. Therapeutic work on self and interpersonal problems occurs increasingly during the control and regulation phase, because it is these problems that trigger the dysphoric states that lead to impulsivity and self-harm.

Earlier discussion of the construct system (Chapter 2) distinguished between the *content or substantive* pathology (maladaptive self and interpersonal schemata and maladaptive interpersonal patterns) and the *structural or organizational* pathology (core self and interpersonal problems) that define personality disorder. This chapter considers the treatment of substantive problems. The main treatment goals are (1) to modify maladaptive self and interpersonal schemata; (2) to change cyclical maladaptive patterns of interpersonal behavior; and (3) to change maladaptive ways of thinking, or cognitive styles, such as self-invalidating thinking and those

described by cognitive therapy such as catastrophizing, all-or-none thinking, and overgeneralizing (Beck & Emory, 1985), that contribute to self
and interpersonal problems.

The attainment of these goals depends on changing *repetitive maladaptive behavior patterns* that involve habitual ways of thinking, feeling, or acting, or combinations of the three. Patients first must become adept at *pattern recognition*. Most patients readily accept the idea that there is a
"pattern" underlying their behavior. The word is reassuring, for it suggests
that there is order and meaning to behavior and experience. Educating patients about these patterns helps them to distance themselves from events
and promotes self-observation. At the same time, pattern recognition promotes integration by connecting events, behaviors, and experiences that
were previously assumed to be unconnected.

These patterns take many forms. The simplest are recurrent ways of
acting, thinking, or feeling, such as the self-invalidating style. Others are
simple A-B-C sequences (see Chapter 4), such as the behavioral sequence
leading to self-harm. Pattern recognition involves linking components of
causal chains. Such patterns are often first apparent during assessment. For
example, one patient with dissocial features was difficult to assess because
he was vague about his reasons for seeking help and the reasons for his referral. He also had difficulty describing the major events in his life. Whenever the clinician tried to elicit details, he said that he did not know and
that he was confused. Attempts to clarify matters evoked irritation. After
this pattern had occurred several times, the clinician commented that
whenever she asked about problems, the patient said that he did not know
and that he felt confused. She added that if she continued trying to understand what had happened, the patient became frustrated and irritated. The
clinician wondered if the patient had noticed this pattern. The patient
laughed and said that he had not realized that he acted in this way, although he could see it now. More complex patterns involve self-schemata,
affects, and interpersonal behaviors. Especially important are cyclical maladaptive interpersonal patterns, in which the individual acts in ways that
perpetuate the pattern. For example, the feeling that a significant other
does not care may arouse fears of abandonment and rejection that lead to
a state of rage. In this state, the individual makes angry demands of the
other person that cause him or her to withdraw. This response confirms
the underlying fear of abandonment and perpetuates the cycle.

SCHEMATA AND CYCLICAL MALADAPTIVE PATTERNS

The concept of schema is the cornerstone for understanding and treating
cyclical maladaptive interpersonal patterns. It will be recalled from Chapter 2 that schemata have three components: a set of characteristics (cog-

nitions, feelings, actions) that are assumed to go together, an explanation of why these features co-occur, and important memories related to the schema.

Characteristics of Schemata

Schemata differ along four dimensions: specificity and abstraction, centrality, permeability, and range of application. With regard to the degree of *specificity and abstraction*, specific or lower-level schemata are organized into more general or higher-level schemata to form a hierarchy (Horowitz, 1998). Specific beliefs such as "No one cares about me," and "Nobody wants to spend time with me" may be combined to form the higher order schema "I am unlovable." Similarly, specific characteristics, such as kindness or impulsivity, are linked to form representations of the self or another person. The most general schema is the person's overall conception of the self—what was referred to earlier as the person's theory of the self. More abstract schemata are difficult to change because they are supported by subordinate schemata. The most effective way to modify them is probably by modifying the subordinate schemata. To use the previous example, it is easier to challenge specific beliefs such as "No one cares for me" than the higher-order schema "I am unlovable."

Schemata also differ in *centrality* or importance. Central or core maladaptive schemata, such as "I am unlovable" or "I am defective—there is something fundamentally wrong with me," are critical to understanding the individual's worldview and interpersonal relationships. Core schemata tend to be grouped into five thematic areas (Cottraux & Blackburn, 2001):

Love (e.g., "I am unlovable")
Ability and competence (e.g., "I am useless and incompetent")
Morality (e.g., "I am bad")
Normality (e.g., "I am flawed" or "I am not normal like other people")
General worth (e.g., "I am worthless")

Other core schemata are organized around themes of attachment, abandonment, and trust.

Maladaptive core schemata tend to evoke strong emotions. They are usually treated as facts and used in an all-or-none fashion, without being challenged or questioned (Layden et al., 1993). For example, the schema "I am disgusting," held by a person with personality disorder, is a categorical statement: exceptions are not acknowledged or tolerated, nor is the belief contingent upon events. In contrast, with a less disordered individual, the same belief is conditional. For example, the individual may conclude that "I am disgusting if I do something repugnant."

Schemata vary in *permeability*—that is, the degree to which they are flexible and open to change (Kelly, 1955). The maladaptive core schemata of mistrust and abandonment, which are the basis of cyclical maladaptive patterns, are highly impermeable. Considerable effort is expended in maintaining these schemata, and they do not yield readily to the usual methods of cognitive therapy.

Finally, schemata differ in *range of application* (Kelly, 1955). Some are applied to a wide range of situations, whereas others are more narrowly focused. Maladaptive core schemata are applied in a rigid and stereotyped way to a wide range of situations and individuals. A task of therapy is to promote more discriminating application of these schemata.

Schema Functioning and Stability

To understand how repetitive, maladaptive patterns may be changed, we need to examine the way schemata function and the role they play in maintaining these patterns. Schemata organize experience, influence what is noticed and becomes the focus of attention, and determine what is discounted and ignored. For example, suspicious individuals who believe that the world is hostile and that people are out to trick or harm them are hypervigilant: They notice minor slights or expressions of hostility that are consistent with these beliefs, and they ignore behaviors that are not consistent with them. Schemata also lead to actions that tend to elicit the very reactions from others that the person fears or wishes to avoid. The suspicious person evokes cautious and hostile reactions, which, in turn, confirm beliefs that people are hostile and untrustworthy. These cognitive and behavioral processes make schemata relatively stable (Figure 11.1). The clinical significance of these processes is illustrated by the following vignette.

> Sandra, a woman in her late 20s with a long history of drug and alcohol abuse, chronic interpersonal difficulties, and dysphoric affects, had a personality profile typical of emotional dysregulation, with the additional trait of suspiciousness. In DSM-IV terms, she met the criteria for borderline personality disorder with paranoid traits. Many of her interpersonal problems were related to her deep suspiciousness about other people's motives and her beliefs that people could not be trusted and that everyone was hostile toward her. She did not recognize how these beliefs influenced the way people reacted to her.
> Sandra arrived for one session angry and frustrated. Earlier that day while walking in a local park, she had been hit by a passerby on two separate occasions. One person, she contended, had deliberately bumped into her, and the other, a woman, had actually thumped her on the arm as she passed by her. These incidents were interpreted as confirmation that everyone was against her. Almost gleefully, Sandra told the therapist, "You see, I'm *right*. People are against me. Two

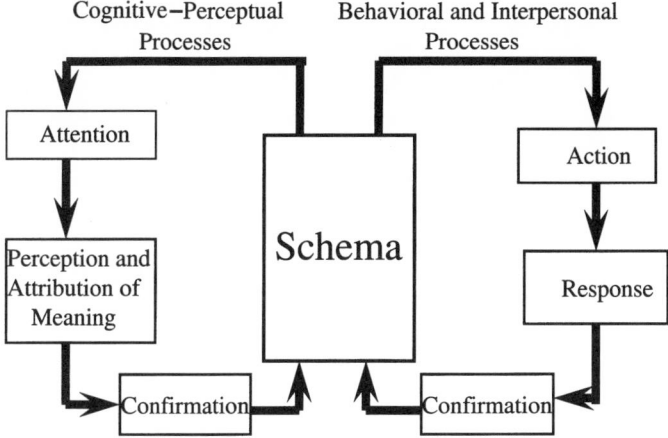

FIGURE 11.1. Processes maintaining schema stability.

people hit me for no reason." The therapist commented that one such incident may, perhaps, be understandable, but two were difficult to explain.

Further discussion of the incidents revealed that before the walk, Sandra was feeling angry about the way her life had turned out, and she felt hostile toward everyone. These feelings were triggered by an acquaintance behaving in a way that made her feel rejected. She decided to go for a walk to take her mind off things. When the woman thumped her as she went past, someone walking behind her asked whether she had been hit. Sandra confirmed that she had. The other person expressed surprise and concern. Sandra went on to tell the therapist that normally she would have reacted strongly and pursued the person who hit her. On this occasion, however, she successfully resisted reacting. She added that she realized she must emanate intense hostility that people readily recognize. When this possibility was discussed, Sandra explained that she always walked on the outside of the path around the lake, in a determined way that made it clear that she did not intend to move out of anyone's way. On this occasion she was also scowling. This realization caused Sandra to wonder whether she helped to create the hostility that she saw in others. Further discussion led her to wonder whether her belief that the world is hostile and that everyone was opposed to her was correct.

This incident illustrates how we all help to create the world in which we live—a process referred to earlier as evocative person–environment interaction (see Chapter 3). Sandra's schema that the world is hostile was self-perpetuating (Figure 11.2). She was always on the lookout for events that confirmed her beliefs, and she usually delighted in pointing them out to her therapist, saying, as she did on this occasion, "You see, I'm *right*" (Hellinga, 1999). Sandra's walk around the lake also illustrates the persistence of schemata in the face of contradictory evidence (Singer & Salovey, 1991). Information suggesting that not everyone was hostile to her, such as the concern expressed by another walker, was ignored. The actions of the people who hit her were generalized to confirm the belief that everyone was against her. Alternative explanations were not considered. Finally, the angry, unyielding way in which she walked provoked anger in others. Their responses increased her sense of injustice and rage. Thus the cyclical pattern was perpetuated. Initially, Sandra did not recognize how she communicated her hostility to others. She externalized all blame and responsibility. The therapist's comment that two such instances were difficult to explain helped Sandra reflect on her actions and see how she produced reactions in others that she sought to avoid. This vignette suggests that effecting change in maladaptive cognitions and interpersonal patterns may involve, in addition to reframing these beliefs, helping individuals act in ways that do not elicit confirming responses from the interpersonal environment.

Sandra's schema played an important role in initiating events that led to her deliberate self-harming acts. She was hypersensitive to anything related to the schema. Actions that others would consider neutral or minor were interpreted in the light of this schema. Her social life was chaotic because she rapidly evoked conflict in her relationships. Interpersonal problems frequently triggered the dysphoria that led to self-harm. Although

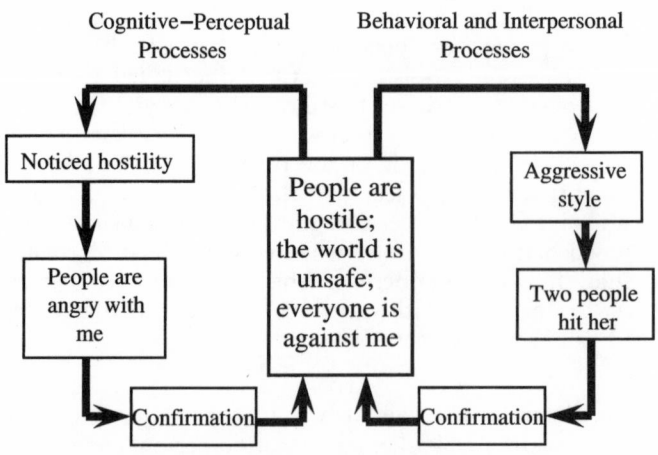

FIGURE 11.2. Illustration of schema functioning.

behavioral interventions reduced the frequency of these acts, the dysphoria continued. It was only when Sandra recognized this pattern and began to challenge and change it that the self-harming behavior finally ceased. This took well over 1 year of individual treatment.

Schemata are also maintained through active avoidance of experiences and situations that are likely to activate them (Young, 1990, 1994). This avoidance prevents encounters with evidence that may be inconsistent with the schema, a phenomenon that is also important in maintaining maladaptive sequelae of trauma. Considerable time and energy are expended in avoiding anything connected with feared or painful experiences and in suppressing painful thoughts and experiences. Examples of schema avoidance mechanisms include the defense mechanisms described by psychodynamic psychotherapy. Whereas psychoanalytic theory assumes, however, that defenses are unconscious mechanisms, schema avoidance is often deliberate, as when the patient says, "I don't want to think about that" or deliberately diverts attention from a given topic. Feelings associated with the schema may also be avoided by engaging in impulsive behavior. Schema avoidance requires continual attention and hinders exploration. Because some experiences are separated or split off from other aspects of self-awareness, avoidance leads to divisions arising within self-knowledge that compromise the integrity of the self.

Restructuring Schemata

The methods used by cognitive therapy to change schemata primarily involve either schema extinction and replacement or schema modification (Beck et al., 1990; Cottraux & Blackburn, 2001; Layden et al., 1993; Young, 1990, 1994). The most fundamental method, *schema extinction and replacement*, requires the individual to stop using a maladaptive schema and replace it with a more adaptive alternative. An example would be for the paranoid individual to stop using the suspiciousness schema and replace it with one of trust. However, because radical restructuring is difficult to achieve, especially with maladaptive core schemata or schemata linked to heritable traits, most changes involve *schema modification*. Schemata may be modified by promoting more *flexible application* of them. For example, the paranoid individual usually distrusts everyone, regardless of the situation. Although radical change is unlikely, because the schema is part of the trait of suspiciousness, it may be possible to help the individual become more discriminating in his or her distrust by *incorporating other attributes* into the schema. A consistent therapeutic relationship, for example, may create the idea that the therapist can be trusted. Over time, the belief that "no one can be trusted" gradually changes into "most people cannot be trusted" and perhaps even into "some people can be trusted sometimes."

Maladaptive schemata may also be changed by *reframing the way situa-*

tions are interpreted. As noted in Chapter 9, successful treatment of self-harm involves developing a new understanding of triggering events. For example, the patient who feels rejected because people cannot always help her due to other commitments may be shown how to reframe these events by recognizing that the other person's decisions had nothing to do with the patient, and everything to do with prior commitments. Other forms of schema modification involve *changing the environment*—that is, seeking situations that provide experiences that reinforce the incorporation of new elements into a maladaptive schema or strengthen a more adaptive schema. For example, a patient who feels incompetent may be encouraged to identify and spend time engaging in activities that he or she can perform well. This strategy can be a powerful way to change schemata at critical junctures in treatment.

The treatment of people with personality disorder also involves the synthesis of new self and interpersonal schemata. This is the final phase of treatment, which focuses on the development of more integrated schemata to represent self and others, and the emergence of a new understanding of the rules that guide interpersonal behavior. This is the topic of Chapter 13.

CHANGING SCHEMATA AND MALADAPTIVE PATTERNS

The cognitive and behavioral components of maladaptive patterns are so intertwined that it is difficult to disentangle schemata from associated behavioral strategies and the reciprocal responses of others. For this reason, changing schemata and maladaptive interpersonal patterns is discussed as a single topic. Schema modification lends itself to the stage of change approach. The sequence begins by identifying a schema and associated interpersonal pattern and exploring how it is expressed in treatment and everyday life. Subsequently, specific behavioral and perceptual–cognitive components of the schema are challenged to promote the acquisition of alternative beliefs and constructs, and changes are then generalized to everyday life.

Schemata Identification and Recognition

The task of identifying schemata and maladaptive patterns initially lies with the therapist, because they are usually used automatically, with limited awareness on the patient's part. Once schemata and maladaptive patterns are identified, it usually takes time for patients to recognize the many ways they enact these patterns. Recognition is facilitated by using the two-step process for managing maladaptive patterns discussed in Chapter 4: (1) identify the global pattern and help the patient understand and accept the way it contributes to problems; and (2) focus on helping the patient recognize the nuances of the pattern and the specific ways it is manifested inside and outside treatment. The *first step* is usually straightforward. For example, the therapist may note a possible pattern of submissiveness that includes the schema "I must do what others expect of me," which leads to subservient acts and consequent feelings of being neglected and exploited. When evidence has accumulated, indicating that the pattern is prevalent, the patient's attention is drawn to the pattern in the context of discussing a relevant event, such as an incident in which another person was abusive or when the patient agreed to unreasonable requests. This strategy focuses attention on the pattern and connects the feelings, actions, and events involved.

Schema avoidance may hinder recognition and acceptance. Avoidance typically occurs when a hypothesized schema is identified before the patient is ready or when the alliance is in a compromised state. Recognition and acceptance are more likely to occur if the therapist waits until the pattern is obvious and then helps the patient to recognize the pattern for him- or herself. For example, when a patient describes an abusive incident, it may be more effective to note how the incident was similar to previous incidents rather than interpret the pattern directly. Thus the therapist might comment: "This incident sounds a lot like the one you mentioned in our last session. On each of these occasions it seems as if people feel that they can push you around. Have you noticed this?" The therapist may then wonder aloud why this pattern keeps happening. This approach allows the therapist to monitor acceptance of the idea and to change tack if it is likely to be rejected or increase reactivity. If the idea is rejected, the therapist acknowledges that he or she may be wrong and reconsiders the hypothesis. If it still seems applicable, the idea can be presented again later, after collecting more evidence.

Although the recognition of broad patterns such as submissiveness is an important step, it is unlikely to lead directly to change because it is difficult to translate an understanding of a global pattern into specific changes. Change involves recognizing and challenging specific expressions of the pattern in treatment and everyday life. This is the *second step* in the recognition process. It takes time and many repetitions before patients can recognize the nuances of key patterns and the automatic ways in which they express these patterns. The following vignette illustrates how basic schemata escape attention:

A severely depressed patient with dependent and avoidant personality disorders and obsessive–compulsive traits complained that his family was not supportive and criticized him for being depressed. They thought that he should be able to overcome the problem and that everything was his own fault. The patient also blamed himself

282   PRACTICAL MANAGEMENT OF PERSONALITY DISORDER

for being unable to control the depression and the problems it caused. Exploration revealed that these thoughts were part of a cluster of beliefs that included: "I must be in control," "Everything is my responsibility," "I should be able to cope with everything," and "If I can't cope or things go wrong, it's my fault." The patient recognized that this self-talk was similar to the statements his mother made throughout childhood, statements that his family echoed in the present.

After spending several sessions discussing how this schema affected his mood, the patient described a recent meeting with a business advisor. A few months earlier the patient had been dissatisfied with the service provided and had transferred his business to someone else, but now he had to contact the advisor once more. The advisor was abrupt and blamed the patient for the problems that had arisen. The patient became intensely anxious and depressed. These feelings lasted for several days. When the therapist asked about his thoughts when the incident happened, the patient insisted that he had not thought anything—the sadness simply occurred, and he did not know why. While discussing the incident, the patient suddenly got exasperated and said, "He was right—everything was my fault." It was only when the therapist linked the patient's conclusion to his family's comments and his own self-talk that the patient recognized that this was another example of the schema. It took many more incidents of this type before the patient was able to recognize and challenge the pattern as it occurred.

Pattern recognition is often facilitated by an active focus on the way the pattern is expressed in the micro-events of therapy, as illustrated by the following vignette:

Christina had been in the individual therapy for about 1 year after presenting with severe self-mutilation, low mood, and frequent suicidal crises associated with transient psychotic symptoms. She gave a history of childhood sexual and physical abuse. The self-harm receded over a period of about 6 months, in response to containment and affect-regulation interventions combined with an SSRI antidepressant and intermittent use of an atypical neuroleptic. Treatment was initially complicated by the fact that the patient felt that the hospital staff had been critical and abusive during hospital admissions and her visits to emergency rooms. As treatment progressed, the patient began to recognize that the escalating dysphoric states culminating in self-mutilation were usually triggered by memories of abuse or being treated abusively. She also began to recognize a pattern of submissiveness that made it easy for her to be abused. She noted that, "If I abuse myself, I make it easier for others to abuse me." She also began to understand that her submissiveness led to the neglect of her own needs, to feelings that no one really cared about her, and to people taking advantage of her. This sequence, in turn, contributed to the depressive symptoms. Although Christina recognized the broad pattern, it was difficult for her to recognize how she acted submissively in everyday situations. The therapy began to concentrate on helping Christina recognize the various ways in which she acted submissively and how she relied on others to confirm her ideas and offer reassurance. The following dialogue illustrates this focus on the details of the pattern.

CHRISTINA: I am feeling much better. I no longer want to hurt myself. Even with all the things that happened this week, I didn't even think about hurting myself. I am much better. Do you think I'm better?

THERAPIST: You obviously handled things very differently this week from the way you did only a few months ago. It sounds as if things went well.

CHRISTINA: But do you think I'm better?

THERAPIST: You also sound pleased with the way you handled things. That's important. It is not what I think that matters; it is what *you* think that counts.

CHRISTINA: But I want to be sure that I'm *right*.

THERAPIST: I understand that, and it would be easy for me to give you an answer, but it is more important that we talk about why you don't trust your own feelings and how this makes you rely on me to decide how you feel.

CHRISTINA: But I'm not really sure . . . I feel better but I don't *know* that I'm better.

THERAPIST: You say you feel better and then you doubt yourself and ask me to decide for you. Over the last few weeks, we have talked about how you feel that everyone tells you what to do, that people push you around, and that even hospital staff treat you abusively. We also talked about your submissive pattern and how you feel that you should do what other people want, and you wondered whether you did things that allowed other people to abuse you and tell you what to do. Can you see how you have just done the same with me? You looked to me to tell you how you feel, even though you had already decided that you feel better. Perhaps it's these simple things that make it easy for others to control you and treat you abusively.

CHRISTINA: I didn't think about that at the time, but I see it now. Do you think that I will ever be able to stop doing these things?

THERAPIST: Have you noticed that the same thing has just happened again? In the past you've been able to take the things that we talk about and use them. Why wouldn't you be able to do the same with this pattern? You seem to lose sight of these achievements and look to me to tell you whether you will be able to do it again. You are relying on me to decide what you can and cannot do.

CHRISTINA: I have, haven't I? ... (*Pause*). I don't think about it. I just do it without thinking.

THERAPIST: That's what's important about the pattern. It's automatic. It is also very subtle. It's part of the way you think. This is why it is important that you get very good at recognizing the way you give power to others in these very simple ways.

This dialogue illustrates more than just Christina's submissiveness. It also illustrates self-invalidation and difficulty accepting the authenticity of her experiences. The strong transference, apparent in the dialogue, is used to illuminate a cognitive style that contributes to her submissiveness. In the process, the relationship component of the transference is downplayed. Here we see the value of *engaging pathological patterns in the treatment interaction* to ensure that patients recognize how pathology is woven into the fabric of their thought and experience. The danger with this approach is that it may be too intrusive and evoke anger or withdrawal. These consequences are avoided by careful attention to the alliance and expressive behavior, including tone of voice. The approach is only used when the alliance is excellent and the conditions for using specific interventions are clearly met. Any decrease in the alliance signals the need for an immediate switch to the strategy for dealing with alliance ruptures (Chapter 7) and containment interventions (Chapter 8).

Schema recognition is also facilitated by encouraging patients to note everyday events and list the ways a given pattern is expressed. The list can then be used to identify targets for change. One patient kept a record of submissive acts during a 1-week period. She commented: "I was horrified when I realized the many ways I'm submissive. Yesterday in the supermarket line, I let the person behind me go first because she seemed impatient. It's as if *I* never matter." This insight engendered an immediate commitment to change and, without prompting, the patient wondered how she could avoid acting in these ways.

Schema Exploration

Pattern recognition merges with exploration and change. As the previous example shows, once the details of a maladaptive pattern are recognized, it is almost automatic to challenge some of the component behaviors and consider alternatives. However, other aspects of the exploration process warrant comment.

Psychoeducation

The groundwork for schema change was covered in the discussions of the role of dysfunctional cognitions in amplifying distress (discussed in Chapter 9). Schema exploration provides an opportunity to extend this understanding. It is useful to explain that a schema is a strong belief expressed through a variety of thoughts to ensure that the idea of a schema as a cluster of beliefs linked by a common theme is understood. It is also useful to point out that people are often unaware of their schemata and their effects, even though these have a powerful influence on all aspects of their behavior. This information begins to direct patients' attention away from symptomatic distress to the need for fundamental changes in the way that they think about themselves, their lives, and their relationships.

A useful way to teach patients about schemata is to summarize information about the behavioral and cognitive processes that contribute to their persistence. Summaries integrate diverse experiences and items of self-knowledge. A *schema diagram*, such as the one shown in Figure 11.2, is a useful way to impart this information and seamlessly incorporate a psychoeducational component into treatment. During the session described in the vignette, the therapist drew this diagram and discussed it with Sandra. Together they explored other examples of the schema in action, until Sandra understood how it operated and how it influenced her behavior. Diagrams are useful because they capture schema functioning in a concrete form that is readily understood and easy to remember, and they force therapists and patients to clarify the details of maladaptive patterns. The patient is encouraged to collaborate in constructing the diagram, so that it becomes a joint understanding rather than something produced by the therapist. A diagram helps patients to distance themselves from their own reactions and to *process* information rather than simply *react* to events.

Besides working on core schemata in treatment, patients also can develop schema diagrams between sessions to consolidate their understanding and promote transfer to everyday life. However, discussion of therapeutic work to be done between sessions should be approached cautiously, because it is easy for the therapist to be seen as a demanding authority figure. Terms such as *homework* are best avoided because they often have negative connotations. After discussing a given schema, it may be sufficient for the therapist to comment: "You may find it helpful to take the diagram with you and think about the way you act in this way in your relationships with other people so that you fully understand how this pattern affects your everyday relationships." Subsequently, the therapist may inquire whether the approach was useful and discuss any problems the patient encountered as he or she made use of the diagram (or perhaps even expanded it) between sessions.

Focus on Antecedents and Consequences

The value of exploring the antecedents and consequences of maladaptive behavior was raised when discussing self-harm. It is also useful to delineate the A-B-C sequence underlying maladaptive schemata and patterns so that the events that initiate a given schema or pattern are recognized and consequences for everyday relationships are understood. This exercise links discrete events with common themes. Reactions such as feeling neglected, abused, exploited, and taken for granted; that others are making unreasonable demands; and powerful needs to take care of others are no longer seen as separate "islands" of unfathomable experience but as part of a general and explicable pattern of submissiveness. Exploration of the A-B-C sequence leads naturally to education about the way that schemata function and their role in maintaining cyclical maladaptive interpersonal patterns.

Exploring Cyclical Patterns

Maladaptive interpersonal patterns were described as a sequence involving a cognitive–affective state organized around (1) one or more core schemata, (2) the patient's behavior when in this state, (3) others' perceptions of these behaviors and their responses to them, and (4) the patient's impressions of these responses (see Chapter 5). An extension of the schema diagram may be used to explore each component of the sequence. For example, Sandra, the patient described in the vignette about the walk in the park, who held the schema, "No one gives a damn about me," came to recognize the following sequence:

Schema:	"No one gives a damn about me."
Associated affects:	Anger and distress
Behavioral component:	
Own responses toward others:	Acted toward people as if they were unimportant
	Cold and distant
	Arrogantly dismissive
Others' responses:	Treated her as if she did not matter
	Ignored her
	Anger
Perceptual–cognitive component:	
Selective attention:	Only noticed acts that could be interpreted as rejecting or neglectful of her needs
Selective inattention:	Did not notice acts of caring and concern
Attributions:	Assumed people were not interested in her problems
	Interpreted their responses as confirming the belief that "no one gives a damn"

Sandra was comfortable exploring the behavioral component of the pattern; she was willing to look at how she behaved toward friends and acquaintances and how her behavior changed when she felt that they did not care. She came to recognize how she evoked reactions that reaffirmed her fears. However, initially she was not comfortable exploring the cognitive component, and she actively avoided thinking about her perceptions of other people because they were too distressing. Gradually, it emerged that these thoughts were avoided because they activated an even more distressing schema, "No one loves me." As feelings became more manageable, Sandra began to consider the possibility that she may sometimes misperceive people's actions and intentions. This new self-knowledge reduced her tendency to externalize responsibility for problems.

Exploring the Origins of Schemata and Maladaptive Patterns

Although the current approach assumes that change is primarily due to modification of maladaptive processes as they occur in the present rather than through insight into their origins, patients often need to understand the origins of their problems. This need means that it is necessary, at some point, to explore important historical events and the ways in which specific individuals influenced the patient's development. An understanding of these factors gives meaning and perspective to problems and helps patients understand how developmental experiences have influenced their lives. This understanding often reduces guilt about the current state of their lives and helps them to take reasonable responsibility for their actions. An understanding of history also may contribute to the development of a more adaptive theory of the self. It is useful to note, however, that *the goal is to provide a perspective on current functioning* rather than in-depth exploration or catharsis.

Exploring Schema Relationships

Schemata are not separate cognitive entities; rather, they are linked into *hierarchical structures* or belief systems. Hence the activation of one schema may arouse others. This "domino effect" is illustrated by the vignette of Sandra's walk in the park. The episode began when a friend's action evoked the schema "People reject me," which aroused the schema, "People are hostile; the world is against me." The intense affects associated with this schema activated the more distressing schema, "No one loves me," which, in turn, evoked the even more distressing core schema, "I am unlovable." The connections among schemata create a network that resists change. Change is also difficult because core schemata are not readily accessible and arouse intense affects that lead to avoidance.

Horizontal links also exist among schema at the same level of generality and among schemata and maladaptive ways of thinking, such as externalizing and catastrophizing cognitive styles. Specification of these relationships can have a powerful effect on the change process by reframing the patients' understanding of their experience. This is illustrated by the following vignette, taken from the treatment of Natasha, the patient first discussed in Chapter 5.

> At the time in question, Natasha had been in twice-weekly treatment for just over 1 year. Slow but consistent progress occurred, using a combination of interventions, including medication. The main psychotherapeutic effort focused on building a relationship, containment, and cognitive-behavioral strategies to reduce self-harm and control affects. Natasha found relaxation and attention-shifting exercises effective ways to regulate distress and control intense rage over how she was treated by her partner and friends. A little progress was also made in changing the catastrophic thinking that increased her distress. These measures led to some decrease in affective lability and an end to deliberate self-harming behavior. However, the general distress continued, and Natasha was unable to return to work. Her life was a constant crisis. Natasha attributed her difficulties to having an abusive partner and problems with friends. She spent considerable time wishing that things were different and planning ways to get the people around her to change and treat her differently. She had little understanding of how she contributed to these problems. She did, however, recognize that she related to others in a submissive way but saw this pattern as unavoidable, given her predicament. She thought that it was the only way to deal with her partner.
>
> She began one session by saying that she had suddenly realized the extent to which she always assumed the worst. A few days before she had been in a state of panic because her daughter was staying in a country where a serious accident had occurred. She had worried about her daughter's safety, even though she was living a long way from the location of the accident. Natasha had been very upset and had told a friend about her worries. The friend was supportive but noted that she always assumed the worst, even when it was very unlikely. This observation made Natasha think about how she catastrophized everything when she was upset. She suddenly realized that she had to change. The chance comment by a friend occurred in the context of treatment focused on preparing Natasha for this understanding. This is a good example of the development of self-understanding, described by Shapiro (1989), in which the patient suddenly realizes the true significance of something that has always been known.
>
> When the links between the panicky feelings and the catastrophizing thinking were discussed, Natasha noted that the panic occurred when she felt useless and incompetent and unable to cope—which, in turn, caused her to feel hopeless and expect the worst.

Discussion of this pattern made Natasha realize that she always blamed everyone else for her problems, but "often it is me—I am the one doing this to myself, I am the one who has to change." She then laughed and said somewhat ironically, "It's taken me a year to realize this. All this time I've blamed everyone else and tried to get *them* to change."

These insights allowed Natasha to connect two maladaptive ways of thinking, catastrophizing and externalizing responsibility, and to link them with the schema of incompetence. In the process, the significance of these patterns changed. The realization that she externalized responsibility enabled her to recognize the pervasiveness of her catastrophic thinking and that it could be changed. As these ideas were discussed, further insights emerged. Natasha suddenly commented, "This is why I feel so hopeless and why I am so passive. If I think that other people are responsible for my problems, then there is nothing that I can do about them. I may as well give up." This insight enabled Natasha to understand how externalizing responsibility and submissiveness were linked and how they contributed to her despondency and despair. She also recognized that seeing herself as incompetent (a core schema) made her more submissive, and vice versa: She felt that she had to rely on others because she could not do things for herself.

This session again illustrates the contribution that chance events make to change. Although there are many features to this material, some of which are discussed in a later chapter, the point to note here is the value of linking schemata, interpersonal patterns, and other cognitive processes. The example also shows how different processes and structures reinforce each other. Externalization limited understanding of catastrophic thinking, increased passivity, and provided a way to express submissiveness and passivity. Externalization also supported, and was supported by, the core schema of incompetence, which, in turn, also reinforced the submissiveness. Although integrating different behaviors in this way facilitates change, the danger is that the amount of information involved may prove overwhelming. This possible inundation is reduced by offering broad summaries and asking the patient to comment and elaborate on them. As noted, it also helps to use a diagram. As Natasha discussed her insights, the therapist drew a diagram of the connection between the different components and then discussed the diagram with her (see Figure 11.3).

Exploring the Relationships among Schemata and Maladaptive Behaviors

An important part of exploration is to describe the relationship between core schemata and maladaptive behaviors such as self-harm. These rela-

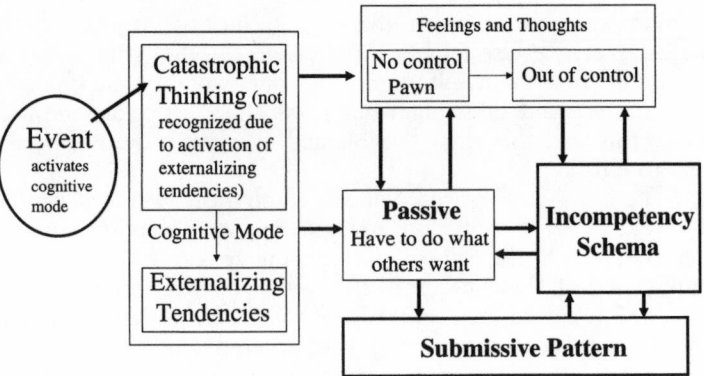

FIGURE 11.3. Externalizing and catastrophic thinking, incompetency schema, and submissive pattern.

tionships are rarely a simple matter of an event activating a single maladaptive schema that in turn initiates a maladaptive response. In most cases, the event triggers a cascade of reactions. With Natasha, one trigger was *any* unexpected event. The unexpectedness evoked the feeling of being unable to cope and the core maladaptive schema, "I am incompetent." When activated, the incompetence schema contributed to submissive behavior and caused intense distress, which was then increased by catastrophic thinking. This cognitive style was also aroused directly by unexpected events and contributed to the sense of being unable to cope. The incompetence schema, in turn, evoked an even more distressing core schema, "I am bad." This schema was also activated by events that evoked memories of childhood trauma and abuse. The badness schema caused considerable self-hatred that led to cutting as a way of punishing herself.

An understanding of the relationship between core schemata and deliberate self-harm helped Natasha to understand the reasons for these acts and the ways in which they were triggered. This new understanding increased her control over them and allowed her to make more effective use of the techniques discussed in previous chapters. Subsequently, attention was focused on modifying the incompetence and badness schemata by helping her (1) understand how they had developed out of repetitive abuse and trauma, and (2) incorporate new beliefs that modulated their expression. The same approach was also used to help her understand events that triggered intense rage, which was also a consequence of abuse.

Exploring Conflicting Schemata

Psychodynamic, interpersonal, and cognitive theories recognize that adversity often leads to conflicting schemata and conflicted relationships.

These conflicts differ according to trait patterns. With the emotionally dysregulated pattern, conflict exists between wanting care and attention, and distrust. This conflict is readily apparent during crises, when patients demand care yet are distrustful, angry, and rejecting of help. Similarly, inhibited or schizoid–avoidant individuals may want relationships and a normal lifestyle, and yet they are fearful of intimacy and revealing personal information because they are afraid that others will use it against them. At times of crisis, they are reluctant to seek help and cautious about revealing their distress. The existence of these inconsistent patterns makes it difficult for other people to satisfy the patient's needs. Hence these conflicts are continually reinforced in everyday relationships and readily activated in treatment. These conflicting patterns need to be identified and clarified in order for the individual to develop more effective relationships. An understanding of these problems early in treatment helps the clinician prevent them from interfering with the therapeutic work.

Nonverbal Schemata

A common problem in treating patients with severe personality disorder is that they cannot find words to describe some common states and feelings. The events that trigger these states are often unclear, and it is difficult to identify the schemata involved. These reactions seem to be related to gross childhood abuse or neglect. Abuse seems to lead to more reactive states, whereas neglect apparently leads to more muted behavior and despair. It is usually suggested that these reactions involve nonverbal schemata linked to abuse and neglect that occurred early in development, before verbal facility was well established. The difficulty with articulating these states may also be the product of intense adversity overwhelming cognitive processes, so that the schemata involved are largely nonverbal.

Exploration of, and change in, nonverbal schemata begins, as with any schema, by finding a label to represent these states, followed by identification of triggering events. Considerable gentle persistence is required when dealing with patients' reluctance to examine these painful feelings. Exploration is also difficult because patients often insist that these feelings occur spontaneously, "out of the blue." In many cases, the triggers are themselves nonverbal, such as a physical stimulus associated with abuse, someone getting too close physically, being touched, a nonresponsive facial expression, or even a particular smell. Recognition may be aided by attending to images and impressions that flash rapidly across the mind as these reactions occur. Within-therapy events are especially valuable sources of information, because they provide an opportunity to examine reactions as they occur. Therapist behavior often inadvertently triggers nonverbal schemata. In one patient, they occurred when she thought that the therapist was not listening. This perceived disinterest evoked painful feelings of despair that were eventually related to abandonment and unlov-ability schemata and memories of a distant and depressed mother who rarely responded to her young daughter. In another patient, the approach-ing end of a session evoked feelings of being unimportant, which origi-nated in being left in her room for long periods when a young child.

Identification of triggers shows the patient that these reactions are not spontaneous and hence can be understood and controlled. Triggers also contain valuable clues about the schemata involved. When exploring non-verbal schemata, it is especially important to keep emotional arousal with-in tolerable limits because cognitive control is limited by the schemata's nonverbal structure.

Schema Change and the Acquisition of Alternatives

Cognitive therapy describes cognitive, interpersonal, behavioral, and emo-tional methods for changing maladaptive schemata (Beck et al., 1990; Cottraux & Blackburn, 2001; Padesky, 1994; Young, 1990, 1994). The most useful cognitive method in early and middle stages of treatment is to challenge and dispute beliefs and schemata. Interpersonal methods based on the treatment relationship are especially useful in changing core mal-adaptive schemata. Behavioral methods involve translating schema change into actual behavioral change and acting in ways that elicit new inputs from the interpersonal environment, which, in turn, weaken maladaptive schemata or strengthen adaptive schemata. Emotional methods involving the activation of feelings and catharsis are powerful ways to effect schema change (Young, 1994), and similar methods are the cornerstone of psycho-dynamic therapy, although their use in treating patients with personality disorder is circumscribed.

Although an impressive array of cognitive interventions is available, standard interventions are not as useful in treating patients with severe personality disorder as they are in treating patients with other disorders (Layden et al., 1993). The role of cognitive interventions in the early and middle stages of treatment is limited, because they require a degree of collaboration and motivation that is often lacking. Even motivated pa-tients experience considerable pessimism about the likely outcome of treatment and hence find it difficult complete cognitive therapy assign-ments. Moreover, the didactic nature of many cognitive interventions, their reliance on a Socratic process, and the assignment of tasks to be completed between treatment sessions tend to evoke strong reactions from patients who feel that they are being told what to do. Additional problems occur because core schemata arouse intense emotions, making it difficult to engage in typical cognitive work. For these reasons, *most inter-ventions appear to work best if they are incorporated as an experiential part of treatment.*

Cognitive Strategies

Cognitive interventions are best introduced through the use of general techniques for challenging dysfunctional thoughts and schemata, which involve examining supporting and disconfirming evidence. A natural extension of descriptive exploration is for the therapist to ask about the evidence for a given belief. When a belief is recognized to be ill-founded and the patient is able to modify it accordingly, it is natural for the therapist to inquire whether the patient could repeat the process the next time the thought, or one like it, occurs. Techniques to dispute schemata and beliefs can be introduced when an event is described that illustrates maladaptive thinking, and when retelling does not arouse feelings that make it difficult to examine thought processes dispassionately. The method is particularly effective when used to *examine and challenge schemata as they are activated during treatment*, because the experience is more vivid and intense.

Examine Supporting Evidence. Challenging a belief arising from a maladaptive cognitive style, such as catastrophic thinking, begins by critically examining the information on which the thinking is based. The goal is to (1) introduce flexibility in the way information is interpreted, and (2) help the patient develop an understanding that maladaptive schemata and beliefs are often based on incomplete evidence or erroneous thinking. In the case of Natasha, for example, an incident had occurred in which she became distressed at the thought that her daughter could have been hurt. The evidence for this belief was that several people had been killed in a natural disaster in the country where her daughter was staying, and she had not heard from her daughter for several days. This evidence was examined by asking Natasha about the population of the country, so that she could see that the chances of her daughter being one of the people hurt were one in many million. Moreover, the accident occurred in a region far from were the daughter was living and was one that she did not plan to visit. It also transpired that the daughter telephoned weekly on a set day and was not due to call for 2 more days. This review helped to consolidate the friend's comment that Natasha always thought the worst. It also showed Natasha how to dispute catastrophic thinking for herself.

This approach is less effective with maladaptive core schemata, although it complements other change methods, especially those based on the therapeutic relationship. With core schemata, a review of supportive evidence may extend over long periods of treatment in order to cover the different stages of the person's life. For example, the evidence used by a patient who maintained that "I am bad" included (1) being sexually abused as a child, (2) being told that she was bad by her family, including her mother, (3) the anger her family showed toward her, (4) being depressed, (5) cutting herself, (6) the fact that men make passes at her, (7) any problem with her children, and (8) being abused by her husband. Over time, each piece of evidence was examined, challenged, and reframed. For example, the patient cited as evidence that she was bad the fact that she had been abused and treated violently by many people, so, she concluded, "I must deserve it, and I must be bad for everyone to treat me in this way." The therapist reframed this evidence by saying, "You were brought up in an abusive family and learned to pick abusive men." The patient responded, "Oh! I had not thought of it that way. That means that I may not be bad, I simply made bad choices." The comment revealed a weakening in the previously fixed nature of the schema, which was then increased by reframing other supporting evidence. Each reframe was also a step toward examining the factors that influenced the patient's choice of men. In subsequent sessions the concept of person–situation interaction was used to help her understand how she selected men who had abusive potential and the things she did to provoke such behavior.

The process of reviewing evidence across different epochs of the patient's life also provided opportunities to *reframe childhood experiences* and explain the dynamics of trauma. To change the core schema, it was also necessary for the patient to recognize the ways in which her family of origin was dysfunctional and how this environment led to maladaptive ideas about herself, which the family continued to reinforce in the present. Although reviewing and disputing evidence supporting core schemata has limited immediate impact, it raises doubts about the certainty of these beliefs and contributes to a readiness to change that enhances the effects of other interventions.

Those who like to use more structured cognitive techniques can use the information provided by a review of supporting evidence as the basis for applying the continuum method, in which patients are asked to rate their core schema, in this case, "badness," on a scale from 0–100 (Cottraux & Blackburn, 2001). Ratings can be repeated following reframing interventions such as the one described. Patients can also rate others, including abusers, on the same scale and rate core schema in each of the situations used as evidence to support the schema. For example, the patient mentioned above could be asked to rate how "bad" she is in each of the situations mentioned. The goal is to show patients how they judge themselves in a more extreme way than they judge others and that once global categories have been broken down into more specific components, they may rate themselves less extremely.

Examine Contradictory Evidence. The vignette of the walk in the park showed that schema stability also depends upon ignoring or discounting contradictory information: in this case, the concern and support offered by other walkers. An examination of contradictory information complements challenges to supporting evidence by encouraging patients to ask the question "Am I missing anything?" whenever distressing thoughts occur. Educating patients about the factors that contribute to schema stability highlights the importance of this question. The search for disconfirming evidence is most effective in disrupting the behavioral sequence if it occurs early in the process of schema arousal, before emotions become overwhelming.

Many patients find it hard to recognize how they discount contradictory information. Their attention needs to be drawn to this information without invalidating them. This task may be achieved by noting that a particular schema is understandable, given the patient's experiences, while also pointing out the contradictory information. In the case of the patient with the schema, "I am bad," the therapist repeatedly drew her attention to actions that she considered good and caring and pointed out how these acts were inconsistent with such a categorical belief about herself. Over time, she noted that other people, including family members, regularly sought her help, that she went out of her way to be helpful, people confided in her, and that she was the only person to help a certain family member with problems. This information gradually modified the maladaptive schema.

Interpersonal Strategies Based on the Therapeutic Relationship

Unlike traditional cognitive therapy, which relies on interventions that do not make direct use of the relationship to effect change, the treatment of patients with personality disorder uses the therapeutic relationship as a major vehicle for changing core schemata (Young, 1994) because core schemata that originate in adversity are difficult to change by purely verbal methods. The treatment process and the relationship offer two strategies to effect change: treatment provides a *continuous corrective experience* that challenges these belief systems, and the therapeutic interaction offers many opportunities for more direct interventions geared toward identifying, exploring, and changing maladaptive schemata and interpersonal patterns. As noted in Chapter 7, ruptures to the alliance and validation failures are also valuable opportunities to address maladaptive schemata. When group therapy is part of the treatment plan, further opportunities arise when maladaptive core schemata and interpersonal patterns are expressed in group interaction.

A clear understanding of how the structure and process of treatment facilitate change enables the therapist to maximize the opportunities provided by within-therapy events. Table 3.1 (see page 68) summarizes the factors that are likely to modify core schemata. Briefly, a consistent therapeutic process, an ongoing collaborative relationship, a consistent emphasis on the alliance, and a validating stance are likely to modulate schemata related to distrust, abandonment and rejection, neglect, defectiveness/

flawedness/unlovability, cooperation/control, predictability, and reliability; and an emphasis on building motivation and competency are likely to modulate schemata related to passivity, powerlessness, and incompetence/mastery.

As treatment progresses, the therapeutic landscape is increasingly dominated by core schemata originating in adversity. During the earlier stages of therapy, schemata relating to trust, cooperation, and worth exert a major influence. Once these issues are addressed sufficiently to form a reasonable alliance, attention rapidly focuses on distress and related problems. When the acuteness of these problems settles, self and interpersonal problems become more apparent and maladaptive core schemata come increasingly to the fore to directly influence the treatment relationship. It is not that they were not present previously, rather that they were overlaid by more pressing problems.

As noted in the previous chapter, the resurgence of these issues often occurs in the context of treating the consequences of early trauma and deprivation. This development represents a nodal point in treatment. Problems with the alliance often emerge in new form, and old patterns and maladaptive behaviors may return, so that progress seems to halt and the patient often feels stuck. These problems appear to be reactivated by a realization of what change really means and the effect it is likely to have on one's life and relationships. Issues related to trust and intimacy get expressed in new ways. This shift allows detailed examination of events that activate core schemata, the evidence used to support them, and the way disconfirming evidence is ignored in the here and now of treatment. These specific interventions, combined with a therapeutic process that consistently counters core schemata, are probably the most effective way to change maladaptive core schemata. Here, an emphasis on providing (1) a consistent therapeutic process, and (2) a supportive, validating stance takes on new significance. Whereas earlier in treatment these components were used to manage core pathology and support other interventions, they are now used as change mechanisms in combination with more specific cognitive and psychodynamic interventions.

The focus on the therapeutic relationship is consistent with psychodynamic therapy. Within the psychodynamic framework, behavior and attitudes toward the therapist—the transference—are pointed out and clarified, and linked to relationships with other people in the contemporary situation and past relations. With the current approach, attention is also focused on the relationship with the therapist as an opportunity to examine schemata in action. This focus ensures that patients fully understand their patterns and the nuances of their expression. In this sense, treatment draws upon components of the psychodynamic approach, including the shared practice of drawing parallels between behaviors in treatment and relationships in everyday life. However, unlike traditional psychodynamic therapy, cognitive interventions are also used to explore and change maladaptive core schemata and cognitive styles that underlie transference relationships.

Cognitive methods in which evidence relating to core schemata is reviewed and disputed in the context of the relationship also provide an opportunity to deal with schema avoidance as it occurs. These methods gain added potency when combined with a discussion of disconfirming evidence provided by the process of therapy. Figure 11.4 represents this process schematically. A maladaptive core schema is activated by an event in therapy or an internal factor. If this activation involves the misinterpretation of evidence, an opportunity arises to explore the way thinking errors contribute to schema arousal. The schema then leads to attitudes and behaviors toward the therapist (transference) that can be examined to show how schemata influence behavior. Again, the patient's application of the schema to the therapist and therapy may involve thinking errors. In the process, emotions linked to the schema and associated cognitive distortions are addressed. Finally, attention is given to the way in which evidence that is inconsistent with the schema, such as that provided by the overall process of therapy, is discounted. For example, ideas of distrust, fears of being ridiculed or rejected, or feelings of intense shame are inconsistent with experiences of a consistent, nonjudgmental, validating relationship.

Where the approach differs from some forms of psychodynamic therapy is in the significance attached to linking the transference to past relationships, especially parental figures. Here it is assumed that change derives primarily from recognizing schemata and behavioral patterns *in action*

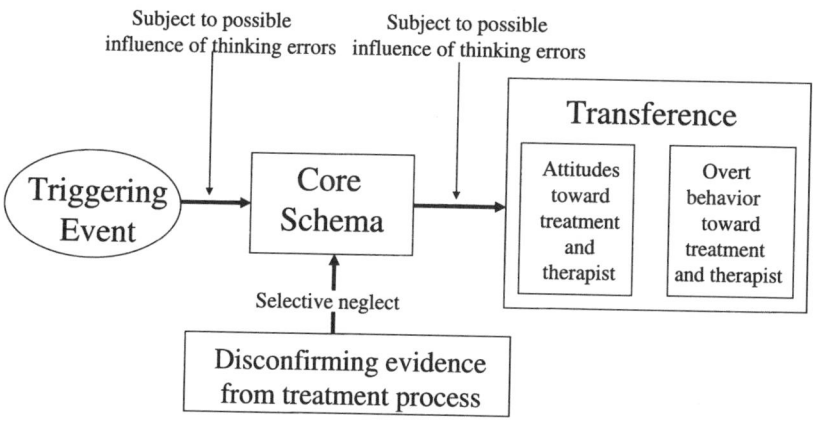

FIGURE 11.4. Interpersonal strategy for schema change based on the treatment relationship.

and challenging and changing maladaptive cognitions. Links to the past may or may not contribute to this process. For some patients a historical understanding provides meaning that is useful; for others, it may not be a central focus.

Behavioral Strategies

Behavioral interventions are aimed at changing those habitual ways of behaving that help to maintain maladaptive schemata and introducing new ways of behaving that support more adaptive schemata. These methods include challenging behavior avoidance, using graded tasks; acting against schema-based rules to test the reality of fears and negative expectations; making environmental changes; and behavioral rehearsal and role playing (Cottraux & Blackburn, 2001; Young, 1994). Patients are often remarkably reluctant to practice behavioral changes, even though they are essential for lasting schema change. Typically passivity, anger, and fear of the consequences, including people's reactions, obstruct the process.

Challenging Behavioral Avoidance. Many maladaptive core schemata are self-perpetuating because schema-based fears are rarely challenged. This avoidance is observed in inhibited (schizoid–avoidant) individuals who are so fearful of embarrassment and possible rejection that they avoid social contact. Hence they have little opportunity to learn that embarrassment or rejection are not inevitable consequences of social interaction and that these events can be handled if they occur. Change occurs through *graded exposure* to appropriate situations as a way of testing the validity of the patient's fears and negative expectations. As the treatment of trauma shows, graded exposure is a potent change mechanism. Inhibited people who have difficulty talking to others because they are afraid of being ridiculed, for example, may be encouraged to talk to another person for a few moments in a no-risk situation and note how the other person responds. Over time, the range of situations may be extended and the duration of conversation increased. Or, submissive individuals who go to great lengths to avoid acting assertively, lest they anger anyone, may be encouraged to act more assertively and note the effects on other people and feelings about the self. Again, assertive behavior may be gradually extended to include relationships with significant others and matters of increasing significance to both parties. These activities involve deliberately *acting against schema-based rules*.

Review Behaviors Eliciting Confirmatory Evidence. Maladaptive schemata and patterns are also maintained by actions that elicit confirming responses from others. Change is more likely to occur if the patient learns to recognize what he or she does to elicit such reactions. This is often a difficult step, particularly with patients who externalize responsibility and blame others for their problems. Unless the idea is introduced gradually, it is easy for patients to feel that the therapist does not recognize the terrible things that have happened to them.

Environmental Changes. Achieving enduring change may, at some point, involve making situational changes, such as avoiding people and environments that support maladaptive schemata and seeking out those that support more adaptive schemata and behavior. For example, patients who believe that they are incompetent may be encouraged to seek out situations in which they feel more competent. For one such patient, the incompetence schema triggered crises that typically lasted several days. Several methods were used to change the incompetence schema, including encouraging the patient to identify situations in which she felt useful. Although she initially maintained that such situations did not exist—an example of the absolute quality of core schemata—the therapist noted that the patient liked animals, talked positively about her ability to care for animals, and had a detailed knowledge of their care and welfare. At one point, she mentioned that she had been wondering about volunteering at an agency that cares for animals. She was encouraged to volunteer at a local animal hospital. There she found that her contributions were valued. As a result of these experiences, the schema "I am incompetent and worthless" was modified to incorporate the idea "I am good with animals, and I can make a useful contribution to animal welfare." She also began to notice other situations in which she was able to use her knowledge of animals, and this recognition further consolidated the schema change.

Behavioral Rehearsal and Role Playing. Rehearsing new behaviors in treatment is often helpful when there is considerable avoidance and fear of change. The sequence of behaviors involved in making a specific change can be rehearsed in imagination or by role playing. Group therapy provides many opportunities to role play changes with a variety individuals. An example of this method was provided in Chapter 4, in the vignette about the dependent patient who underwent cosmetic surgery. Behavioral rehearsal may take many forms, as illustrated in the following vignette:

One extremely submissive patient, who had a DSM-IV diagnosis of dependent personality disorder and a history of repetitive abusive relationships, was unable to set any kind of limit in her dealings with people. This inability had led to a series of relationships that always ended with her feeling abused, used, and suicidal. One particularly abusive relationship had lasted, on and off, for many years. Typically her partner left her for another woman, only to return months or even years later. She always took him back, whereupon the cycle of physical and verbal abuse resumed. She had not seen him for over a year when he recently tried to reestablish the relationship. She was determined not to get involved with him again but was afraid that if she met him, she would not be able to say no. She had been in this situation many times and felt she could not trust herself if she met him. She decided to write a letter to him, making it clear that the relationship was over, and she asked if she could discuss the letter with the therapist.

She drafted a letter and brought it to the next session. The letter stated that the relationship was over, but it was written in an apologetic way, with many qualifying statements that left doubts about her determination. It also contained many reasons for ending the relationship that added to the hesitant, apologetic tone. The therapist pointed out the wording and tone of the letter to help the patient see how difficult it was for her to assert herself in a way that left no doubt about her intent, particularly when she felt that the other person would not like what she had to say. She had not recognized the degree to which submissiveness had permeated her language. She noted that she used a hesitant style that made it easy for others to ignore her wishes and reject her point of view. She also hedged her main point to a degree that created uncertainty about whether she was determined to carry out her intention to terminate the relationship.

Working on the wording helped her to understand more about the dynamics of submissiveness and how actions that she thought were very assertive were really so tentative that it was easy for others to ignore her wishes. This process enabled her to understand why the relationship had dragged on for years and how she acted in ways that triggered abuse. The discussion also provided an opportunity for her to learn how to analyze social situations and apply problem-solving methods to relationships.

The important feature of rehearsal is the opportunity to concentrate on the fine details of behavior. Problems occur at this level as much as at the general level of understanding themes and patterns.

Emotional Strategies

Achieving change in core schemata involves defusing some of the intense emotions they evoke. Although emotive techniques are likely to be used later rather than earlier in treatment, they still need to be used cautiously. As with the exploration of trauma, previous regressive and dissociative behavior, a history of severe abuse and deprivation leading to primitive object relationships, poor affect tolerance, and limited psychological mindedness are reasons for minimizing the use of these techniques. These factors need to be borne in mind particularly when treating patients with higher than average intellectual level and good verbal skills; therapists tend to overestimate the ability of these patients to manage the stress involved. Parallels with the treatment of trauma also extend to using a graduated approach, with a strong emphasis on affect tolerance and regulation, especially when dealing with anger and rage associated with early trauma and deprivation. Feelings of confusion and dissociative behavior are reasons to switch to containment interventions. With this graduated approach, the goal is to achieve tolerable doses of catharsis to drain some of the intensity of emotions while maintaining affect regulation. Specific techniques, such as imaginative recall and role playing, may be useful in some situations, but often all that is needed is the standard approach of dynamic therapy: focusing attention on the feelings associated with schema arousal and the memories evoked and dealing with any avoidant or defensive behavior.

Consolidation and Generalization

Translating emerging understanding of maladaptive schemata and interpersonal patterns, and the changes to these patterns made in therapy, into lasting behavioral change is often difficult and frustrating. These schemata are well entrenched, having been confirmed repeatedly over time. Moreover, the situations of the person's life often reinforce these patterns and undermine efforts to change. Consequently, patients can become discouraged when understanding does not lead automatically to change, and by the sheer effort required to change.

Transforming Understanding into Behavioral Change

Patients need active help and support to apply new learning in their everyday life and to learn how to interact with others in ways that elicit responses that support new directions rather than confirm old patterns. On occasion, the frustration generated by the change process reactivates patients' anger about the way that they have been mistreated, and outrage at the injustice of having to work so hard to overcome problems created by the abuse or neglect of others. Frustration, anger, and outrage can threaten to undermine the commitment to change, as illustrated by the case of Natasha described previously and continued here:

> During the session, when connections were made between catastrophic thinking, externalization, submissiveness, and feelings of incompetence, Natasha was almost euphoric about suddenly understanding some of the repetitive problems in her life. She came to the next session, however, depressed and discouraged because things were not radically different. Although the therapist had noted, at the end of the previous session, that it usually takes time to translate under-

standing into change, Natasha had expected an almost magical transformation of her life, especially in her relationship with her partner.
When these expectations were discussed, Natasha began to see how
unrealistic they were and that her reaction was another example of
catastrophic thinking. She noted that, in fact, some modest changes
had occurred, but she had dismissed them because they were not as
extensive as she had hoped. She reverted to a core schema that
"nothing would ever change." On several occasions she had recognized that she was engaging in catastrophic thinking and managed to
control her distress by challenging these thoughts. These events were
highlighted to promote a sense of mastery and strengthen motivation. Natasha also noted that although she was disappointed that
major changes had not occurred in her relationship with her partner,
she had begun to set limits, and once or twice she had been able to
tell him that she found some things unacceptable. To her surprise,
he accepted this statement and responded by being a little less demanding. As a result, there had been less friction between them.

This process continued for some weeks. Gradually, Natasha became more adept at challenging catastrophic and externalizing modes
of thought. However, there were also periods of intense discouragement when Natasha needed considerable support and validation of
the difficulties that she was experiencing. Progress continued slowly,
eventually culminating with Natasha's return to work. The work
arena had been a major problem area for her. She had felt too depressed to contemplate work and thought that it would be disastrous
to return. When she recognized that this stance also had elements of
catastrophic thinking, she was able to challenge the thoughts. She
also realized that being unemployed made her dependent on her
partner and that part of her reason for not working was that she was
passively resisting his demands that she find employment. When she
returned to her job, she performed far better than she had expected.

After about 6 weeks the initial enthusiasm about her success
wore off, Natasha felt discouraged, as though "everything would fall
apart" again. The struggle filled her with intense rage, much of it
focused on her current partner. She was furious that she had to
struggle because of the abuse she had suffered throughout her life.
Sometimes she was so angry that she refused to use the cognitive
strategies she had learned. Over subsequent weeks, treatment focused
on validating the anger and reframing it by helping her to understand how it affected her present situation and that she was dealing
with it by using old ways of thinking. As the rage abated, Natasha
became more reflective and began to apply her new understanding
more consistently.

This vignette shows the importance of helping patients accept that although understanding is a necessary part of the change process—one can
only change behaviors that are recognized and understood—it does not lead
automatically to change, and that change is usually gradual: it takes *time* to

learn how to dispute habitual modes of thought as they occur and acquire the skills needed to relate to others in ways that minimize the reinforcement of maladaptive patterns. In Natasha's case, time had to be spent learning how to relate to her partner more assertively, without creating additional problems, and how to communicate her needs more directly rather than assume that others knew what was on her mind. In the past, she had reacted to others' demands, even when they were unrealistic, either by submitting to them or passively frustrating them. This latter reaction tended to exacerbate interpersonal conflicts and undermine her efforts to change. Over time, she learned to recognize her passive oppositional style and became more assertive. This translation of understanding into change took many months, during which it was necessary not only to focus on specific problems but also on bolstering and maintaining her commitment to change.

Situational Issues

Lasting changes in personality are most likely to occur if accompanied by changes in the life circumstances that contribute to maladaptive schemata, cognitive styles, and interpersonal patterns. The significance of social and interpersonal factors on the stability of personality is shown by research that indicates that changes in such personality features as self-esteem, in children and adolescents, are greatest during life transitions such as graduation and moving (Harter, 1993); it is also shown by attempts to force changes in the individual through brainwashing and similar methods, which are most effective when the person's social ties are disrupted (Baumeister, 1986). To help people change we need to help them manage their social environment differently and even to change it substantially. It is not just that people become enmeshed in maladaptive relationships that are consistent with their personality and reinforce maladaptive patterns, but also that there are clear expectations from the social environment that people stay the same. In general, we expect the people around us *not* to change; this absence of change allows us to predict their behavior and thereby exercise a measure of control over our social world. We choose to relate to people who have qualities with which we are comfortable, and we become very uncomfortable when they act differently. This consistency in the social environment and the expectations that people stay the same are powerful obstacles to change. The people in patients' lives are likely to continue to treat them in the same way, despite their efforts to change. Moreover, patients often feel guilty about the changes they make because of the potential impact on others.

To consolidate change it is often necessary to encourage patients to seek situations that are conducive to the changes being made or to learn how to relate to the environment, especially other people, so as to avoid confirming old schemata or undermining new ones. At this stage, it is often necessary to spend a considerable amount of time validating the problems encountered and dealing with the reactions of other people. In some cases, conjoint interviews with significant others are needed to help them adjust to the changes in the relationship.

Journals and Other Records

Implementing and generalizing the new learning are often impeded because the patient does not recognize that changes have occurred. Initial changes are often dismissed because they are less dramatic than the patient had hoped (as happened with Natasha) or simply because they happened so gradually as to escape perception. It is often useful to review the process of treatment with patients help them recognize how they are handling situations inside and outside therapy differently. Keeping a journal makes it possible for patients to refer to events that occurred earlier in treatment and see the progress they have made.

Attributions Regarding Change

The value of patients' learning to understand the reasons for any changes that have occurred, and the value of attributing those changes to their own efforts and collaborative work with the therapist, were noted in Chapter 4. Reviews of therapeutic progress provide opportunities to foster the kind of adaptive attributions that will help to ensure continued improvement and implementation of new learning after treatment. Such reviews also provide a further opportunity to deepen the collaborative nature of the alliance by examining specific instances of change that were the product of the joint efforts of patient and therapist.

COMMENT

It may be useful, at this point, to summarize the methods that can be used to change maladaptive core schemata, given their significance in personality pathology. Change begins with the two-step process of recognizing broad patterns and specific manifestations, with particular attention given to within-therapy events. The most important change mechanism is the continuous corrective experience provided by the structure of treatment, the therapeutic frame, and the treatment relationship; these offer an ongoing experience that runs counter to expectations based on the maladaptive schemata. This process is supplemented with more direct interventions that use the experience of the therapeutic relationship to challenge the beliefs. Here generic mechanisms take on additional significance by providing (1) the basis for modifying core maladaptive schemata, and (2) the input required to develop more adaptive beliefs.

CHAPTER 12

Exploration and Change

Treating Maladaptive Traits

Traits form the basic scaffolding of personality. They influence the development and functioning of most parts of the personality system and shape reactions to most situations. The central role of traits in conceptions of normal and disordered personality is recognized in the DSM-IV definition of personality disorder as characterized by inflexible and maladaptive traits. It might be expected, therefore, that therapies for personality disorder would devote considerable attention to managing and treating maladaptive traits. If traits influence reactions to events, they are also likely to shape responses to treatment. And, if maladaptive traits cause significant impairment and distress, treatment should address these problems. However, most current treatments hardly mention the topic. There are several possible reasons for this omission. Many traits are involved in the relationship patterns that are addressed by cognitive and psychodynamic treatments. Hence changes to schemata or object relationships are assumed to change trait functioning. Also therapy tends to focus on specific incidents and narratives the patient provides about self and others, rather than on broader dispositions. However, these incidents are often manifestations of traits. Hence trait descriptions provide a useful way for therapists to group events and summarize diverse incidents and behaviors for themselves as well as their patients. These summaries help the clinician to conceptualize the treatment process and summarize critical themes.

It is also important to address traits directly because maladaptive expressions influence the clinical picture, and traits such as anxiousness, affective lability, and impulsivity influence the effects of stress and adversity. For this reason, lasting change often depends on modulating the effects of these characteristics. Furthermore, a focus on traits reminds us of the limits to which some aspects of personality can change.

We need to work with traits in two ways. First, the individual's salient traits need to be taken into account when planning therapy and selecting interventions. This means tailoring treatment to fit patients' personality styles in addition to their problems and psychopathology. In general, the emotional dysregulation pattern and, to a lesser extent, dissocial traits involve high levels of behavioral expression. The problem is that these patients are too reactive, so that an important, ongoing task is to contain behavior and reduce reactivity. With the schizoid–avoidant pattern, the opposite problem is encountered. Since these individuals are relatively unresponsive, the task is to increase behavioral production—a far more difficult task.

Second, treatment needs to incorporate interventions aimed at changing the maladaptive traits. This need is the theme of the present chapter. Many of the traits discussed here were considered earlier, in relation to their contribution to dysphoric affects, maladaptive behaviors, and interpersonal patterns. However, the management of these traits needs further consideration; evidence that traits are stable raises questions about the extent to which maladaptive traits can be changed with treatment and what change means in this context (see Chapter 3). The principle underlying the approach adopted is that treatment should focus on modulating trait expression and helping individuals to find more constructive ways to express their basic traits. The way in which this modulation may be achieved becomes apparent when we examine how the environment influences trait expression.

ENVIRONMENTAL EFFECTS AND THE STRUCTURE OF TRAITS

Environmental Influences

Behavioral–genetic studies demonstrate that genes and environment have approximately equal effects on traits. However, the nature of these effects differs. Genetic factors give rise to the basic structures of personality and influence the organization of traits into personality patterns (Livesley et al., 1998; Livesley, Jang, & Vernon, 2003). Environmental effects operate more at the level of specific traits by influencing (1) *the degree to which a genetic predisposition is expressed* and, (2) *the actual behaviors through which a trait is manifested.*

The same genetic loading is unlikely to produce the same level of a particular trait in all individuals. For example, the expression of a genetic predisposition toward anxiousness may be reduced if the child has a secure attachment relationship and is raised by parents who spend time listening to the child's fears and teaching him or her to manage anxiety; or conversely, the expression of this trait will be increased if the child is less secure or exposed to trauma and abuse. Similarly, the expression of inhibited traits is affected by attachment status (which is influenced by relationship factors): Behaviorally inhibited children who are insecurely attached show more autonomic arousal to strangers than inhibited children who are securely attached (Nachmias, Gunnos, Mangelsdorf, Parritz, & Buss, 1996). These ideas suggest that *one strategy for treating maladaptive traits is to modulate the degree to which a trait is expressed.*

For a given level of genetic predisposition, phenotypic expression varies within a fixed range. Within this range, the environment may amplify or dampen the expression of the genetic predisposition. At the extreme levels of genetic predisposition found in personality disorder, this range may be limited; that is, the environment may have less effect than at more moderate levels of genetic predisposition. This possibility suggests that the highly emotionally labile person will probably always be emotionally reactive and subject to mood swings, although the magnitude of these changes may be reduced by teaching the individual how to regulate emotions. Similarly, the highly inhibited individual is unlikely to become even modestly extraverted but may be helped to feel more comfortable when dealing with people.

The environment also influences the actual behaviors through which a trait is expressed. Not all individuals with high levels of stimulus seeking behave in the same way (see Figure 12.1). A successful entrepreneur may use this trait adaptively by taking calculated risks that lead to business success. Others may pursue high-risk activities such as adventure sports. Patients with personality disorder, however, may express the same level of stimulus seeking through a chaotic and reckless lifestyle, as was the case with the patient discussed in Chapter 1. Similarly, some highly inhibited

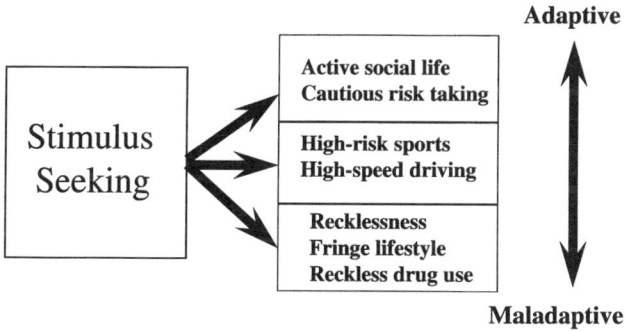

FIGURE 12.1. Effect of environment on trait expression.

individuals may capitalize on their introversion and disinterest in social contact to focus on intellectual pursuits and achieve success in realms that do not require interpersonal involvement. Others, however, may express this quality through an isolated and passive lifestyle that offers little satisfaction. This range of possibilities suggests that *a second strategy for managing trait-related behavioral problems is to help the individual find more adaptive ways to express his or her basic traits.*

The environment also influences trait-based behavior in the broader sense that traits require a suitable environment before they can be expressed. To take an obvious example, friendliness can only be expressed in social situations. This basic reality suggests that it may also be possible to influence the expression of maladaptive traits by *modifying the environment.* In some patients, it may be possible to reduce maladaptive behavior by encouraging them to avoid environments that encourage or evoke these behaviors. Clinicians do so routinely, especially in the early stages of change, by encouraging patients to avoid situations that are conducive to dysfunctional acts. A more important implication of this idea is that some patients may benefit from receiving help in finding or creating environments that allow them to express basic traits in more adaptive and personally satisfying ways. This strategy is especially pertinent for patients at the extreme ends of a continuum of trait expression. For example, many highly introverted or inhibited individuals are best helped by receiving encouragement to create a satisfying lifestyle that is consistent with their basic dispositions, rather than attempting to modify traits that are extremely resistant to change.

The Structure of Traits

To convert treatment strategies based on environmental effects into specific interventions, we need to understand more about the structure of traits. As social–cognitive theorists have pointed out, traditional trait theories do not explain the processes through which an underlying disposition becomes expressed in observable behavior (Zelli & Dodge, 1999). Traits are complex structures: a long chain of biological and psychological events links genes to behavior. Over time, genes interact with the environment to establish what might be called *biopsychological systems*—the biological and psychological structures and processes that produce the trait-based behavior that we observe and seek to change. These systems may be described *biologically* in terms of neural networks and transmitter systems (e.g., impulsive–aggression appears to involve the serotonin system [Coccaro, 2001; Coccaro et al., 1989]) and *psychologically* in terms of the cognitive and emotional processes that mediate trait-based responses by influencing what is noticed and the way events are interpreted, and activate response tendencies that increase the likelihood of impulsive–aggressive behavior (see Figure 12.2). The implication of this model is that both pharmacological and behavioral interventions may modulate trait expression.

The behavioral or psychological component of traits consists of cognitions, behavioral tendencies and overt behaviors, and associated emotions. During development, environmental factors, under the influence of genetic predisposition, become encoded as a set of cognitions that influence the way the individual perceives and responds to situations. These encoded factors may be described using the concept of schema used earlier to describe the self and interpersonal systems. For example, the schemata that are part of sensation seeking incorporate beliefs about action, excitement, vulnerability, and normality. The invulnerability schema may include ideas such as "Harm is something that happens to other people" and "Nothing bad ever happens to me," and the schemata dealing with normality and routine may include beliefs such as "Normality is boring" or "I'm too special to tolerate a normal existence." The activation of these schemata increases the probability of thrill- and excitement-seeking behavior. Feelings of anticipation, excitement, or boredom accompany schema arousal, and feelings of thrill, satisfaction, and pleasure result from overt action. The tripartite structure of traits accounts for much of their stability. To change maladaptive traits, we need to modify this structure. The cognitive component is probably the most amenable to restructuring, using the methods for modifying schemata discussed in the previous chapter.

Table 12.1 lists typical schemata associated with the basic traits defining the four personality patterns. The list is not exhaustive but rather illustrates some of the more dysfunctional beliefs and expectations that require restructuring. It should be noted that some schemata are likely to be associated with several traits. For example, fear of feelings may be a feature of

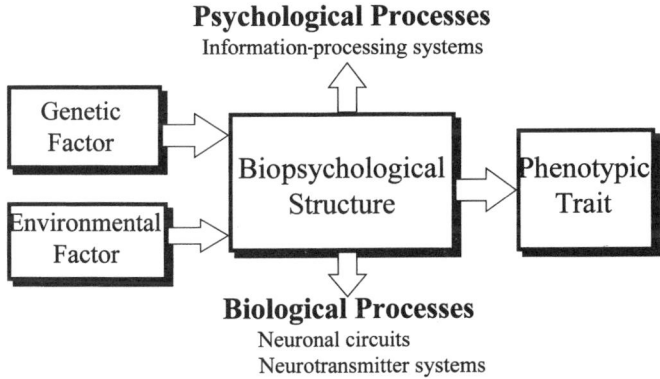

FIGURE 12.2. The biological and psychological structure of traits.

affective lability, anxiousness, restricted expression, and compulsivity. Similarly, most maladaptive schemata are associated with several DSM-IV personality disorders; and few are specific to a given disorder (Petrocelli et al., 2001).

GENERAL STRATEGIES FOR MODIFYING TRAIT EXPRESSION

Viewing traits as relatively stable characteristics that the individual has to learn to use constructively, and which the environment influences with regard to range and mode of expression suggest four treatment strategies (Livesley, 1999, 2000, 2001a, 2001c):

1. Increase trait acceptance and tolerance.
2. Attenuate trait expression.
3. Facilitate more adaptive forms of trait behavior.
4. Promote the selection and creation of environments compatible with adaptive expression of salient traits.

These overlapping strategies are readily applied using the stages of change approach. The first step is to identify maladaptive trait expressions by using either structured assessment methods, such as questionnaires, or clinical observation. Subsequently, the more maladaptive ways in which a given trait is expressed are identified using the two-stage process used to explore maladaptive patterns, and the dysfunctional cognitions involved in maladaptive behavior are explored. Cognitive interventions are then used to restructure dysfunctional beliefs. It is probably not sufficient, however, to rely solely on cognitive methods; behavioral interventions are usually needed to change trait expression.

Strategy 1: Increase Trait Tolerance and Acceptance

The first step in modulating traits is to facilitate more adaptive use and to promote acceptance and tolerance of these qualities. Most patients are remarkably intolerant of many of their basic qualities. As a result, they often seem to be at war with themselves, continually struggling to deny key components of their personality—a process that is both exhausting and time consuming. In contrast, most healthy individuals are comfortable with their traits, even ones they would like to change, and find them to be normal ways of being. Internal conflict may be reduced and acceptance increased through psychoeducation: explaining the genetic basis of traits and providing information on how the environment influences the expression of biological predispositions. The goal is to help patients recognize that traits are part of their biological heritage—and hence they need to own

TABLE 12.1. Schemata Associated with Basic Traits

Emotional dysregulation

Anxiousness

Apprehensiveness: pervasive sense of anxiety and apprehensiveness; defines the world as anxiety provoking; worries about doing anything new or different.

Guilt: considers self as bad; almost always feel as if he or she has done something wrong; often feels guilty without knowing why.

Punishment: expects to be punished for mistakes; thinks he or she deserves to be punished.

Rumination: actively reviews previous mistakes and embarrassments in great detail; repeatedly relives embarrassing moments.

Inhibition: feels uncomfortable about doing anything new or different.

Affective lability

Dyscontrol: believes affects are uncontrollable and that he or she is unable to do anything to make self feel better.

Fear of affect: fear of affective experience; unable to tolerate emotions.

Exaggeration: reacts initially to all problems as if they were crises; usually thinks that problems are insoluble.

Cognitive dysregulation

Superstitious beliefs: superstitious, believes in telepathy, the supernatural, and related ideas.

Submissiveness

Competence: doubts ability to cope effectively with people and situations; lacks confidence in abilities; considers self to be incompetent; feels unable to protect self; believes that he or she is helpless and needs continual support and help.

Approval dependence: satisfaction and self-esteem depend on the approval of others.

Conflict avoidance: believes that it is necessary to submit to the wants and wishes of others to avoid conflict.

Assertiveness guilt: feels guilty about asserting own interests and wants.

Anger intolerance: believes that he or she is unable to cope with the anger or disapproval of others; expects anger or disapproval to lead to rejection; feels guilty if someone is angry with him or her.

Retaliation: expects others to retaliate for any attempt at self-assertion.

Self-deprecation: devalues self, especially in relation to others; thinks self is not as important as others.

Martyrdom: values making sacrifices for others; always places others' needs first.

Insecure attachment

Security: believes that security, well-being, and coping ability depends upon the physical presence of significant others; needs people to be available to offer support whenever required.

Abandonment: fears being left or abandoned; expects separations, rejections, or abandonment to be painful and catastrophic.

(continued)

TABLE 12.1. (*continued*)

Availability and responsiveness: believes that people cannot be relied upon; fears that people will not be available, respond appropriately, or understand his or her needs and problems.

Aloneness: fears solitude; considers the physical presence of others to be essential for happiness.

Oppositionality

Preservation of independence: goes to great lengths to preserve independence; sensitive to any encroachment on independence.

Passive–resistant: blocks others' requests in a passive and indirect manner; does not believe that direct disagreement is desirable.

Unappreciated: believes that he or she is not sufficiently appreciated.

Resentment: resents receiving advice or instruction from anyone; perceives advice or instruction as an infringement of personal liberty.

Social apprehensiveness

Apprehensiveness: expects to feel anxious and uncomfortable in social situations.

Social worth: considers self to be worthless and uninteresting.

Probable negative evaluation: expects people to criticize, embarrass, or humiliate him or her.

Intolerance of negative evaluation: excessively fearful of negative social evaluation, leading to social withdrawal.

Dissocial behavior

Callousness

Remorselessness: is not concerned about the effects of own actions on others; guiltless.

Egocentricism: believes that own needs are more important than others' and that he or she should receive priority.

Exploitation: considers exploitativeness and manipulativeness to be valuable and acceptable ways to attain goals.

Sadism: enjoys the pain of others.

Contempt: has little regard for other people.

Irresponsibility: takes responsibilities lightly; does not think that responsibilities should have a limiting effect on actions.

Rules: believes that rules and laws should not be allowed to stand in the way of getting what he or she wants.

Rejection

Judgmental: hypercritical of others.

Authoritarian attitudes: believes that people need to be told what to do and what is best for them, and that most people suffer from a lack of self-discipline.

Rigidity: has rigid beliefs that are difficult to change; holds categorical opinions on most things; considers it a sign of weakness to change his or her mind.

Dominance: believes that it is important to control and dominate others.

Stimulus seeking

Invulnerability: believes that risk taking is not likely to have harmful consequences;

ignores or downplays possible harmful consequences of own actions; thinks bad things only happen to others.

Dependence on stimulation: considers everyday life to be dull and uninteresting; risk taking is necessary to add interest to life; stimulation is necessary for contentment and happiness.

Impulsive decisions: does things suddenly, on the spur of the moment; does not think things through before acting.

Narcissism

Recognition: places emphasis on being recognized as special and different from others.

Attention: needs attention; happiness and well-being depends on receiving attention.

Discounts disapproval: discounts or becomes angry at disapproval.

Gratification of others: believes that it is necessary to entertain and amuse people to gain their attention, approval, and admiration.

Specialness: considers self to be special, unique, and destined to be important.

Entitlement: believes that he or she is entitled to special treatment and should not be treated in the same way as other people; considers him- herself to be above the rules that apply to others.

Inhibitedness

Intimacy problems

Intrusion: fears intimacy; believes that relationships are intrusive.

Autonomy: expects intimate relationships to interfere excessively with independence.

Interpersonal disinterest: values social isolation; values the fact that he or she does not need other people; disinterested in people.

Alienation: feels alienated from others; defines self as different from other people.

Sexuality: fearful of sexual involvement.

Restricted expression

Expectations of harm: avoids expressing affect or revealing personal information lest others use it against him or her; does not think it safe to reveal personal information.

Self-reliance: believes that it is best not to rely on other people, because they may use the information to one's disadvantage.

Embarrassment: embarrassed by own emotional expression.

Exposure: feels exposed when expressing feelings or revealing personal information.

Social reaction: believes that others do not like affective expressions.

Control: avoids emotional expression because feelings may become uncontrollable; fears loss of control.

Social avoidance

Isolation: prefers solitary pursuits.

Social ineptness: believes that he or she is socially inept.

Apprehensiveness: expects to feel anxious and uncomfortable in social situations.

Social worth: considers self to be worthless and uninteresting.

(continued)

TABLE 12.1. (*continued*)

Probable negative evaluation: expects people to criticize, embarrass, or humiliate him or her.

Intolerance of negative evaluation: excessively fearful of negative social evaluation, leading to social withdrawal.

Compulsivity

Perfectionism: expects perfect performance at all times; rarely satisfied with own performance; feels like a total failure if he or she does not do something perfectly; horrified at the idea of making a mistake.

Criticism: fears the criticism of others if a mistake is made; expects condemnation; considers others to be intolerant; worries about being criticized.

Structure: believes that structure is necessary to cope effectively and that he or she needs order and rules to work effectively.

Order: values order and cleanliness.

Containment: seeks to contain and control situations; needs to have all aspects of life under control at all times; worries about things getting out of control.

Disapproval: disapproves of the lack of cleanliness, organization, and tidiness shown by other people.

Catastrophe: the failure of structure, order, and perfectionism associated with catastrophic expectations; beliefs that if things are not kept in tight control, the outcome will be a disaster.

Other traits

Suspiciousness

Threat: considers the world to be threatening and opposed to self.

Mistrust: mistrusts the motives and intentions of others.

Vigilance: believes that it is necessary to be watchful and on-guard at all times, otherwise one may be taken by surprise.

---

them—without conveying the idea that traits cannot be changed. This balanced communication is achieved by explaining how the environment influences traits, so that the patient understands that, within limits, it is possible to change the way traits are expressed.

A useful step toward building tolerance and acceptance is to encourage patients to identify ways in which their traits are beneficial. Most common traits probably emerged sometime in the evolutionary process because they conferred an adaptive advantage: They helped our remote ancestors solve adaptive problems presented by their environment and to survive long enough to pass on their genes. Many of these advantages apply to the present. This idea suggests that *traits are not intrinsically maladaptive* (Livesley, 2002). They are only maladaptive when the individual has learned to express them in ways that cause problems or lack the flexibility that characterizes adaptive trait functioning. This realization often facilitates change; the person does not need to change a global quality that he or she feels is a fundamental part of the self, but rather more specific aspects of his or her behavior.

The adaptive advantages of some traits are readily apparent. This is the case with compulsivity: moderate levels of orderliness, precision, and conscientiousness are useful in a wide range of situations and occupations. Similar considerations apply to most traits. Even apparently problematic traits, such anxiousness and affective lability that cause so many problems, can be useful. One rather inhibited woman, who had high levels of affective lability that led to periods of intense dysphoria and despondency, learned to be more tolerant of these feelings when she recognized that they contributed to her work. She was an aspiring writer and the despondency added a dimension to her writing that was not present when her mood was more normal. Previously, she feared feeling despondent and whenever her mood dropped, she would ruminate over problems. Once she realized that the feelings could be used constructively, she ruminated less (and wrote more), which had the effect of moderating her despondency.

Another patient, a struggling potter, had a similar experience. She had extremely labile moods as part of the emotional dysregulation pattern. Like the previous patient, she feared mood changes and regularly told herself that she could not cope with them and that she would have to kill herself if they continued. As problems with self-harm receded, and she began to resolve some persistent interpersonal problems, the affective lability settled sufficiently for her to recognize that it actually helped her work. Rather than fearing periods of elevated mood because they evoked the fear of losing control, she began to enjoy the spontaneity that these periods added to her life, and she certainly enjoyed the freshness to her art that had not been there previously. Even low mood was useful: she thought it added depth and substance that complemented the freshness and spontaneity. This development made it easier for her to tolerate and manage mood changes, and also had a settling effect that reduced the intensity of the changes.

It is often easier to recognize the adaptive significance of traits when the environment is taken into account. As noted earlier, traits are context-dependent. Hence, a given trait may be valuable in some situations but not in others. This is apparent if we consider the cluster of inhibited traits. Although problematic in social situations, there are situations in which it is an advantage to be self-reliant, capable of considerable self-absorption, and have little need for social contact. An understanding of the way context influences the usefulness of trait-based behavior changes the tendency to evaluate traits in all-or-none terms.

Strategy 2: Attenuate Trait Expression

This strategy is based on the idea that the environment dampens or amplifies trait expression. The goal is to reduce the frequency and intensity of trait expression by (1) restructuring the way triggering events are perceived, (2) modifying amplifying factors, (3) teaching skills to regulate and control trait expression by enhancing incompatible behaviors, and (4) using medication to modulate specific traits.

Restructuring Perception of Triggering Situations

The biopsychological structure mediating trait behavior is an information-processing and decision-making system that scans input from the internal and external environments for information that is relevant to a given trait. For individuals at the extremes of a trait distribution, the threshold for interpreting situations as relevant to the trait is low and hence the trait is frequently activated. Presumably, this is what the DSM means when referring to personality disorder traits as inflexible and maladaptive. Thus, anxiousness is triggered when situations are perceived as potentially threatening or harmful. Anxious behavior would decrease if fewer situations were perceived as harmful. The simplest way to achieve this goal would be to avoid threatening situations—a course taken by many traumatized individuals (see Chapter 10). Although in this case, the avoidant behavior produces additional problems, there are situations and traits for which avoidance may be adaptive. For example, a patient with a high need for stimulation may show a high frequency of maladaptive thrill seeking simply because he or she spends a lot of time in situations that provide many opportunities to act in this way. Hence early in treatment it may be useful to encourage individuals to avoid these situations as an initial step toward containing seriously disruptive behavior and creating the temporary stability needed that to effect other changes.

More lasting change is likely to be achieved in reducing the tendency to see situations as relevant to a given trait by restructuring the way situations are perceived. For example, individuals with high levels of anxiousness may learn to view previously threatening situations as less harmful, or suspicious individuals may be helped to challenge automatic tendencies to believe that others are attempting to harm them. This strategy essentially involves applying the methods of schema change (discussed in the previous chapter) to question the evidence on which trait-based action is based. Most clinicians do this automatically, but there is merit to thinking specifically about modifying traits: (1) such a focus ensures direct and concentrated attention to specific maladaptive traits and encourages the systematic use of multiple interventions; and (2) it also reminds the clinician to moderate expectations of change and to consider other strategies in addition to restructuring.

Modifying Cognitions that Amplify Trait Expression

Some traits are expressed frequently because cognitions that are intrinsic parts of the traits increase their behavioral expression. For example, for those individuals with high levels of narcissism who enjoy being the center of attention (not all do, some have traits that are only concerned with grandiosity), the satisfaction achieved enhances self-esteem and activates thoughts about how others appreciate them and want to hear more—which, in turn, increase the probability of further attention-seeking behavior. Thus each narcissistic act increases the likelihood of further acts. With other traits, amplifying cognitions are separate from the trait. For example, the dysphoria that is part of emotional dysregulation (Chapter 9) is increased by ruminating and catastrophizing modes of thinking. This amplification occurred with Natasha (Chapter 11): when Natasha learned to challenge catastrophic thinking, she was able to recognize situations that were previously threatening as inconsequential, and the frequency with which the underlying trait of anxiousness led to overwhelming distress decreased.

Similar maladaptive thoughts increase the frequency with which other traits are expressed. For example, highly submissive individuals typically hold a variety of "ought" and "should" types of beliefs that create a sense of duty and obligation to do as others wish. For example: "I ought to do what others want," "It's selfish not to help other people," or "I should always look after other people." These beliefs have an absolute quality to them, so that changing them involves helping the individual to take context into account. Hence the value of looking after others is acknowledged in combination with the need to recognize that this obligation depends on the circumstance. A similar amplification of submissiveness occurs when the individual cannot refuse even unreasonable requests due to a fear of retaliation and an inability to tolerate the other person being angry. Statements such as "I can't cope with people being mad at me" and "It's not nice to get people mad" also undermine any attempt to act assertively. Reducing submissive behavior requires changes to these underlying dysfunctional beliefs. Similar modes of belief-based thoughts accentuate traits such as social apprehensiveness and fear of intimacy.

Enhancing Incompatible Behaviors

The example of submissiveness illustrates a related intervention to modulate trait expression: namely, the development of incompatible or complementary behavior—in this case, assertiveness skills. People fall back on trait-based actions when alternatives are not available. Excessively submissive individuals can be taught how to act assertively without causing additional interpersonal problems. Similar opportunities exist to modulate social avoidance and social apprehensiveness by teaching social and communication skills. Relaxation training is another way to teach alternative responses that are incompatible with strong emotions in stressful situations.

Medication

Medication may also help to modulate expression of a small number of traits. The rationale for this pharmacological intervention is provided by studies showing that specific neurotransmitter systems mediate trait expression (Coccaro, 2001): Studies have shown that SSRIs reduce hostility and impulsivity in patients with borderline personality disorder and that neuroleptics may also be useful in managing impulsivity. Although impulsive behaviors are usually considered symptoms, they are often expressions of an underlying trait linked to sensation seeking. Even more convincing evidence that medication may influence traits is a study showing that paroxetine decreases hostility and increases affiliative behavior in normal individuals (Knutson et al., 1998).

Application to Affective Lability and Anxiousness

This strategy of attenuating trait expression is particularly relevant to managing anxiousness and affective lability, the core traits defining the emotional dysregulation or borderline pattern. It is useful to address these traits directly because they are also prominent features of most forms of personality disorder and contribute to vulnerability to stress. The anxiousness component, in particular, is a feature of most Cluster C disorders and many cases of Cluster A disorders.

In people with personality disorder, the activation of these traits contributes to dysphoric states and leads to maladaptive responses. Healthy individuals with moderate to high levels of these traits usually react to emotional arousal by adopting various adaptive responses, such as distraction and problem solving, to reduce distress (see Figure 12.3). In contrast, the schemata associated with these traits in patients with personality disorder are less adaptive and increase distress: namely, tendencies to exaggerate problems and ruminate over how bad and intolerable things are, fear of affects, and preoccupation with losing control. Table 12.1 lists some of these beliefs. These traits can be managed with a combination of interventions used in conjunction with the strategy of building tolerance and acceptance of these traits, using the treatment relationship to support and contain

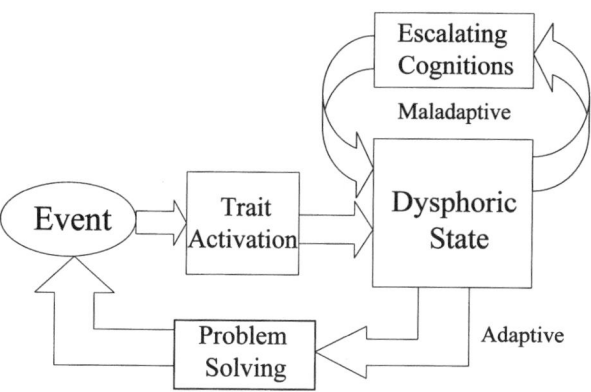

FIGURE 12.3. Adaptive and maladaptive responses to affective trait activation.

emotional expression. Change begins by drawing patients' attention to how these beliefs contribute to problems, followed by a restructuring of the beliefs. In addition to reducing cognitions that amplify trait expression, it is also useful to teach behaviors that healthy individuals use to modulate emotions, such as distraction and problem solving. At the same time, medication may be used to dampen trait expression. Although the value of SSRIs in managing affective lability is unclear, these medications often lead to improvement in other mood symptoms and impulsivity, which, in turn, helps to dampen the more extreme levels of reactivity. Acquiring anxiety management and affect-regulating skills also help patients decrease their reactivity and reduce instances of escalation.

Strategy 3: Promote More Adaptive Trait-Based Behavior

This strategy is based on the idea that the primary effect of the environment is to influence the way in which traits are expressed. The intent is to increase adaptive expression rather than attempt to reduce the overall level of the trait. The case of the patient with an extremely high level of sensation seeking, described in Chapter 1, illustrates this way of working with traits.

> In the incident described in the vignette, the patient complained that treatment was boring. Previously, her life was in a constant state of turmoil that was exciting. Self-mutilation, a fringe lifestyle that led to many fights and arguments, and constant interpersonal problems were among the many events that filled her life with dramatic focus. As the crises subsided and her behavior became more settled, the patient was left with the problem of how to satisfy her need for excitement. For a while this need threatened treatment, and

there was a danger that she would revert to her previous lifestyle and behavior patterns. Attempts to reduce sensation-seeking behavior were unsuccessful, and it was difficult to find more adaptive ways to meet her needs for excitement and stimulation.

One day, the patient announced that she had solved the problem by taking up a high-risk sport, which she was pursuing with great enthusiasm. She pushed herself to the limit, accompanied by rich fantasies of ever more risky ventures. This athletic outlet added spice to her life and satisfied her immediate need for excitement. The threat to therapy subsided.

One form of actual self-harm was replaced with another, although the sporting activities were probably marginally less maladaptive. In traditional psychodynamic terms, symptom substitution had occurred. But this explanation does not take into account the biologically driven need for stimulation. Over time, a decrease in thrill seeking and risk taking was achieved by challenging her beliefs of invulnerability and reframing ideas that accidents happen only to others. Subsequently, alternative ways of meeting the need for stimulation that were less dangerous were explored. As other symptoms improved, the patient began to think about what to do with her life. She decided to pursue career opportunities that proved challenging and satisfying. Equally importantly, these activities generated constant activity that was stimulating. As the significance of these changes became apparent, her interest in high-risk sports decreased, and she pursued them with less unbridled enthusiasm. This progression took about 2 years to achieve.

This case provides a somewhat typical example of working with a trait rather than attempting to change it. The approach follows from an understanding of the genetic basis for sensation seeking and how the environment influences the choice of behaviors for expressing traits. The change achieved did not occur simply by finding, rather serendipitously, alternative exciting and stimulating activities. It also depended on restructuring maladaptive schemata that mediated maladaptive forms of sensation seeking. The approach worked because the patient was strongly motivated and highly intelligent, which allowed her to pursue a stimulating career.

Modifying Maladaptive Schemta

The maladaptive forms of sensation seeking shown by this patient were mediated by two schemata: a belief in her own invulnerability and an intense fear of normality. The invulnerability schema involved strong beliefs that harm happened only to others, and her almost magical belief that she was protected by a superhuman force. Challenging and restructuring these beliefs employed the usual techniques of schema change discussed in the previous chapter. Contradictory evidence was sought by looking at the effects of self-harm and extreme risk taking and the fact that complications arising from one incident suggested that she did not, after all, live a charmed life. Other evidentiary sources included a minor accident and an incident with some of her friends, who also lived a fringe lifestyle, in which one of them was seriously attacked.

Similar restructuring was undertaken with regard to her fear of normality. She thought that she should not have to live the normal life of ordinary individuals and that normality was intolerably boring. Not surprisingly, she had a moderately high score on the trait of narcissism. This schema was more difficult to restructure than the schema of invulnerability, and eventually the career she pursued provided an adequate outlet.

Promoting More Adaptive Behavioral Expression

Change is more likely when cognitive interventions are combined with actual behavioral interventions. Maladaptive dependency behavior, for example, may be managed in this way. Dependency incorporates two dimensions: *anxious attachment* that involves fear of losing, or being separated from, attachment figures and caregivers; and *submissiveness* involving problems with assertiveness, subservience, and need for advice and reassurance. These traits are strongly associated with the emotional dysregulation pattern, although they may occur independently of other traits defining the pattern, as occurs with DSM-IV's dependent personality disorder.

For these patients, crises and parasuicidal behavior often serve multiple functions, including satisfying the need for care and support. A graded approach to change, based on the recognition that these are heritable traits, involves encouraging the patient to find progressively more adaptive ways to meet these needs. Encouraging the patient to seek help before a crisis state is fully established is a good beginning point that may involve restructuring beliefs such as: "People have to be coerced to provide help," "It is not possible to ask for help directly," "I should not need help," and so on. It also involves helping these patients identify more effective ways of eliciting the care and attention that they believe they need. Modification in behavior may involve changing how they approach people for help, telling someone close that problems are brewing, asking for support, and so on. In addition, beliefs that they lack the resources and cannot manage on their own could be challenged in efforts to modulate the frequency of trait expression.

Later in treatment, the relationship between these traits and episodes of abuse and victimization may be explored to help patients recognize how dependent care-seeking behavior may lead to abuse. This focus provides further opportunities for patients to learn how to seek help and reassurance in ways that elicit collaboration rather than control and do not leave the patient open to exploitation. These dependency behaviors often include the need to take care of others. Again, rather than relinquish the need to provide help people, patients may learn how to provide this care of others without neglecting their own needs and to do so in a way that enhances, rather than diminishes, self-worth.

Strategy 4: Select and Create Conducive Environments

Most applications of psychotherapy and most of the interventions discussed so far, are concerned with promoting more successful adjustment to the environment by changing maladaptive behavior, cognitions, or emotions. The proposed strategy is the antithesis of this approach. The intent to help patients (1) establish a personal space that supports adaptive rather than maladaptive action, and (2) create lifestyles and personal worlds that allow them to express their personality in ways that are rewarding and fulfilling. This idea is more of philosophical position than an intervention strategy. It is also a position that some therapists may find disconcerting. However, the idea follows from empirical evidence on the stability of personality and an understanding of personality–environment interaction (see Chapter 3). People do not react passively to their environment; rather, they shape the inanimate and animate environment to which they relate to create a *personal niche* (Willi, 1999). Most healthy individuals work to create a physical and social environment that is congenial to them. Once established, the niche provides the structure that organizes their behavior and provides the opportunity and support for the expression and satisfaction of their abilities, interests, needs, and traits. We can think of the niche as a structure in the environment, which people create over time, that sustains and nurtures their interests, offers opportunities to express their basic nature, and provides opportunities for fulfilment and growth.

People feel secure and comfortable when their personal niches have the structure and resources to permit their unique form of self-expression, and the flexibility to accommodate changing needs and circumstances. Unfortunately, people with personality disorder are not especially effective in creating niches that allow personal expression and fulfillment. Rather they create niches that limit and constrain, and that encourage maladaptive expressions of basic traits. This pattern was seen with the patient who had high levels of sensation seeking and who established a personal niche that encouraged maladaptive risk taking and frequent interpersonal problems. A similar situation occurs with dependent and submissive individuals who feel obliged to submit to other people's demands and continually find themselves in abusive relationships that leave them feeling exploited and drained, as illustrated by the following vignette:

Jenny was 39 when she sought treatment, primarily because she felt depressed. Psychiatric problems had started in her early teens, when she became depressed, suicidal, and started to self-harm. Over the years, she sought psychiatric help intermittently, but her problems continued. In DSM-IV terms, she was diagnosed as having dysthymic disorder and dependent personality disorder with avoidant traits. Using the dimensional system adopted here, Jenny had high levels of anxiousness, submissiveness, and insecure attachment and more moderate levels of affective lability.

At the time of the current treatment, Jenny was unemployed and living alone. She was the eldest of six children, raised by professional parents who were largely absent from the home. Jenny assumed much of the responsibility for caring for her younger siblings, and she continued to feel tremendous responsibility toward them and her now aging parents. Her time was filled looking after her parents and helping her siblings, who were married with children and treated her as a general babysitter and helper. Jenny felt enormous demands from her family. They expected much of her and always complained that she was not doing enough, although, in fact, she was so busy that she had little time for herself and lived a relatively isolated life, apart from interaction with her family.

Because the self-harm had increased prior to referral, leading to several hospital admissions, therapy focused first on the self-harming behavior and attendant dysphoria. A combination of medication and cognitive-behavioral interventions led to a substantial decrease in deliberate self-harm and modest improvement in mood. Jenny began to wonder about her future and whether she should seek further education so that she could obtain reasonable employment. Whenever she thought about these issues, she always came across the stumbling block of whether she would have sufficient time. Her family was ambivalent about her plans. On the one hand, they offered tentative support and criticized her for not working; on the other, they continued to make excessive demands of her time. They were also very critical of her efforts to obtain further education and to find employment and berated her for having psychiatric problems. Her life continued to involve a constant shuttling between babysitting for family members and helping with medical problems and caring for her parents.

This degree of care and attention to others fit well with Jenny's basically dependent and submissive style. Childhood experiences of comparative neglect by parents and the need to care for her siblings amplified predispositions toward submissiveness and insecure attachment. She felt an intense sense of duty and obligation toward her family. Although she recognized they did not appreciate what she did and complained that she was selfish and not doing enough, she felt intense guilt whenever she thought about building a life of her own. Caring for others also brought her satisfaction, and she evinced an almost masochistic pleasure in sacrificing herself for her family, for this sacrifice contributed to her self-esteem. As she frequently pointed out, "It's important to look after people. That's what I believe I'm here for."

This vignette shows how Jenny had created a personal niche that provided an outlet for dependency and compulsive caregiving. Jenny had clearly learned to express these traits in a rigid and fixed manner and had difficulty setting limits and maintaining boundaries. There are, however, other dimensions to the situation. The problem that Jenny faces does not lie only within herself. The environment that was both imposed on her and created by her is highly structured in terms of demands and expectations. Although many opportunities are provided to express basic traits, the niche does not provide satisfaction and fulfilment. Goals based on a sense of obligation are rarely satisfying. Instead, the situation creates feelings of exploitation and frustration and obstructs the fulfillment of other needs.

Although Jenny could be helped to modulate her submissive and caregiving behaviors, there are likely to be limits to which these traits can be changed. She did not really want to change these qualities; she valued putting others first, and caring for others was an important source of self-worth that was central to her sense of self and identity. Yet, the ways these traits were expressed also detracted from her identity because she felt that she could never be herself or satisfy other important needs. However, limited motivation, the significance of submissiveness and caregiving for self functions, and the enduring nature of these traits limited the potential for change. Consequently, treatment began to focus on helping Jenny restructure her life by finding more satisfying ways to express these traits and to place limits on caregiving by challenging and restructuring schemata that maintained these behaviors. At the same time, she was encouraged to restructure her environment to provide outlets for these qualities that did not leave her exhausted and overwhelmed.

> An opportunity to move in this direction occurred when Jenny talked about a child with disabilities in her neighborhood, whom she saw regularly and had befriended. The child seemed appreciative of the time Jenny spent with her, and Jenny thought that it would be rewarding to work with people who have these problems. The idea of volunteering at a residence for people with handicaps was discussed. She was enthusiastic about the idea. She made contact and shortly afterward started working as a volunteer. For some months, she accompanied residents on field trips. She found the work satisfying and appreciated the praise that she received from members of staff and the gratitude of the residents and their families. This work began to channel Jenny's need to care for others and provide an outlet for her feelings of responsibility for others. It also started to place limits on this behavior. The demands from her family continued. Jenny still felt obliged to meet them, but there were occasions when their needs conflicted with her volunteering commitments. With help she was able to point out to family members that there were times she could

not come to their assistance. These were perhaps the first occasions when she had actually said no.

Some months later, an opportunity arose for a part-time position as an aide in the residence where she volunteered. Much to her delight, Jenny was asked if she was interested and accepted the job. Her hours increased, which meant that she had to learn how to place further limits on her family's demands. She was able to do so because she did not feel that turning down their requests meant that she was failing people. She was still providing care and attention to others but now in a more controlled manner. Gradually, her lifestyle became more organized. She also began to recognize that to work effectively, she needed to ensure that she had adequate recreation and rest. Over a period of about a year, as the work gradually increased to full time, Jenny was able to create a new personal niche in which she was able to express both dependency needs and the need to care for others in a less rigid way that was rewarding. Her self-esteem, dysthymic symptoms, and low mood slowly improved.

Work on personal niches does not preclude the use of other change mechanisms designed to modulate traits. The establishment of a more congenial environment often facilitates other interventions by ensuring an adequate outlet for basic tendencies. The creation of personal niches that are containing and rewarding is especially important in managing very vulnerable individuals or those with traits at the extreme poles of variation, who have limited capacity for change. This point is illustrated by the following vignette:

Peter was in his late 30s when he presented for treatment, largely at the behest of a partner with whom he had lived for the previous 2 years. The problem, he explained, was that he did not talk very much or show any feelings, and his partner was finding this lack of communication difficult. They both wondered whether he could be helped. The DSM-IV diagnosis was schizoid personality disorder, and dimensional assessment revealed an inhibited pattern with high levels of restricted expression, intimacy problems, and social avoidance. He had some depressive symptoms and felt intense despondency about his situation. However, he was not unduly concerned about his difficulty with people. He simply felt he did not have much to say to people, nor did he really want to talk to them, and he never showed feelings. In fact, he was not quite sure what people meant by *feelings*. He was content with the life that he had with his partner, although he found her demands for communication and emotional expression puzzling and irritating. They caused him to withdraw, and at times he literally hid. He was, however, worried about the future. He was not comfortable with his current life situation. He found his job unrewarding and unsatisfying because it did not match his interests or values. Unfortunately, he was not sure what he would like to do instead. He said that he had never really been sure. He simply drifted from job to job, situation to situation, without any clear plan or purpose. He thought the relationship he was currently in would end because his partner found it impossible to accept that he was not demonstrative or communicative. This possibility did not bother him unduly; it was much more his lifestyle that caused him to feel despondent.

He really wanted a lifestyle in which he could live alone, but he felt that this desire was wrong because everyone disagreed with him about it. This dissonance added to his despair. He was quite clear in his preference for a solitary life and said that he had been happiest when he had lived in total isolation in the wilderness. This he had done several times in his life, once in his late teens and another time about 10 years earlier. On each occasion, he spent several months alone, hiking in a remote area where he saw no one. He thought that if he could have a life like that, he would be content. During the early months of treatment, the relationship came to an end when his partner realized that Peter did not want to change. This ending caused momentary sadness but little else. He continued to worry about the fact that he was still not doing what he wanted.

It was fairly clear that the opportunities for change were limited because of the extreme level of traits delineating the inhibitedness pattern and Peter's lack of motivation to change these qualities. What he really wanted was a lifestyle that would allow him to express these qualities and not feel guilty about doing so. The methods for increasing trait tolerance described earlier were followed. Particular attention was spent on helping Peter understand the structure and origins of his personality characteristics and how the intrusiveness of his mother, combined with violent arguments between his parents, reinforced natural proclivities to withdraw. Acceptance of his basic personality pattern increased, which allowed him to show more flexibility in thinking about what he might do. He decided he would like to go back to living in a remote area and began exploring job opportunities in this direction. Eventually he found the position of a research assistant for an ornithologist; the job involved spending the spring and summer months alone in an isolated part of the country, making observations as part of a study that the ornithologist was conducting from his university base. Peter was delighted with the prospect. He would be in a part of the country that he loved, doing a job that he found interesting and satisfying because he had an interest in wildlife. He would be totally alone, supplies for the period would be taken in initially and thereafter he would be self-contained.

The last time Peter made contact with his therapist was several years later. He said he had continued doing those sorts of jobs and had managed to find a series of positions that allowed him to work in much the same area, doing similar things. He was content.

COMMENT

In this chapter we have explored some of the themes discussed in earlier chapters, this time from a different perspective that is mindful of the limitations of change. Implicit in the general approach to treating maladaptive traits is the idea that it is more effective to help individuals establish a social context that is conducive to their more salient personality characteristics than to try to change those characteristics. This idea may appear to conflict with therapies that are more concerned with changing inner structures and processes. Such an approach to change is effective when these processes and structures are relatively plastic. When they are not, it seems therapeutically maladaptive not to pursue other methods. Nevertheless, some therapists may understandably feel uncomfortable with the idea of helping patients adjust to their personality traits as opposed to trying to change them. This approach does not imply that attempts should not also be made to modulate these traits or to help patients find ways to use their traits more constructively. However, to attempt more radical change in extreme levels of traits raises unrealistic expectations that can impose considerable stress and guilt. It seems better to help patients understand that some of the qualities they considered negative are not only acceptable ways of being, but can also be beneficial and fulfilling in the right context.

CHAPTER 13

Integration and Synthesis

Treating Core Pathology

The model of personality disorder on which treatment is based distinguishes between the *contents* (substantive component) and *organization* (core component) of the self and interpersonal systems. The treatment of substantive problems was discussed in Chapter 11. This chapter considers the treatment of core self and interpersonal pathology—the defining features of personality disorder. Unfortunately, there are even fewer empirical studies on the treatment of these problems than on other components of personality pathology, so that suggestions for interventions are based largely on a conceptual analysis of the problem and what clinicians have found useful.

The ultimate goal of longer-term treatment is to develop more differentiated and integrated self and interpersonal systems. The specific goals include:

1. Establish clearly delineated interpersonal boundaries.
2. Promote differentiation in self and interpersonal schemata.
3. Promote more cohesive and integrated representations of self and others.
4. Promote autonomy and agency.
5. Facilitate an improved understanding of the rules governing human behavior.
6. Facilitate the development of a more adaptive "theory of the self."

CORE PATHOLOGY AND THE NATURE OF CHANGE

Before considering how to promote more adaptive self and interpersonal systems, it may be helpful to review ideas about core pathology and the processes giving rise to integration, discussed in Chapter 2, because these form the basis for the interventions proposed.

Structural and Functional Sources of Integration

The self and interpersonal systems develop through simultaneous processes of differentiation and integration. *Differentiation* occurs as cognitions and emotions are refined over time and global impressions give rise to more specific schemata. The emergence of the self depends on the formation of an interpersonal boundary. This boundary is created by distinguishing experiences arising from the self from those arising from the environment. Differentiation increases self-knowledge—the raw material for constructing the self system—and leads to the recognition that one is the author of one's thoughts, feelings, and actions, a development that is fundamental to self-directedness. Problems with differentiation lead to poor interpersonal boundaries, global and imprecise self and interpersonal schemata, and impoverished representations of self and others. Poor differentiation may be due to (1) neuropsychological and emotional deficits that limit the ability to discriminate among stimuli, (2) repetitive failure of significant others to help the child label his or her experiences appropriately, and (3) invalidating experiences that negate the child's experience.

Integration has structural and functional components arising from the organizing effects of basic *cognitive* and *conative* processes (self-directedness). The *structural component* arises from the connections produced within self-knowledge by cognitive mechanisms that organize information into categories (represented by the concept of schemata) that are arranged into a hierarchy. These connections create a coherent body of knowledge that gives rise to a sense of stability and historicity. Cohesiveness is the experiential consequence of these links and the ease with which self-knowledge can be accessed. The culmination of cognitive integration is the elaboration of a "theory of the self" that makes sense of the individual's self-knowledge and life story. Problems with integration lead to fragmentary images of self or others. These fragmentations may be due to (1) problems integrating information, caused by compromised neuropsychological functions; (2) emotionally laden information that overwhelms cognitive mechanisms; or (3) information that is too disparate to integrate.

The *functional component* of integration arises from the organizing effects of goal directedness. Goals give meaning and purpose to life, which contribute to a subjective sense of wholeness. Complex long-term goals also promote integration by linking subgoals that need to be attained along the way and by drawing together motives, interests, abilities, and other attributes in the interests of goal attainment. The idea that the integration stems from two fundamental behavioral mechanisms suggests that changes in core pathology may be achieved by (1) forging more integrated conceptions of self and others through the establishment of links among the different elements of knowledge about the self or another person, and (2) by interventions that promote agency and self-directedness.

The Nature of Change

Changes to core pathology involve a different kind from change from those discussed in previous chapters, which largely involve modifying already existing behaviors and structures by (1) developing more adaptive ways to manage affects and impulses, (2) modifying self and interpersonal schemata, (3) enhancing self-esteem, (4) modifying rigid maladaptive interpersonal patterns, (5) resolving conflicted feelings about the self and others, (6) modulating trait expression, and so on. These changes may be thought of as *substitutive changes*; the essential feature is the replacement of maladaptive behavior with more adaptive alternatives, using the stages of change approach. Changes to core pathology involve an additional component: the synthesis of integrated and cohesive self and person concepts and an intuitive understanding of human behavior. *Synthetic change* is not just concerned with modifying already existing structures and processes but also with promoting new structures. Here the usual application of the stages of change model is less directly relevant. Instead, emphasis is placed on *integration* and *synthesis*, which are achieved through the cumulative effects of numerous interventions that promote more stable representations of self and others and a new form of self-directedness. Substitutive and synthetic changes are not totally distinct—substitutive changes establish the conditions for integration and remove obstacles in its way.

GENERAL EFFECTS OF TREATMENT

Although there are few empirical studies of methods to promote integration and synthesis, it seems that most changes to core pathology occur gradually, as an indirect consequence of the treatment process and changes to other domains of psychopathology. Specific interventions to promote integration and synthesis play a more secondary role. The basic structure of treatment creates a therapeutic process that gradually changes core pathology. The therapeutic frame, the treatment relationship, and general treatment strategies provide a stable experience of the self that forms the basis for a more stable representation of the self and a more integrated representation of the therapist. A validating and empathic stance contributes

to these developments by affirming and consolidating changes as they occur. As stressed repeatedly in previous chapters, the patient learns much
more than is imparted by the therapist's interventions (Chessick, 1977).
The therapist's consistency and calm nonjudgmental way of handling situations and feelings, his or her avoidance of getting caught in the patient's
maladaptive patterns, and his or her commitment to the process provides a
model that the patient can use to construct a new understanding of the
self and relationships.

Collaborative Description, Self-Knowledge, Self-Observation, and Self-Reflection

The process of collaborative description is basic to the long-term process of
integration and synthesis. Although the descriptive process is basically
concerned with clarifying problems that are targets for specific interventions, it also increases and reformulates self-knowledge. Integration occurs
as suppression and avoidance are reduced and self-knowledge, formerly
warded off, is connected and reframed. The repetitive process of linking
feelings, thoughts, and actions gradually imposes structure and organization
onto self-experience.

Collaborative description also contributes to integration by encouraging self-observation and self-monitoring. As noted in Chapter 4, patients
with personality disorder are often excruciatingly self-aware, but the evaluative component of self-observation is often missing. Self-observation and
self-reflection transform self-experience into self-knowledge. They allow
one to (1) examine and reorganize self-knowledge, (2) identify issues about
the self that are unclear, and (3) recognize inconsistencies that need to be
reconciled. Without self-reflection, integration is not possible. The integrative effects of improved self-observation are enhanced by encouraging
patients to be curious about the nature of their experience and their own
minds and by supporting recognition of the complexity of their mental
processes and personality.

Guided Development

Because the self is a complex system, it is tempting to assume that interventions to treat self pathology must be equally complex. But this may not
be the case. Although the self is complex, the information on which it is
based is more straightforward. The self emerges from numerous everyday
interactions with the social environment that provide the input for the
adaptive mechanisms that organize and integrate information and establish
self-directedness. Most of these events are minor; few are memorable.
What matters is the consistency of this information and whether it provides the input required to organize self-knowledge and support conative

mechanisms. Change in core pathology probably depends on a similar process occurring during treatment, thereby providing opportunities to correct pathology and facilitate more adaptive developments. Consistency, repetition, and effective use of routine events may be the key components of change, suggesting an approach to treating core pathology that is deceptively simple. The simplicity lies in using routine events, occurring in treatment sessions and everyday life, to effect change. The challenge for the therapist is to recognize the therapeutic opportunities these events offer. Consider the following example, drawn from the treatment of Natasha (see Chapter 11):

> In the weeks before the current session, the major theme had been her submissive pattern, discussed earlier, that contributed to her dysthymic symptoms and led to a series of abusive relationships. Natasha clearly recognized the pattern and worked hard to identify the many ways in which she behaved submissively. As these became clearer, she began to contemplate how she might be less submissive with her partner, who was a demanding and verbally abusive person. During one session, she described a situation in which she had been more assertive. A few days previously, she was in a restaurant with her partner, who told her what to order and began criticizing her. In the past, she reacted to such situations by submissively accepting what he said and then getting upset. On this occasion, however, she told him to "lay off," that she wanted to make up her own mind what to eat, and that she was not prepared to put up with him continually putting her down. When he reacted by saying that she could never make up her mind—and, anyway, she did not know anything—she responded by quietly telling him that she had had enough and that if he continued in this manner, she would leave. When he continued, she simply got up and left without a fuss.
>
> Since the main focus of treatment at that time was her submissive behavior, the event was explored initially from this perspective and used to reinforce more assertive behaviors and enhance self-esteem. Subsequently, however, it was also discussed in terms of its implications for changing self pathology. Natasha had frequently referred to a lack of direction in her life and her profound passivity. She also repeatedly questioned the validity of her beliefs and feelings and noted that often they did not feel real or genuine. When the therapist asked how she felt about the way she had managed the situation, she said, "I felt good about it. It felt like the right thing to do." This statement seemed to reflect more than mere pleasure at succeeding in behaving differently. It also seemed to reflect that her actions had felt genuine to her. In the past, she would have been submissive because she was afraid of doing anything else, but it had not always felt comfortable or right to act in this submissive way. The therapist noted the change and how it seemed to feel genuine and real. This comment led to a discussion about the fact that she

had been able to do what she felt was right rather than what another person had expected, and how doing what she thought others
wanted led her to do things that did not seem genuine or consistent
with the person she wanted to be.

This event was used not just to reinforce assertiveness but also to validate the *feeling of authenticity*, which is an important quality of adaptive
self-functioning that occurs when individuals act in a way that they feel is
in accordance with their nature. Although most therapists would intuitively respond in these ways, an understanding of the structure of the self
and dimensions of adaptive self functioning helps therapists to recognize
core-related opportunities that arise when focusing on other issues. Simple
repetition is important for change, so seizing each core-related opportunity
is an important therapeutic task.

The therapeutic process described in this vignette involved more than
just collaborative description of the event in the restaurant; it also involved highlighting, validating, and promoting those aspects of the incident that were relevant to enhancing authenticity and agency. We can
think of this as a process of *guided development*. Ideas about the nature and
structure of the self are used as a guide to identify events and encourage
actions that may be used to effect core change. With Natasha, this involved encouraging her to seek out situations in which she thought that
she could behave in a way that felt authentic and taking an active interest
in these new developments and their outcome. The approach seems to reflect the way the self emerges in the normal course of development. It is
also consistent with the views of several psychoanalytic therapists, who
contend that self pathology (identity disturbance) is best modified by
noninterpretive work that largely involves supporting and validating new
ideas, feelings, and actions (see Gunderson, 1984, 2001; Masterson, 1976).

Modifying Impediments

Integration and synthesis are facilitated by changing behaviors and cognitive processes that impede the construction of an adaptive self system.
Multiple schemata and cognitive processes hinder integration and limit
self-directedness: self-invalidating, catastrophizing, and externalizing cognitive styles, passivity and low motivation, and assumptions about the unpredictable and uncontrollable nature of interpersonal events. Changes to
these modes of thought create conditions conducive to more adaptive developments. For example, reducing the strength and frequency of the self-
invalidating style contributes to the person's differentiation and integration by increasing his or her certainty and clarity of self-experience.

Traits can also hinder self-development. Affective lability and anxiousness, for example, give rise to unstable emotions and ever-changing ex-

perience of the self that hinder the development of a stable self representation. They also lead to an unstable social landscape in which the reflected appraisals of others continually change, leading to inconsistent and unstable experiences of the self in relationships with others. Modulation of these traits is a prerequisite for feelings of stability and continuity. Other traits, such as maladaptive sensation seeking, can also contribute to a chaotic lifestyle that offers little in the way of consistent experiences that would permit the development of a stable self.

The effects of substitutive changes on impediments to self development may be increased by educating the patient about the ways in which these characteristics hinder self-understanding and by exploring their effects on self-experience. The idea is to extend the changes made in specific behaviors to core structures and processes.

Promoting Authenticity

Authenticity is experienced when the individual feels that he or she is acting in accordance with his or her basic nature and expressing his or her true self (Sheldon, Ryan, Rawsthorne, & Ilardi, 1997). This authentic experience is most likely to occur when individuals have reasonable access to self-knowledge and a reasonable grasp of the different aspects of their personality. Schema avoidance and suppression of self-knowledge undermine authenticity, so that any intervention that increases self-knowledge and helps the individual to incorporate warded off or suppressed aspects of the self can potentially enhance authenticity. Psychoeducation may help patients understand the significance of dealing with suppressed material, even though painful. For example, telling one patient about the way schema avoidance and suppression of self-knowledge affects the self helped her to understand that the distressing feeling that she was artificial and that nothing about her was real occurred because she did not allow herself to experience important but painful events that had happened to her, and that it is not possible to feel genuine or authentic when important aspects of experience are denied.

Once experienced, authenticity contributes to integration; the feeling that one is acting in accordance with one's basic nature produces a sense of cohesion. It seems, therefore, that a certain level of integration is needed to generate authenticity and that, once experienced, authenticity increases integration. This reciprocal feedback is characteristic of complex dynamic systems such as self and personality.

Authenticity is also experienced when (1) individuals feel that they are the authors of their own actions (Wild, 1965), (2) that these actions are internally caused (deCharms, 1968; Ryan, Deci, & Grolnick, 1995), and (3) that the individuals had a choice (Sheldon et al., 1997). As illustrated by the vignette of Natasha in the restaurant, any event when the patient feels a sense of agency can be highlighted to reinforce feelings of genuineness. Since authenticity is experienced when people act in accord with their basic traits, experiencing it depends on the individual first recognizing and accepting these traits. Situations and relationships that offer opportunities for individuals use these traits adaptively are conducive to authentic experience, whereas situations that force persons to act in ways that are at odds with their basic nature are not. Treatment therefore should involve a *search for situations and roles that help individuals express their inherent qualities*, as discussed in the previous chapter. As noted earlier, however, many patients continually try to mold themselves to the perceived expectations of others, rather than seeking satisfying forms of self-expression. Change requires therapists to take an active interest in, and affirm, any initiative toward self-expression.

PROMOTING DIFFERENTIATION

Problems with differentiation involve defective interpersonal boundaries and poorly differentiated self and interpersonal schemata. Boundary problems are most apparent in emotionally dysregulated patients. Difficulty differentiating their own experiences from those of other people leads to self-images that change according to the reactions of others. Similar problems may occur with inhibited patients, although the problems are often less apparent. Instead, the most salient feature is often an impoverished self-concept and a sense of inner blankness or emptiness. A poorly differentiated self structure is also observed in some emotionally dysregulated patients, as illustrated in Chapter 2 by the patient who described herself simply in these terms: "I would not kill anyone. I like dogs—in fact, all animals. I like music. I like the color green."

Development of Interpersonal Boundaries

In everyday life, an understanding of interpersonal boundaries and how boundaries are maintained is probably learned implicitly by watching others and modeling their example. Similarly in treatment, boundaries are unlikely to be learned from specific intervention but rather by modeling the way the therapist establishes and maintains a consistent treatment process. As one patient noted toward the end of long-term treatment, "I really appreciate your consistency. I didn't always like it, and lots of times I did things just to make you inconsistent. It didn't work very often and that was good. I've never had a stable relationship before, and it helped me to be more stable and develop boundaries."

Education about interpersonal boundaries and discussion of specific instances of boundary problems facilitate the process. Most patients readily accept that they have poor boundaries and many have an intuitive understanding of the problem. Metaphors may help to clarify what needs to be done to change. Patients readily understand the image of their skin as permeable, so that what people say or do gets through to them and that they readily take others' thoughts and feelings as their own. This image helps them to understand the need to develop a protective skin so that others' reactions can run off them and have less impact.

Differentiation of Self-Knowledge and Person Concepts

Differentiation of self-knowledge is primarily a consequence of the general process of exploring problems and psychopathology. Additional interventions play only a limited role in the process.

"Unpacking" the Meaning of Experience

Many experiences and memories of patients with personality disorder have a global, impressionistic quality with few details. Shapiro (1965) referred to this way of thinking as the hysterical cognitive style. Differentiation of self-knowledge is increased by "unpacking" the meaning of these cognitions and focusing on details and nuances. Emotions may have a similar global quality; this globality occurs when (1) patients are unable to describe feelings because the schemata involved are preverbal, and (2) complex feeling states are reduced to a single dimension so that they can be expressed in ways that are tolerable for the patient. Dissocial and some emotionally dysregulated individuals, for example, are often uncomfortable with feelings that make them vulnerable and rapidly convert these feelings into anger. Change involves helping patients appreciate the complexity of their experiences. Achieving this goal is often aided by detailed examination of reactions to everyday events. A benefit of keeping a journal is that it provides a constant source of material with which to explore the nuances of thoughts, feelings, wants, and memories related to specific events. The process can be extended to promote differentiation of person images by inquiring about the way other people reacted to the event and the patient's impressions of their reactions. This exercise fosters empathy and self–other differentiation by helping the individual recognize that different people may perceive and react to the same event differently.

Differentiation of the impoverished self and person representations of inhibited or schizoid–avoidant individuals is a considerable challenge. Here the problem is not the occurrence of global schemata and poorly differentiated affects but, rather, the comparative absence of schemata and feelings. Although most interventions produce only modest benefits, the best approach seems to be a detailed analysis of everyday experience, which generates material in a nonthreatening way and helps these individuals "take the role of the other" and begin to develop empathy. This exercise also seems to be useful in building empathy in those with dissocial traits.

The Significance of Preferences and Wants

Self-descriptions by young children provide interesting clues about some simple origins of stability and cohesiveness, two central attributes of core personality. They are largely lists of likes and preferences, such as the games they like to play, favorite toys, people they like, and things they like to eat (Livesley & Bromley, 1973). Likes and preferences create continuity and give direction to action by representing simple goals the child likes to achieve. This function of likes and preferences suggests that validation of them may be useful in treating severe self pathology. This idea is supported by the remarkable uncertainty that patients express about identifying even simple wants. As with the young child, it is helpful to focus on concrete examples to create rudimentary feelings of stability, as the following vignette illustrates:

> The patient, a man in his late 30s, had severe psychiatric problems, including self-injury, dating to early adolescence. His personality was characterized by inhibited and emotional dysregulation patterns, and he had been variously diagnosed as having (DSM-IV) antisocial, borderline, or avoidant personality disorders, and sometimes all three. During one session, he mentioned how difficult it was for him to decide on anything, because there was nothing that he really liked. Even if he decided on something, a voice inside his head told him to do something different. He linked this voice to his mother. Although she had died some years previously, it was like having her still alive inside him, always criticizing and telling him what to do. For example, he liked a particular kind of candy, but he rarely bought it because his mother had preferred a different variety. Whenever he bought candy, he always followed Mother's choice. Although the matter may be considered trivial, it offered an opportunity to validate and strengthen the patient's preferences as a step toward helping him define himself with greater clarity and assurance. As the issue was discussed over several sessions, it was possible to strengthen the patient's ability to follow his own wants. Gradually, he became more confident about his preferences and more comfortable challenging his mother's voice within.

The example illustrates the role of preferences, however inconsequential, in self-development and the value of repeatedly affirming simple likes as an initial step toward building confidence in decisions and creating a nucleus of consistency that can be extended. The intervention enacts the developmental process whereby young children define themselves through likes and dislikes.

PROMOTING INTEGRATION: SELF-STATE DISJUNCTIONS

Multiple, poorly integrated self-states are a feature of severe personality disorder (Horowitz, 1998; see aslo Ryle, 1997). Different self-states are also associated with "neurotic" conditions (Horowitz, 1979) and normal personality functioning, but the subjective experience of cohesiveness is not impaired because the self-states are more integrated, less extreme, and the transition from one state to another is more gradual and explicable. With personality disorder, states may be distinct so that it is difficult to recall events and experiences in one state when in another, and transitions from one state to another are often abrupt. This is especially the case with emotional dysregulation and dissocial patterns where differences between states are accentuated by intense affects. The state-dependent quality of experience and memory contributes to the fragmentation of the self.

When the emotional component is less intense, as is the case in inhibited individuals, self-states are often organized around apparently incompatible traits rather than emotions. As Akhtar (1992) noted, apparently inconsistent traits that the individual cannot reconcile contribute to identity diffusion. This condition is illustrated by the following vignette:

> The patient, a man in his early 30s, was distressed by the feeling that there were "two sides" to him—one passive, and the other aggressive and hostile. These states were experienced as unrelated, and the patient ruminated at length over which "is the real me." Experiences and beliefs also differed across states. In the passive state he was extremely self-critical, despising everything about himself because nothing had any meaning and everything seemed pointless. In the aggressive state, in contrast, he was competitive, anxious to achieve, highly motivated, determined that no one would get in his way, and contemptuous of other people, believing that they lived a worthless existence. At times, the contempt flowed into anger and occasionally violence.
>
> As he struggled to make sense of these competing qualities, he began to talk about his abusive and critical parents. Nothing he did was ever good enough, and he was frequently told that he would never amount to anything. Faced with this barrage he withdrew, passively accepting that they must be right. The opposite poles of this relationship—the critical abuser versus the passive, self-denigrating recipient—matched salient traits, which then developed into self-states that were experienced as unrelated.

Ideas about self-states, or states of mind, developed by Ryle (1997) and Horowitz (1979, 1998) provide the basis for understanding the fragmentation of the self and ideas for effective treatment strategies. The following case example illustrates how these ideas may be used in treatment and how Ryle's suggestion that self-states be represented as a diagram showing the relationship among states promotes integration.

Sarah, a 39-year-old woman with a long history of problems related to emotional dysregulation, arrived for treatment 10 minutes late, as she had on several occasions in previous weeks. Almost immediately she said that while on the subway to the therapist's office, she felt angry and annoyed. A few days earlier she had talked to a friend about the way people who did not use public transport did not understand how difficult it is to get to places on time. This comment was clearly a reference to a discussion with her therapist about the problem of getting to treatment on time. The therapist noted the connection and Sarah expressed anger at the therapist's lack of understanding about being late. After further discussion, the therapist acknowledged the problem of relying on public transport but also reiterated the reality that her lateness reduced the time available for treatment. Sarah then described her feelings in more detail. She said that she had become anxious, frightened, and eventually angry when she realized that she was going to be late again. It was the unfairness of the situation that made her so angry.

Without prompting, she revealed that her first thought, when she realized that she would be late again, was that the therapist would probably be annoyed and not wait for her. She added that she had always been terrified of being abandoned. Currently she was terrified that Jim, her husband, would leave her. This fear caused many of their marital problems. Whenever something happened that made her think that Jim would leave, she became terrified and then filled with uncontrollable rage that could last for days. She said that, when in this state, "I go on and on at Jim until he gives up and falls silent." Then she becomes terrified that she has driven him away. Nevertheless, she continues to attack him and demand that he prove that he would not leave her. Jim initially reacted with concern but as the rage continued and nothing that he did made a difference, he withdrew. Sarah interpreted his withdrawal as evidence that he did not care and that he would abandon her, like everyone else. This perceived confirmation of her basic fear added fuel to her rage.

This information revealed a self-state of rage that is triggered by fear of abandonment. Activation of the abandonment schema led first to fear and terror and then to anger and rage. In this state, Sarah was needy and demanding and attacked those upon whom she depended, especially her husband. These reactions were represented as a diagram that was shown to Sarah. She then noted that the fear preceding the rage also occurred when she was uncertain either about her relationship with another person or how someone was likely to behave. This uncertainty made her feel vulnerable and triggered the abandonment schema. Sarah then spontaneously commented that her mother had been very unpredictable and difficult to understand. She never knew whether she would be pleasant, angry, withdrawn, or cruel.

Her mother often said cruel things. For example, a few days earlier, during a telephone conversation, she had told Sarah that when she was pregnant with her, she had not wanted to have her. Sarah thought that her mother's attitude explained her own suicidal thoughts and ideas, such as, "I should not be here," "I should die," and "I should not have been born." Sarah continued by describing ever-present thoughts of suicide and how she regularly took to her bed, often for several days at a time, because she felt over-whelmed. In this state she felt numb and unable to do anything. This description introduced a second self-state. As this state was explored, Sarah noted that the overwhelmed state often followed the state of rage. Interestingly, she referred to these states as her "core pattern."

At this point, the therapist showed Sarah a diagram of the "rage" and "overwhelmed" states. Rapport, which had been increasing slowly during the session, increased further. Sarah added details about the terror that she felt whenever she was perplexed by someone's behavior or felt abandoned, so that the diagram became a collaborative effort. She also noted that feelings of confusion and abandonment sometimes led directly to the overwhelmed state, without triggering the rage state.

When the therapist asked how her husband reacted to each self-state, Sarah said that Jim usually reacted to her rage initially by trying to be calm and concerned, but later, in the face of her incessant assault, he would become angry, leading to an escalation of their collective rage. Eventually he would withdraw. When she was over-whelmed and depressed, he also showed concern and worry. When his concern produced little response, however, he would withdraw. Thus both states led eventually to the same response. This information was incorporated into a final diagram of the self-states and the relationship between them (shown in Figure 13.1).

Having identified her husband's responses, the therapist noted that those responses seemed to be the very thing that Sarah feared. Sarah responded that she seemed to cause the situations that, in turn, caused her problems. The therapist used this comment to emphasize the cyclical nature of the pattern and the ways in which she contributed to the abandonment that she so feared. Sarah said that she had been aware of the components of the cycle but had not seen them as connected. After a few moments, she added that the diagram helped to explain several things in her life. In particular, it explained the failure of one of her long-term relationships. She then revealed an almost 20-year history of an on–off relationship with Arthur, someone she had loved deeply.

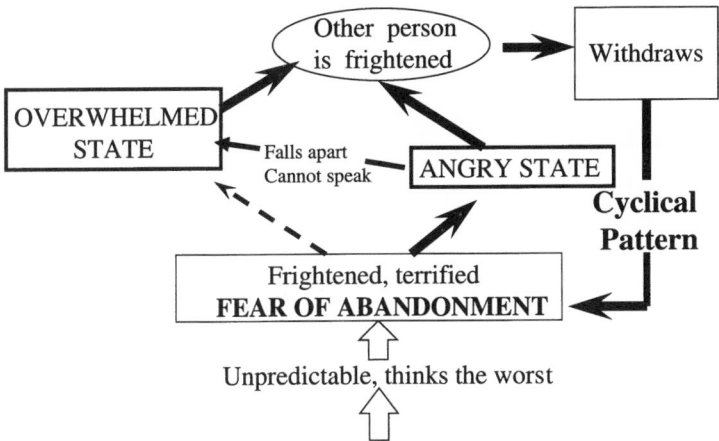

FIGURE 13.1. Core self-states in action.

On one occasion, while on holiday with Arthur, she had become very distressed and overwhelmed after getting some bad news.
In this state, she told Arthur she did not want him. To her surprise,
he booked her into a hotel in the town that they were visiting for
the day. She was horrified that he could abandon her in a strange
place. She now realized how she had provoked the abandonment. A
similar incident occurred a little later, when she told Arthur that she
could not stand the uncertainty of their relationship. He asked if she
wanted to leave. She said that she did. He offered to drive her to
the train station. She accepted and never saw him again. At the
time, she thought that if he could abandon her by sticking her into
a hotel or on a train, he did not truly care about her. She now realized how she tested him and that she was doing the same with her
husband.

The remainder of the session was spent elaborating on this pattern. The time was also used to strengthen the alliance by focusing
on the collaborative nature of the process and how this work had
made sense of major events in her life. Sarah noted that Jim thought
that she was better since she had started therapy. The therapist wondered what she thought. She agreed; things were much improved.
Her mood was more stable and she had not been fighting as much
with Jim. She thought that these changes had occurred because she
was dealing with "important things." However, recognizing the pattern made her realize the "depth of Mother's influence" and that
"there is not much else to me."

This case illustrates the use of collaborative description to explore self-
states. Few interpretations were offered. Instead, Sarah was encouraged to

describe her experiences to the point where she was able to recognize the maladaptive behaviors that contributed to her difficulties.

Exploration of Self-States

Exploration of self-states involves detailed descriptions of the thoughts, feelings, and actions that characterize each state. States are triggered either by specific events or mood changes that activate a basic schema, leading to a cascade of other schemata, feelings, and actions. In Sarah's case, the trigger for both the rage and overwhelmed states was any event that activated rejection or abandonment schemata. Sarah was hypersensitive, perceiving rejection, abandonment, and criticism in events that others would dismiss as insignificant. On occasion, biologically based mood changes also triggered these states because they made her more sensitive to rejection. Once activated, the schemata led to actions that evoked responses from others that confirmed the pattern.

Sometimes other people's behavior is less important in maintaining these patterns because patients react to what they *believe* others are thinking and do not check the validity of these assumptions. For example, a patient with an inadequacy–incompetency schema believed that he was unlikely to achieve anything in life and that everyone thought that he was a failure. This schema triggered a self-state comprised of dysphoric affects, passivity, resignation, and inertia. He said that, "When I feel like this, it does not matter what other people say or do. It's what I think they are thinking that matters. I know that they think that I am a failure." The tendency to assume that other people have similar thoughts to oneself is especially problematic in patients with inhibited and avoidant traits, because limited interaction with others gives little opportunity to test this assumption.

A matter-of-fact, nonjudgmental descriptive approach and the use of a diagram can help minimize defensiveness so that patients are willing to accept their self-states and view them more objectively. The approach invites the patient to join the therapist in observing and describing his or her life, without ascribing motives. Change arises from recognizing and challenging components of the pattern, as they occur in everyday interaction, and the integrating effects of connecting multiple aspects of the self.

Interpersonal Behaviors Associated with Self-States

The repertoire of interpersonal behavior associated with self-states is learned in interactions with significant others that usually involve either *complementary* behavior, as when the significant other provides care and the child receives it, or *similar* behavior, as when both express love. From these relationships, the child learns how to behave in both ways—that is, giving and receiving love and care. In adverse childhood relationships, comple-mentary behaviors are extreme as when the significant other is a cruel abuser and the child a passive victim. Again, both behavior patterns are learned, which means that victims of abuse learn the roles of both victim and abuser. The disparity between these roles makes them difficult to inte-grate. The two opposing ways of relating form the basis for self-states that are experienced as separate and unrelated, as occurred with Sarah's rage and overwhelmed states. The behaviors involved in these states are en-acted in rigid ways that lead to unstable relationships; sudden shifts in self-states can cause major behavioral changes as when a victim suddenly be-comes abusive. The purpose of a self-state diagram is to show how these states are connected. Subsequent discussion of the origins of these states consolidates this understanding and begins the process of integration, which is then extended when these patterns are enacted in treatment. The therapist's task is to avoid colluding with these patterns by adopting recip-rocal behavior that confirms the underlying schemata. Unfortunately, as the discussion of crises noted, patients have the knack of evoking recipro-cal responses from others. For this reason, is important to note these pat-terns at an early stage and to monitor their enactment in therapy.

Self-State Description

Often self-states are most conveniently explored as they emerge in treat-ment, as was the case with Sarah. However, structured evaluation can also be used either during assessment or early in treatment. Patients may be asked to provide written or oral descriptions of themselves, as used in stud-ies of impression formation (Bromley, 1977; Livesley & Bromley, 1973). One approach that combines free description with the method described by Ryle (1997) is to provide patients with a booklet that describes the idea of self-states and lists typical self-states observed in people with personality disorder, such as out of control; frozen, paralyzed, shut down, blank; very special, different from everyone else, brilliant; filled with rage; terrified, frightened; loser, a mess; jealous (see the appendix). Using this list as a stimulus or guide, the patient is asked to identify his or her major self-states (usually three to five). They are then asked to describe each state and respond to a series of questions that systematically covers the compo-nents of each state. This information is then used to construct a self-state diagram.

Changing and Integrating Self-States

Achieving changes in self-states involves modifying the schemata, inter-personal patterns, affects, and environmental responses that comprise each state, using the methods discussed in Chapter 11. Here, however, we are concerned with how an understanding the relationships among self-states promotes integration because it imposes meaning and cognitive control on experiences that may have felt chaotic.

Exploration of the self, spread across long periods of treatment, begins by the therapist describing maladaptive schemata and rapidly incorporates the relationship between schemata and interpersonal patterns. Later, the process extends to describing the schemata, relationship patterns, and feelings associated with each self-state. Finally, the connections among different self-states are identified. Thus, over time, the exploratory process mirrors the hierarchical structure of the self and promotes integration by reiterating the connections among self schemata and self-states. The understanding sought is not an intellectual appreciation of the way personality is organized but a more profound recognition of the dynamics of behavior and experience that transforms the individual's understanding of the self. This process was illustrated in the case of Sarah, who understood the major events in her life differently when she suddenly realized that many apparently separate events, feelings, thoughts, and actions were connected.

This process is also illustrated by the case of Natasha, discussed in Chapter 11. After about 1 year of treatment, Natasha suddenly realized that catastrophic thinking increased her anxiety, and that externalizing responsibility led to passivity and helplessness. In the process, she realized that she contributed to the turmoil around her and that only she could change her life. This case was used to illustrate the interaction among maladaptive schemata and cognitive styles. Other aspects to this phase of Natasha's treatment, however, are relevant to integration and synthesis. Here the description her treatment continues from where it was left in Chapter 11:

> Further exploration revealed that the distressed state Natasha frequently experienced was usually triggered by an unexpected event, either positive or negative. Events that took Natasha by surprise made her feel incompetent and unable to cope. Activation of the incompetence schema led to a distressed state that then escalated in response to catastrophic thinking. In this state, Natasha felt overwhelmed and that there was nothing she could do to change things. Externalization of control further increased her distress. The upshot of these feelings was that Natasha "gave up" and withdrew. In effect, she behaved as if she were incompetent.
>
> This behavior evoked a variety of reactions from friends and acquaintances. Some were concerned about her distress and colluded with her externalization of responsibility and her assessment that there was nothing she could do about the situation. This agreement only reinforced her passivity and resignation and confirmed her low self-esteem and feelings of incompetence. Other friends, however,

would become frustrated by her passivity and inability to deal with situations and being to avoid her. This withdrawal also confirmed the incompetence schema.

As the details of this state emerged, Natasha realized that it had occurred frequently throughout her life and sometimes had lasted for months. She also noted that the feeling of incompetence also contributed to the submissive behavior that characterized her relationships, especially with men. In effect, incompetence and submissiveness reinforced each other to form a self-perpetuating structure. Natasha referred to this pervasive self-state as her upset and incompetent state. She noted, however, that she did not always feel this way and that there were times when she felt the opposite—competent, capable, and in control. In this state, she was good at whatever she did, including her job selling large ticket items. Unfortunately, this state never lasted for very long, and the transition between states was abrupt. In the upset state, she was unable to access feelings of competency, and even memories of success felt false.

Recognition of these self-states and the development of a self-state diagram helped Natasha to develop a greater understanding of her life experience and had a settling effect. As she made changes to the different components of the incompetent state, Natasha began to develop control over catastrophizing and externalizing modes of thought. As noted in Chapter 11, these changes took time, and there were periods when Natasha was able to recognize these thought patterns but was too angry to control them. Eventually, she was able to recall feelings of competency when she felt incompetent and hence gained access to more effective coping strategies when in this state. During this time, the therapist continually recalled the competent state and sought to strengthen its components, without exploring the feelings and beliefs about competency. As the distinction between states diminished, Natasha decided to return to work.

The idea of self-states offers a conceptualization of core pathology that suggests strategies for promoting integration. When exploring these states, it is important *not* to treat the states as distinct entities, because this leads to further fragmentation and sets the stage for iatrogenic "multiple personalities." Throughout, the emphasis is on connecting and integrating self-states and on experiencing personality as a coherent whole.

PROMOTING INTEGRATION: TREATING REAL SELF–FALSE SELF DISJUNCTIONS

The second fracture in self-knowledge is a disconnection between the real self and the false self, or the self that is presented to the world. This is most apparent in inhibited or schizoid–avoidant individuals who feel that the self they present to the world is false, a facade that masks the real self, which is hidden or buried and cannot be shown.

Characteristic Features

Those who experience this kind of fracture feel alienated from the world because their experience feels unreal. A common fantasy is that of being an unseen watcher who observes the world from an anonymous viewpoint. One patient, for example, had a time-consuming fantasy of living in a secret control room equipped with cameras and spy holes that allowed him to monitor everything around him. Another fantasized about living within a mobile capsule made of one-way glass that allowed him to be with others without being seen. Real self–false self discontinuity involves a separation of emotions and cognition. Core aspects of self-experience are isolated to protect the individual from feeling vulnerable and threatened. One patient, who was reluctant to reveal personal information and felt that no one could ever see her true self, recalled attending the funeral of her sister when she was very young. She remembered that, as the coffin was lowered into the ground, it was as if she had disappeared into a bottle, where she has remained ever since. The sense of falseness about her identity was reinforced by her parents, who dressed her in her sister's clothes and treated her as if she were the dead sister.

The alienation and restricted expression of feelings involved in this form of self pathology explains the association with the inhibited pattern. Such individuals are socially avoidant. Feelings are rarely expressed, presumably because they may lead to social contact. Beneath the surface, however, many of these individuals are hypersensitive. If the inhibited child experiences abusive and intrusive relationships, withdrawal is likely to be his or her response. This may involve actual social withdrawal or the creation of a facade that hides the real self. The following vignette illustrates this pathology:

> Matthew, a single man in his late 20s, presented with a 10-year history of depressive symptoms and personality problems characterized by social avoidance, restricted expression of feelings (although there was an underlying hypersensitivity), difficulties with intimacy, and passivity that led to difficulties accomplishing tasks. As the mood disorder responded to medication, personality pathology became more apparent. Matthew had always been a solitary person; although he compensated, at times, by engaging in team sports, he was never one of the team. Throughout his life he had pursued many interests but had brought none to fruition, largely because nothing ever seemed important. Most problems were handled in a passive way that caused difficulties with family and acquaintances.
>
> As therapy progressed, Matthew noted that his inability to com-

plete tasks occurred because he was never really sure what he wanted to do. This uncertainty was particularly true in the area of career choice. Although highly intelligent and articulate, he did not know how he wanted to use his talents. Nothing seemed to matter, and there were times when he anguished over his inability to understand himself and what he really wanted. He noted that "nothing ever really seems real to me," and even when talking to the therapist, it "feels as if I'm telling a story about someone else—none of these things really seem to have happened to me." On other occasions, he noted, "It is all a façade. I never let anyone know me." He went on to explain how he thought that this intentional self-concealment accounted for his relationship problems. He went from one relationship to another. None lasted because he felt overwhelmed and drained by ongoing contact.

Matthew felt that he was rarely able to access his real self. Given the lack of authenticity to his experience, it is not surprising that he had difficulty with self-directedness. Nothing felt worth pursuing, so that when difficulties were encountered, he simply gave up rather trying to overcome them.

Intervention Strategies

Achieving change in real self–false self discontinuity is difficult. The low behavioral output and general reluctance to disclose personal information of inhibited individuals are major obstacles to change. In addition, the problem does not lend itself to the kind of descriptive, integrative process used to treat self-state disjunctions. Change seems to depend on the creation of a safe therapeutic environment. Although this environment is required for any successful treatment, it is especially important with this form of self pathology; change requires the patient to relate to another person and to experience and reveal aspects of the self that have always been suppressed and protected. This kind of relationship is not established quickly or easily. Attempts to rush the process or press for affective expression usually provoke further withdrawal.

An important step in treatment is to identify situations in which the patient feels real and genuine. Achieving this goal requires a diligent search, because patients are often unaware of these situations or are reluctant to disclose them. One patient, for example, only felt authentic when playing with his dog. Another felt real only when playing a musical instrument while alone. Focusing on these situations within a supportive relationship begins to create the idea that "I can be myself"; "I can be real"; and "It is safe to be myself."

Life events occurring during treatment are often valuable opportunities to facilitate an experience of the authentic expression of feelings. The patient who felt that nothing about him was real or authentic, except playing with his dog, experienced genuine sadness when his dog died. The dog was the only real relationship he had in his life. When playing with the dog, he felt a sense of contentment and genuineness that was rarely experienced with people. While discussing the event, the patient commented that he thought he was experiencing genuine sadness for the first time and that the sadness reflected the way he really felt. He became aware of feelings that he had not been able to access. The change was not dramatic. To the observer, his emotional response seemed muted, but to the patient the experience was different and he felt aware of an aspect of himself that he had not previously experienced. Equally importantly, the patient felt real when discussing his feelings with the therapist. This discussion provided an opportunity for him to communicate a part of himself that he had not previously shared with anyone, and it began a slow process of becoming more open emotionally and feeling a little more in touch with his own experiences.

PROMOTING INTEGRATION: CONATIVE FACTORS

Although the cognitive links within self-knowledge make a major contribution to integration, they are not the whole story. The self also consists of future possibilities: goals to be attained, lifestyles to be achieved, and the self one hopes to become (Markus & Norius, 1986). This aspect of the self promotes a sense of unity and purposefulness. As with other aspects of integration, self-directedness is seriously disturbed in people with severe personality disorder (Cloninger, 2000). Like authenticity, self-directedness is both a consequence and a condition of cohesion and integration. Feelings of certainty about simple wants and preferences early in life and success in attaining short-term goals establish the conditions for self-directedness to flourish. Once a rudimentary sense of agency forms, it facilitates the establishment of longer-term goals. Invalidating experiences hinder the emergence of certainty about wants and the confidence in self-efficacy on which self-directedness depends. People feel a sense of fulfillment and satisfaction when they are working toward goals that they feel are their own. Personal goals organize and integrate by giving direction and purpose to action. When these goals are achieved through personal action, they build confidence and competence and create the impetus for further action.

The importance of goals and self-directedness increases during treatment. As maladaptive patterns change, patients often become frustrated because they cannot envisage how their lives may be different. Having lived largely in the present, they find it difficult to change perspective. A major task in the middle and latter stages of treatment is to help patients imagine future possibilities and martial resources to achieve them. Goals also become important because in the past, patients often were more pre-occupied with avoiding feared situations and outcomes than achieving pos-itive goals. This fear crippled motivation and initiative. As the fear re-solves, the problem of establishing positive goals and a direction to their lives comes into focus. To help patients move forward at this stage, it is of-ten important to spend time teaching them how to identify simple and practical goals that can create a future focus for their behavior.

The Significance of Real-Life Events

The development of self-directedness is often facilitated by events that force individuals to reevaluate their lives and recognize the importance of having long-term goals. The following incident, taken from the treatment of Sandra, the patient described in the vignette of the walk in the park (Chapter 11), involves a chance event that had a major impact on treat-ment.

> Sandra had a long history of affective lability, a wide range of self-harming actions, seriously disturbed relationships, and substance abuse. When treatment began, she had been unemployed for many years. Three years of individual and group treatment produced reasonable improvement. She no longer abused drugs or alcohol, parasuicidal behavior had ceased, her moods were more stable, and she had greater control over her affects and impulses. At the same time, her understanding of interpersonal problems increased. Her behavior to-ward other people became a little more flexible, but she still found it difficult to form friendships. She also felt stuck, finding it impossible to imagine how her life could possibly be different. As a result, she lived from day to day and remained unemployed. These issues were discussed at length in therapy, without change. The problem was that Sandra could not identify anything that she would like to do. The future continued to be defined by negative goals. She was well aware of what she did not want to do—the kinds of jobs that she did not want, the life paths that she was not prepared to follow, and the relationships she wanted to avoid.
>   Change was initiated by a relatively minor event. Sandra was hypersensitive to noise, which had caused sleeping problems for her. For many years she regularly moved from apartment to apartment in search of somewhere quiet. She had moved into her present apartment about 6 months previously because it was so quiet. After spending a lot of time and effort making the place to her liking, she found, to her dismay, that her neighbors had become increasingly noisy and disrupted her sleep. The only happy part of her life was that she had found a pet that gave her great pleasure. After one disturbed night, Sandra suddenly decided that she had to get a place of her own. Al-though simple in nature, this decision crystallized discontentment

with her current lifestyle. She suddenly felt the urge to make a change; ultimately, she had to plan to buy her own home. Only then would she be in a position to control the noise and ensure that she and her pet had "a happy life." When this issue was discussed, discontent with the current situation crystallized into the goal of having "a place of my own." Initially, the goal was simply to have somewhere she could sleep without disturbance, but the goal expanded as she realized the many things she had to do to purchase her own home. This event proved to be a powerful motivator. Over the course of a few weeks, Sandra found part-time work and began to pursue educational objectives. Her life had changed. Her self-esteem increased because she was able to obtain and hold down a job.

This incident illustrates the energizing and organizing effects of goals (Baumeister, 1989; Pervin, 1992). The organizing impact occurred because "to have a place of my own" meant that the patient had to find a job. Thus the initial decision established motivation and direction. First, she had to find any job that would allow her to establish a credible work record. Then she had to obtain training or education that would allow her to get the kind of job needed to generate the income required to buy her own home. Thus the long-term goal implied several short-term goals that covered a range of activities and interests. More importantly, because the self is partly defined by the person's goals (Carver & Scheier, 1998), the sense of self took on new meaning, and the patient now experienced a sense of purpose that had previously eluded her.

This vignette is a further example of the importance of everyday events in the change process. Problems with noisy neighbors led to a reformulation of future possibilities and the definition of a future lifestyle. The incident also illustrates the importance of an underlying model of personality and the self that alerts the therapist to the way chance events may be used to achieve synthetic change. The example illustrates the value of viewing treatment as a process of collaborative description and guided development. Collaborative description sets the stage for change by building connections within self-knowledge. Guided development builds on these foundations by encouraging and supporting events and everyday experiences that are consistent with more adaptive self-functioning.

Goal Setting

At this stage we are concerned with working with patients to set goals for the ways in which they would like to live their lives. To be effective in promoting purpose and unity, goals need to be positive, inclusive, autonomously conceived, and authentically reflective of the person's real self. Many patients, however, place greater emphasis on goals that they want to avoid. The patient in the vignette initially saw her future only in terms of what she was not prepared to do: not working in an office at a 9-to-5 job; avoiding routine; not having relationships because intimacy was always a problem and relationships never lasted; not having a sexual relationship because "men are pigs"; and minimizing social contact because she really believed that people were against her. These goals led to restriction rather than personal growth, and created a fearful focus on the present rather than a sense of purpose and direction.

The goals that are most effective in integrating personality functioning are broad, inclusive goals with multiple components that require the individual to draw upon a wide variety of interests, talents, skills, and values. The goal of "getting a place of my own" had these qualities. Because it was concrete and specific, it created a clear sense of direction. It could be broken down into specific goals, such as getting a short-term job, seeking information about training and funding to support retraining, applying for courses, and so on. The short-term goals prevented the patient from feeling overwhelmed by the daunting prospect of buying a place of her own. Each subgoal was attainable and there were short-term payoffs that maintained motivation.

For goals to contribute to self-development, they need to be experienced as personal choices freely made, as opposed to being imposed by others or selected to meet others' approval. Goals based on a sense of obligation and responsibility rarely create a sense of unity. Clearly, therapists need to help patients identify the things that matter to them, validate decisions that they make, and help them to understand the origins of feelings of obligation.

PROMOTING INTEGRATION: CONSTRUCTING A NEW "THEORY OF THE SELF"

The ultimate expression of integration is the construction of an overall understanding of the self. As Bruner (1990) noted, individuals try to impose meaning on events and experiences by developing accounts or narratives that make sense of their behavior and the events and situations in which they find themselves. People also try to make sense of their life experience by creating an explanation of themselves that welds together an understanding of their salient qualities, past experiences, and future hopes and aspirations. People who are able to make sense of the pattern of their lives in this way experience a sense of coherence and unity. We can think of this construction as a global schema of the self that combines cognitive understanding and conative striving. Such belief systems can only be constructed when individuals can stand back and reflect upon themselves and their lives and see their ideas not as facts but as constructions that are open to various interpretations. This perspective makes it possible to review experiences and organize and reorganize them to create coherence and consistency within self-knowledge.

Individuals with personality disorder have usually failed to construct well-rounded explanations of themselves and their lives. Some form one-dimensional views of the self that lack depth and richness and are usually organized around a single schema that is often negative, though occasionally grandiose. These schemata are taken to be facts and the individuals' experiences and their understanding of events are then distorted to fit these "facts." Others have disjointed and unconnected images of the self that they struggle to control and integrate. Still others fail to develop any real understanding of any of their defining qualities.

The task of longer-term treatment is to help patients construct and reconstruct a new narrative about the self until an adaptive theory is achieved that provides meaning and coherence. Such belief systems are not constructed easily or quickly. People accept, and indeed cling to, their theories even when maladaptive until a better one comes along. Change occurs gradually, as the possibility of a new understanding of the self emerges from the therapist's descriptions of what has happened to the patient and the patient's own efforts to make sense of his or her life experience. The process begins when the initial formulation is discussed with the patient at the end of assessment. This beginning formulation provides a narrative account of the individual's life and personality that is added to, revised, and reframed during treatment.

The general thrust of descriptive exploration enriches self-knowledge largely through an analytic process that deconstructs the meaning of experiences. The synthesis of a new theory of the self depends on a parallel process that combines and connects emerging elements of self-knowledge. The integrative process is aided by regular summaries that draw together the therapist's understanding of the patient. These broad summaries provide an anchor to the self and help to construct a new self theory by organizing a large number of previously unconnected events, experiences, and actions. As Horowitz (1998) pointed out, integration can "be achieved by establishing a larger belief system that connects meanings and synthesizes the competing elements operating in smaller belief systems" (p. 10). Integration can also be facilitated by providing frequent summaries at the end of sessions, which provide an overview of the issues discussed and link them to previous themes to create connections across sessions. Throughout treatment it is important to invite the patient to contribute to these summaries, to offer their own accounts, so that understanding becomes fully incorporated, and to work collaboratively with the therapist to construct an understanding that allows him or her to view his or her life in a new way that is less distressing. The self, however, is never totally integrated. Conflicting views always exist. Part of treatment is to help patients accept and tolerate a reasonable degree of ambivalence and inconsistency in self-experience.

COMMENT

This chapter has attempted to provide some admittedly sketchy ideas about the treatment of core self and interpersonal pathology. Although this area of therapeutic work is, in many ways, the central issue in treating personality disorder, the pathology involved is poorly understood. Constructs to describe and define these central issues are lacking or so poorly articulated that they are almost impossible to translate into coherent intervention strategies. Our understanding of the mental structures and processes captured by the concept of self is in its infancy and the meaning of concepts such as self-integration, self-cohesiveness, and self-directedness need considerable conceptual and empirical research. Clinically, the concepts seem rich in meaning, conveying important psychological dimensions associated with mental health, but this meaning is, in many ways, a chimera that can lull us into thinking that we understand what we seek to treat. The goal in including a chapter on treating core pathology is as much to draw attention to the problem of self pathology and the need for clearly defined constructs to replace the seductive but tenuous constructs so readily available in the clinical literature, as it is to offer suggestions for treatment strategies that may contribute to change.

CHAPTER 14

Implementation and Concluding Comments

This chapter considers aspects of implementation and treatment planning that were not discussed earlier (see Chapter 6): namely, duration of treatment and treatment modality. With each of these issues, recommendations are based largely on a consideration of the nature of the pathology involved and current opinion. Regrettably, hard evidence is limited. The concluding section provides a brief overview of the principles underlying the approach and considers some final points about the proposed framework.

IMPLEMENTATION AND TREATMENT DELIVERY

For convenience and descriptive clarity, treatment has been presented thus far as if it were best delivered through long-term individual therapy. The approach is, however, sufficiently flexible to use in individual or group therapy. The emphasis on core interventions based on generic change mechanisms makes the approach relevant to all modalities and settings and is independent of the duration of treatment. The specific interventions that supplement this core may be considered separate treatment modules that are used according to circumstance and duration of treatment. Individual treatments will incorporate modules dealing with crises, symptoms (including dissociative behavior and the consequences of trauma), affect and impulse regulation, self and interpersonal problems, maladaptive traits, and core self and interpersonal problems, as needed, to treat the individual as permitted by the duration of treatment. These modules were described in the approximate sequence of implementation, based on the urgency of different problems and symptoms and ideas about the plasticity of personality pathology. However, when patients do not present in a crisis, or emotional dysregulation and parasuicide are not part of the clinical picture, some early modules may be omitted.

Duration of Treatment

Relatively few empirical data are available on the time required to implement different forms of change. Although comprehensive treatment of people with personality disorder is usually thought to take years rather than months, we know little about the time needed to effect reasonable changes or whether the use of systematic structured and eclectic interventions are likely to expedite the process. It seems reasonable to assume, however, that the comprehensive treatment of typical cases requires lengthy work, especially when therapy begins with the patient in a dysregulated state. It takes time to implement and consolidate changes to engrained maladaptive patterns, especially when these are grounded in underlying genetic predispositions and have been honed and reinforced over many years of dysfunctional relationships. This is not the sort of news that the administrators of contemporary health-care systems like to hear, but nature did not organize personality with bureaucracy in mind.

The assumption that change is likely to be relatively slow is supported by evidence that patients with personality disorder show a poorer response to treatment (Reich & Green, 1991). Studies of rates of change in unselected nonpsychotic patients receiving treatment in a mental health center or hospital outpatient clinic show that most of the change occurs in the first 6 months, with approximately 75% showing improvement. This improvement continues subsequently, but at a slower rate, over the next 2 years (Howard, Kopta, Krause, & Orlinsky, 1986; Howard, Lueger, & Shrank, 1992). In patients with major personality disorder, however, these changes are slower: improvement after 1 year is approximately 50% (Kolden & Howard, 1992; Kopta, Howard, Lowry, & Beutler, 1994). Similar results are reported by Perry, Banon, and Ianni (1999), in a review of the effectiveness of psychotherapy. They found that, on average, 52% of treated patients no longer met the criteria for a specific disorder after an average of 1.3 years of treatment. This rate is substantially higher than for untreated individuals.

It also appears that improvement continues after treatment (Bateman & Fonagy, 2001; Hoglend, 1993; Horowitz, Marmar, Weiss, Kaltreider, & Wilner, 1986). Hoglend reported that after nine to 53 sessions of individual dynamic therapy, patients with personality disorder showed less improvement than patients with other disorders, but that after 4 years the difference in improvement between the two groups had disappeared. Change was also greater for patients with personality disorder who received longer treatment.

Duration of treatment is closely related to goals of therapy and the kinds of change that the patient and therapist hope to achieve. When the goals are crisis oriented and the primary goal is symptom relief, treatment may be relatively brief and rely on general treatment and containment strategies. As these goals are extended to include more definitive treatment of symptoms and impulsivity, the anticipated duration of treatment increases. In the initial evaluation of dialectical behavior therapy, changes in self-harming behavior took 1 year to achieve (Linehan et al., 1993). Although considerable improvement in parasuicidal behavior can often be achieved more rapidly, changes in longstanding self-harming behavior linked to severe pathology may take even longer. As treatment goals are widened to embrace changes to interpersonal pathology and maladaptive trait expressions, the duration of treatment increases further, and it may require 2 to 3 years, or even longer, to effect lasting change, especially when the initial presentation includes self-harming behavior. In patients for whom self-harming behavior is not a problem, treatment may begin addressing these issues much earlier. However, even in these cases, change is rarely rapid. Finally, enduring change in core pathology usually requires several years of treatment and, even then, problems often remain.

It should be noted, however, that some short-term treatments can be effective. Ryle (1997; 2001), for example, advocates a short-term cognitive analytic approach, and some very brief interventions may be effective in managing specific problems. The study by Evans and colleagues (1999), mentioned earlier, showed that cognitive-behavioral interventions lasting only a few sessions, accompanied by a workbook for patients to follow, led to fewer reported suicidal acts and lower self-rated depression. The problem is that we have relatively little information, based on methodologically sound studies, on many practical aspects of the treatment of personality disorder. As our understanding increases and new interventions are developed, it is likely that treatment will become substantially more efficient.

Continuous versus Intermittent Treatment

Although most accounts of therapy for people with personality disorder describe continuous long-term treatment, intermittent therapy may be more viable in settings where resources are limited. In these situations, a useful model is the "general practice" approach, in which patients attend for treatment only when in a crisis or acute symptomatic state. The approach is particularly effective when the patient sees the same therapist on each occasion and forms an attachment that provides additional support. Failing the availability of the same therapist, the same treatment model is used on each occasion, and the patient should be encouraged to bond with the *program* providing the service. The understanding that assistance will always be available when needed often has a containing effect that reduces the frequency and severity of crises, especially when patients are encouraged to seek help before a crisis state is fully established. When this approach is used, the focus of treatment can gradually be extended across occasions to address triggering situations and interpersonal problems. The approach is particularly effective when combined with interventions to treat parasuicidal behavior and improve affect and impulse control. As noted, these interventions may not need to be extensive to be effective.

Although empirical studies are not available to substantiate the value of intermittent therapy, it is possible to offer a cogent rationale for delivering treatment in blocks of 20 or so sessions that focus on a specific set of issues, followed by a break of several months. This system differs from the general practice model in that treatment systematically addresses different domains of pathology and the blocks are based approximately on the specific modules. The model has several appealing features. The method incorporates the capacity of short-term therapy to build motivation and concentrate on specific issues. At the same time, long-term treatment is offered, something that is reassuring to many patients. Breaks from therapy enable treatment to capitalize on findings that improvements in personality problems continue after treatment ends (Bateman & Fonagy, 2001; Hoglend, 1993). This pattern of care should also help to diffuse the more intense reactions toward the therapist and minimize pathological forms of dependency that can occur with long-term treatment. It is, however, important that this pattern of care is introduced at the outset and discussed with the patient when negotiating the treatment contract, so that the patient understands that the contract is for long-term treatment. This knowledge provides a sense of continuity and stability that is so important in settling immediate problems and building the treatment relationship.

Treatment Setting and Range of Services

The settings used to treat people with severe personality disorder range from long-term residential treatment through day hospital or partial hospitalization programs to long-term ambulatory care. These are not really alternative ways of delivering treatment but rather the range of services needed for comprehensive care. The exception is long-term residential treatment. There is little evidence to indicate that this type of care is beneficial. However, as noted in Chapter 8, short-term inpatient treatment is often used to ensure safety. A mental health system seeking to provide the range of services needed to treat people with personality disorder should also include day treatment facilities. Evidence from methodologically sound studies indicates that day hospital programs are effective and offer "a comprehensive intervention 'package' and capitalize on the patients' shared group experience. These elements likely work singly and in combination to promote benefit across a range of outcome indices" (Piper & Joyce, 2001, p. 331). Early studies on day hospitalization, in which patients were randomly assigned to day hospital or inpatient treatment, showed that many patients with personality disorder could be accommodated effectively in day programs (Zwerling & Wilder, 1964) and that outcome was not different from inpatient treatment (Dick, Cameron, Cohen, Barlow, & Ince, 1985). More recent studies have shown that day program treatment, involving a psychoanalytic approach delivered in a group program that included community meetings, group and individual therapy, art therapy, and occupational therapy, leads to substantial improvement across a range of outcome variables (Azim, 2001; Bateman & Fonagy, 1999; Karterud et al., 1992; Mehlum et al., 1994; Piper et al., 1993, 1996; Vaglum et al., 1990). This improvement is maintained and even increased at follow-up 3 months later (Bateman & Fonagy, 2001). Given evidence of the value of skill training in enhancing emotional regulation and impulse control, an effective program should also include these interventions. The major strength of a day hospital program is the opportunity to combine multiple interventions that are delivered through group and individual treatment that affords multiple opportunities to promote integration. The latter component is important: an effective program should not consist merely of a series of groups that addresses different domains of pathology but also include components that facilitate the integration needed to treat core pathology.

Day hospital programs are cost-effective (see Bateman & Fonagy, 2003) and useful alternatives to inpatient treatment for many patients that should be used, whenever possible, to avoid the complications that frequently arise when patients are admitted to hospital. Such programs are also useful in managing patients with severe problems who have not responded to regular therapy. With entrenched pathology, an intense therapeutic experience is often helpful in overcoming a therapeutic impasse. Duration of treatment in a day hospital program varied across studies, from 4 to 8 months (Karterud et al., 1992) or 18 weeks (Piper et al., 1993, 1996) to up to 18 months (Bateman & Fonagy, 1999, 2001). A reasonable length of stay appears to be about 20 weeks, providing additional treatment is available subsequently in the form of weekly group or individual therapy. The service is best regarded as part of a spectrum of care, with weekly or twice-weekly individual or group therapy (or a combination of the two) being the main component.

Treatment Modality

Although individual therapy is the commonest modality used to treat patients with personality disorder, the evidence does not show that it is generally more effective than group treatment. Reviews of early studies comparing the effectiveness of individual and group therapy for various disorders and problems yielded mixed conclusions (Bellack, 1980; Luborsky, Singer, & Luborsky, 1975; Malan, Balfour, Hood, & Shooter, 1976); however, more recent reviews and meta-analyses concluded that there is little difference in outcome (MacKenzie, 2001; McRoberts, Burlingame, & Hoag, 1998; Piper & Joyce, 1996, 2001).

Individual versus Group Treatment

The primary theoretical advantage of individual treatment over group therapy is the opportunity to concentrate on the fine details of maladaptive behavior. As noted repeatedly, this focus is critical to facilitating change in maladaptive patterns. This kind of attention to the individual is difficult to achieve in groups that use group process as the major vehicle for change. The inability to focus on fine details of psychopathology is a limitation of group therapy, especially in the early stages of treatment when detailed behavioral analysis is often critical to improve affect and impulse regulation and gain control over suicidal and parasuicidal behavior. A focused behavioral analysis is also important in the later stages of therapy to promote greater integration of the self, and when the therapist's encouragement of new directions is needed to enhance self-directedness. Although this work can be achieved in group therapy, it is easier in individual treatment to tailor therapy to the patient and combine multiple structured and unstructured interventions.

In contrast, group therapy provides a greater range of change mechanisms, and group interaction provides extensive opportunities to identify, explore, and change maladaptive interpersonal patterns. These opportunities are probably the greatest advantage of group therapy over individual treatment. The interventions for treating maladaptive interpersonal behavior, discussed in Chapter 11, are readily adapted for use in groups. Moreover, the multiple interactions among members provide ongoing opportunities to identify the specific ways the patterns are enacted in the here-and-now of treatment. In group therapy, the role of the therapist is less central to the treatment process, and hence the group tends to dilute the more intense reactions toward the therapist that can obstruct treatment and lead to regression and dependency (MacKenzie, 2001). This dilution is particularly helpful in the early stages of treatment, when these reactions often adversely affect the emergence of an effective alliance. The dilution may not be advantageous, however, later in treatment, when reactions to the therapist are used to modify maladaptive schemata, as discussed in Chapter 11.

Regression and dependency are also counteracted by opportunities to engage in the altruistic behavior of taking an interest in the problems and well-being of other members. Furthermore, groups provide additional perspectives on generic change mechanisms. In addition to receiving support, validation, empathy, and encouragement from the therapist and other group members, members also have an opportunity to *provide* support, validation, and empathy to each other, which fosters a new appreciation of these behaviors. In the process, self-esteem and self-worth are enhanced. Groups also provide an additional perspective on maladaptive schemata originating in adversity. In individual therapy, schemata involving trust–distrust, cooperation and collaboration, and attachment/safety are expressed through the therapeutic relationship and modified in the light of therapist activity. In the group, each member also has an opportunity to experience what it is like to be the recipient of distrust or lack of cooperation. Such experience enables a more objective appreciation of the behaviors and their impact on relationships.

Theoretically, groups should be of value in managing resistant egosyntonic actions and patterns as they arise in the interaction within the group. In individual therapy, confrontation of these patterns may elicit strong adverse reactions from the patient, whereas patients are often more accepting of such confrontations from other group members. Groups should also be more effective in fostering social integration and enhancing social skills and in providing a richer array of opportunities to recognize problematic behaviors and rehearse new behaviors in a supportive environment.

It seems apparent that groups offer many opportunities for change that are not available with individual treatment. In particular, the interpersonal focus of the group is especially pertinent in treating a disorder that has a large interpersonal component. Yet the difficulty focusing on the detailed behaviors needed to effect change at critical stages of treatment is a major disadvantage with a group approach that largely has an interpersonal focus. This analysis suggests that if group treatment is used, several groups may be needed to provide comprehensive treatment. One option is to combine a standard interpersonal group and with a group focusing on cognitive-behavioral interventions and skill building. Even better would be a combination of group and individual therapy. This approach will be discussed, following more detailed consideration of group treatment.

Group Therapy

The evidence shows that group therapy is an effective treatment of personality disorder. Studies of group therapy for diagnostically heterogeneous samples show lasting change to the kinds of longstanding interpersonal problems that characterize personality disorder (Pilkonis, Imber, Lewis, & Rubinsky, 1984; Piper, Debbane, Bienvenu, & Garant, 1984). Specific studies of the outcome of group treatments for personality disorder yield similar conclusions. For example, Budman, Demby, Soldz, and Merry (1996) evaluated time-limited group therapy for personality disorder, studying five groups for 18 months (72 sessions). Groups had nine or 10 members (49 patients) with various personality disorders, and at least two patients in each group had borderline personality disorder. Fifty-one percent of participants terminated therapy early (25 patients); 11 of these participants had borderline personality disorder. Patients completing treatment showed consistent improvement on most outcome measures. The authors concluded that BPD patients may need more structure and intensity than the approach offered.

Marziali and Munroe-Blum (1994; Munroe-Blum & Marziali, 1995) reported a randomized comparison of group therapy and individual psychodynamic therapy for patients with borderline personality disorder. Group therapy, based on Dawson's relationship management (Dawson, 1988; Dawson & Macmillan, 1993), consisted of 25 sessions of weekly therapy, followed by five biweekly sessions. Both conditions led to significant improvement. Group treatment, however, was substantially more cost-effective, requiring approximately half the contact hours. Approximately 30% of patients terminated group treatment in the first five sessions. This rate is lower than typically reported for treatments of personality disorder but higher than usual for group therapy. The authors suggested using a limited number of individual sessions to address this problem.

Although considerable additional research is required to evaluate the potential of group therapy in treating personality disorder (as is the case with all other forms of treatment), the studies to date justify its use. Unfortunately, however, there are even fewer empirical studies of the best way to deliver group therapy. Basic decisions about group membership and heterogeneity versus homogeneity of pathology and personality patterns are largely based on anecdotal evidence. The Budman study (Budman et al., 1996) used heterogeneous groups but limited the number of patients with borderline personality disorder in each group. This method is similar to the recommendation of Leszcz (1989), who advocated heterogeneous groups with only one or two patients with borderline and narcissistic disorders and four to six less disturbed patients. Marziali and Munroe-Blum (1994; Munroe-Blum & Marziali, 1995), however, reported good outcome for homogeneous groups of patients with borderline personality disorder. Budman and colleagues reported poorer outcome for patients with borderline pathology than other forms of personality disorder and recommended more structure with these patients. As noted, Marziali and Munroe-Blum made a related recommendation for including a few individual sessions at the beginning of treatment to try to reduce early termination.

Group Composition

There are considerable advantages to forming groups with members who have different personality patterns. The heterogeneity increases the range of interaction in the group and facilitates the recognition of ego-syntonic traits and an understanding of alternative forms of behavior. The exception is the presence of dissocial traits. Although moderate levels of this pattern can be managed to advantage in heterogeneous groups, higher levels create a problem, especially when they involve traits such as vindictiveness and remorselessness, which tend to get expressed in ways that are damaging to other group members. Remorselessness makes it difficult to help such individuals modulate their behavior and recognize its impact on others. For this reason, high levels of dissocial traits are probably best managed in homogeneous groups, as occurs in forensic settings.

Another factor influencing the use of groups and group composition is stage of treatment. Actively parasuicidal patients in acute crisis states are difficult to manage in groups. When these patients are included in heterogeneous groups that include patients in a more settled state, there is a tendency for their crises to dominate the group. The intensity of their distress and the group's perception of the importance of these events lead group members to become preoccupied by the latest crisis. Members feel guilty about discussing their problems, which, in a climate of crisis, may seem less important than acute suicidal or parasuicidal behavior. At the same time, other members use these events as ways to avoid dealing with their own issues. When several members are in this state, contagion effects are common, leading to an escalation of impulsive acts. It seems best, therefore, to ensure that groups are composed of members who are at approximately the same phase in the sequence of change or at least are relatively stable.

Chronically self-injurious patients are probably best treated with individual therapy, or a combination of individual and group therapy, to contain the behavioral disorganization and promote more adaptive alternatives. Once behavioral stability is achieved, they may be transferred to a group if this is the preferred long-term modality. Currently, we lack empirical data on the optimal strategy. For this reason, it is important that rational combinations are explored and evaluated.

Support Groups

One form of group that is a useful part of a treatment service for people with personality disorder is the support group. These groups are a cost-effective way to manage patients who have severe pathology and limited capacity for change, and who would otherwise place significant demands on the health-care system. They are also useful for patients who seek therapy rather than treatment—patients who need or want the support provided by regular contact with a therapist but are not strongly motivated to change.

Interventions are largely based on the general therapeutic strategies that are tailored to a group context. The emphasis is on building group cohesiveness—the group analogue to the treatment alliance (MacKenzie, 2001)—and on promoting attachment to the group and the idea of the group as a secure base. This cohesiveness and attachment are facilitated by emphasizing the stability of the group and its relative permanence, even though members and therapists may change. These groups also work best if there are minimal expectations of changes; therapists feel less pressure to effect change, which frees them to be more supportive. However, gradual changes do occur in overall level of adjustment and quality of life.

Combined Modalities

The evidence indicates that both individual and group therapy are effective in treating people with personality disorder. Theoretical considerations suggest, however, that these modalities should be considered complementary rather than alternative ways of delivering treatment. The value of individual therapy lies in the containing effects of a therapeutic relationship and the time available to focus on specific problems, including behavior that obstructs therapy. Traditional group therapy that uses group processes and dynamics as the vehicle for change provides extensive opportunities to explore maladaptive interpersonal patterns that are characteristic of personality disorder. This analysis suggests that, at least on theoretical grounds, the optimal treatment is a combination of individual and group treatment, a suggestion made repeatedly in the literature (Horwitz 1980; Wong, 1980).

Individual therapy is used initially to contain affects and impulses and to develop the patient's affect and impulse control abilities (the first three phases in the sequence of change). Once a measure of regulation and control is achieved, individual treatment could be supplemented with weekly group therapy, based on a traditional interpersonal approach and emphasizing an understanding of maladaptive schemata and interpersonal patterns as they arise in the here-and-now of therapy. Individual therapy would continue with a focus on the more individual aspects of maladaptive behaviors and cognitions, and later on developing integration and promoting self-directedness.

The limitation of combined treatment is that it provides more opportunities for psychopathology to be expressed in ways that create conflict between modalities. When care is split across therapists, even if they are part of the same service, there is also the potential for conflict and confusion among therapists and between therapists and patient. These problems are minimized by following an explicit treatment model that is supported by frequent and open communication among therapists and careful monitoring of therapist compliance to the treatment model. Problems are also reduced when the same therapist is responsible for both group and individual treatment.

With this approach, group interaction is used as a major change mechanism. That is, the group is not used simply to deliver treatment in a cost-effective way—the kind of approach that has been characterized as individual therapy in a group setting. Instead, group process is used to build cooperation and collaboration by promoting group cohesion, and group interaction is used to explore and change maladaptive interpersonal behavior.

Family and Conjoint Therapy

Suggestions are also made for treating people with personality disorder in family and couple therapy (MacFarlane, in press). Although few studies have been reported, such treatments appear to be effective (Gurman & Kniskern, 1981). It seems unlikely, however, that family therapy will be the primary treatment for most patients. It is, however, likely to be an important adjunctive treatment in many cases and essential for some. As part of a comprehensive treatment plan, family therapy may be needed to (1) help patients resolve the more enduring consequences of earlier relationship problems; (2) help other family members cope with difficulties and stresses arising from having a member with severe personality disorder; and (3) modulate current family dynamics that are increasing the patient's current level of distress, sustaining problem behaviors, or constituting obstacles to change.

CONCLUDING COMMENTS

In many respects the approach to treatment that has been described is similar to what competent therapists do intuitively. This similarity is not accidental. The intent was to systematize eclectic practice and provide a rationale for a pragmatic approach to treatment that seeks to use what works rather than following the requirements of theoretical models that have little empirical support. At present, there is no evidence to suggest that one form of treatment for personality disorder is better than another. There are sound reasons, however, for combining interventions that systematically address the various domains of pathology that constitute personality disorder. In developing an approach to treating personality disorder, the intent has been to base ideas for principles, strategies, and interventions on what we know about personality disorder rather than what we think we know. And yet it must be recognized that our knowledge is scant and hence the treatment proposed suffers from the significant limitation of an adequate empirical basis. At times, it has been possible to draw upon the results of empirical studies to identify appropriate methods and ideas. But all too often it has been necessary to rely on inferences about what may be useful from our knowledge of the disorder and general findings of therapy outcome for related conditions. These are unavoidable limitations of any treatment, given current knowledge. Strategies and especially interventions are likely to change with advances in understanding. The framework itself, however, is perhaps a little more robust, because it is more securely based on empirical findings about the nature and origins of personality pathology.

Inadequate empirical foundations are not the only limitation. The approach also lacks a coherent theoretical foundation. It has been argued that this lacuna is unavoidable, given the lack of a satisfactory theory of personality disorder, and that it is better to base treatment on a framework for understanding personality disorder and therapeutic change than impose constraints on treatment by adapting a theoretical model that is subject to substantial limitations. Nevertheless, the lack of a theoretical structure risks inconsistent and disorganized treatments, as therapists struggle to combine multiple interventions. The problem is heightened by the nature of personality pathology, which itself can lead to a chaotic approach as therapists struggle to manage frequent crises, diverse problems, and patient demands. Inconsistent treatment is not an easy problem to address and one that all therapies face, regardless of their theoretical base. However, there is a real danger that the therapist will be supportive and validating at one moment and confronting at another, focused on skill building at one moment and on exploration of problems at another.

Three principles for organizing therapy were introduced to address this problem. The first was the distinction between general strategies and specific interventions and the proposal that specific interventions are only used when the conditions created by the general strategies are met. Hence specific interventions are used only when (1) the alliance is satisfactory, as indicated by a good rapport, (2) there is adherence to the frame, (3) the patient feels validated, and (4) there is a commitment to change the behaviors that are the focus of any specific intervention that is being contemplated. The therapist always seeks to support and validate; any confrontation of pathology occurs within this context, and specific interventions (ranging from skill building to schema change) are used only when conditions established by the general strategies are met. This is an important principle that substantially reduces inconsistency by creating an intervention hierarchy.

The second principle is that the overall process of treatment may be divided into five phases: (1) safety, (2) containment, (3) control and regulation, (4) exploration and change, and (5) integration and synthesis. Underlying these phases is the idea that treatment is based on a continuum of interventions, ranging from more structured behavioral and cognitive interventions, combined with medication, to less structured interventions derived from interpersonal and psychodynamic approaches. It is not that cognitive and behavioral interventions are not used in the middle and later stages of treatment. Rather they are increasingly supplemented with less structured techniques as interpersonal and self themes become predominant. This continuum reflects (1) the way in which interventions drawn from different approaches are used, and (2) the emphasis placed on enhancing emotional regulation skills before systematically tackling more sensitive, emotion-arousing material. However, this sequence is not invariant, nor is change an orderly linear progression. Instead, considerable movement back and forth across phases of therapy is inevitable. Thus in the middle and later stages of therapy, as trauma and significant interpersonal problems are addressed, it is often necessary to use containment interventions to regulate intense affects and continue skill building to consolidate these skills and ensure that they become part of the patient's normal coping repertoire. Nevertheless, the phases of treatment imposes an order on the overall process of therapy that helps the therapist to organize treatment over time.

The third principle, the stages of change, describes the way in which specific behaviors change. In contrast to the sequence of treatment, which indicates how and when interventions from diverse approaches may be integrated into therapy, the stages of change model describes how changes to specific behaviors may be approached. It reminds therapists of the importance of tackling specific issues in a systematic way. The model, along with the distinction between general and specific interventions, helps to organize treatment within sessions and over shorter periods of time, within the phases of treatment sequence.

These principles and the idea of the therapeutic exchange as a process of collaborative description provide an overall structure for approaching the treatment of patients with personality disorder. In articulating this structure, the intent is not to offer a definitive approach to the treatment of personality disorder—we are a long way from specifying such a model—nor is it a treatment manual in the traditional sense. It is simply a framework, based on what we currently know, which therapists can use creatively to organize interventions that they find useful and which have been shown to be effective.

Treating personality disorder is difficult, and outcomes are often less than we would like. Treatment failures are also common with most approaches, and the current approach is no exception. Like any psychosocial intervention, the approach relies upon the patient's ability to process information. The presence of any factor that limits this ability, such as neuropsychological dysfunctions or severely limited psychological mindedness, creates a serious obstacle to implementing many of the intervention strategies discussed, with the exception of more structured behavioral interventions.

One of the commonest problems, however, is difficulty establishing a treatment alliance. Paradoxically, the strength of the approach—an emphasis on the relationship, especially the alliance, as the major vehicle for managing and changing core pathology—is also a weakness. As repeatedly noted, the capacity for cooperation is a core deficit in personality disordered patients. Hence treatment may be considered to be moving toward termination once an effective alliance has been established. However, a modicum of cooperation is needed before treatment is possible. Patients need to attend to, and at least begin to work with, the therapist. For some severely disturbed individuals, even this modest requirement is too much. These are usually patients who have multiple problems and major deficit pathology associated with severe deprivation and abuse, and a long history of involvement in the health-care system. These are the individuals who desperately need help but are often unable to use it. The problem is illustrated by the following case.

> Kelly was a 40-year-old, unemployed single woman who had sought treatment repeatedly from many clinicians and agencies. None of the treatments lasted long and none appeared to have any discernible effect. At the time she presented for treatment with her current therapist, she had chronic suicidal ideation and engaged in repetitive parasuicidal behavior that took many forms. Affective lability was a major problem, and her mood was low, although this varied substantially from day to day. Her life lurched from one crisis to another, and she had little support from family and friends, most of whom were exhausted from having to deal with repeated problems over many years. In these crises Kelly was impulsive, suicidal, and angry. She blamed everyone for her problems and was unable to see how she herself contributed to them. Self-harm occurred several times each week and sometimes daily, leading to regular visits to emergency rooms in the city in which she lived. On most occasions she demanded help but angrily rejected whatever was offered. She was also involved with a wide range of agencies and received treatment from several clinicians for a variety of complaints. Community concern was considerable.
>
> The assessment interviews were difficult; Kelly was not very self-disclosing, although she insisted that she needed help. She also used the interviews to ventilate her anger about previous treatments and how the health-care system was reacting to her current problems. She was highly articulate and clearly had high verbal intelligence, although she had little ability to process psychological information. She seemed unable to reflect on anything said to her but rather reacted immediately without thinking about the material.
>
> It was difficult to get details about her past. She described a dysfunctional and abusive relationship with her mother and multiple episodes of sexual abuse in childhood and early adulthood but gave few details about any of these matters. There was also substantial evi-

dence of extensive core pathology. The capacity for object relationships was severely limited, and there was no evidence that Kelly had been able to maintain even one consistent relationship in adult life. Sense of self was severely impaired, with considerable evidence of boundary problems and poorly differentiated self schemata. When asked to describe herself, Kelly embarked on a lengthy description of the terrible things that had happened to her. It was not possible to refocus her, even with supportive, validating interventions. When the possibility of treatment was discussed, Kelly was adamant that she needed help and that she particularly needed help with the suicidal and parasuicidal behavior. It was agreed that she would attend twice weekly. This was considered necessary to contain the impulsivity and repetitive self-harm. Attempts were also made to curtail involvement with other clinicians. Kelly was agreeable to this, saying that it was not helping anyway.

The initial approach of containment and supportive limit setting had little effect, despite consistent application for a substantial period of time. Medication was discussed, and although Kelly insisted she needed medication and initially accepted the idea, she did not take it. For months she demanded medication for dysphoria and sleep problems but rejected all recommendations. She turned everything into a battle, regardless of the stance adopted by the therapist. From the outset, she missed many appointments, usually because she said that she was too ill to attend. Attempts to deal with this noncompliance were unsuccessful. The alliance was nonexistent and, in many ways, the frame of therapy did not exist either, because Kelly simply ignored it. The problem was that Kelly did not really listen to anything the therapist had to say. It was not that she discounted what he said, although she also did that; rather, she steadfastly ignored whatever he said. Sessions were almost entirely monologues. Whenever the therapist managed to get a word in, it had no effect, and the monologue continued as if nothing had happened. Because of this barrage, limit setting was ineffective. It was as if Kelly needed the therapist to be physically present, but apart from that, he did not matter. She did not seem to be aware of the effect her actions had on others, including the therapist, and she did not really attend to anything he or others said.

The crises continued, as did Kelly's involvement with other agencies and organizations. Treatment was further rendered impossible by the fact that Kelly lied about many things in her life, including the many agencies that she contacted for help. There was no basis for treatment and no way to deal effectively with the problem. Even limit setting requires some collaboration between patient and therapist. Eventually treatment was terminated.

Cases like this are salutary reminders of the problems of severe personality disorder and the comparative ineffectiveness of current treatments in these circumstances. It is not clear whether treatment failed because of (1) undue reliance on a supportive, validating stance, (2) the therapist failing to follow the stance consistently, (3) a poor fit between patient and therapist, or (4) the patient's inability to form an alliance. Some would argue that a more confrontational approach, as adopted by some psychodynamic therapies, might have been more successful. However, the evidence suggests that early termination is high with this form of treatment. Moreover, the externalizing style and profound egocentric attitude would probably negate such interventions. Furthermore, this approach had been used by other therapists, without success. It seems likely that a combination of factors was responsible for treatment failure. The patient was not very psychologically minded and had limited capacity for self-observation and self-reflection, despite high verbal intelligence. Her thought processes were also unusual; she did not attend to or process information in the typical way. In some ways her mode of thought recalls Cleckley's depiction of individuals with psychopathy as having "semantic psychosis."

From the outset there was only superficial agreement on the treatment contract and little foundation for an alliance. The case illustrates the importance of the frame for all aspects of treatment and the difficulty establishing the frame and even a rudimentary alliance that can occur with some patients. There seems to be a small number of patients who have severe pathology and longstanding patterns of self-harm and frequent suicidal and parasuicidal crisis who are difficult, if not impossible, to engage in treatment. With such patients, the repetitive crises and involvement with a range of agencies make it difficult to provide the stability and continuity required to break these cycles. This is a Catch-22 situation, in which a stable treatment context is required to disrupt repetitive self-harm, but the frequency of this behavior and the severity of psychopathology prevent the establishment of a stable treatment process.

Fortunately such patients are few. In most cases, treatment can make a substantial difference to symptoms, problems, quality of life, and feelings of self-worth. More importantly, it can also help patients give freer expression of their true selves.

APPENDIX

Self-State Description

INSTRUCTIONS

Most people's ideas and feelings about themselves change from time to time. For some people, these changes are very pronounced; the way that they experience themselves is very different from one occasion to the next. These different ways of experiencing the self are called *self-states*. Each self-state consists of a characteristic set of ideas, feelings, and behaviors. These states are not the same as fleeting thoughts or feelings. Instead, they are different ways of experiencing the self that last for a period of time. Sometimes a self-state may last for days, and at other times it may persist for a much shorter period. Changes from one state to another can also be very sudden—so sudden, in fact, that we may feel confused. On other occasions changes in self-states can be very gradual, as one state slowly gives way to another.

Often the most obvious feature of a self-state consists of the feelings that we experience when in that state. Each self-state involves different feelings and a particular mood. But self-states are more than just moods. They also involve different ways of thinking about and describing the self. These different ways of thinking and feeling about ourselves affect the way we behave, especially the way we behave toward other people. Each self-state usually includes a particular way of interacting with other people. This is why other people are often more aware of changes in our self-states than we are ourselves. Sometimes we behave very differently, depending on the self-state that we are experiencing.

You may find that the idea of a self-state will help you understand the different feelings that you have, and why your feelings can change so much. It may also help you understand why you sometimes behave very differently on different occasions. For these reasons it is helpful for you to identify and describe your different self-states. This means describing the different ideas and thoughts that you have during each state, the feelings that are characteristic of each state, and the typical things that you do in each state. It also means describing the way in which other people behave toward you in each state. You may have noticed that people treat you differently, according to the state you are experiencing at the time.

At first, it may be a little difficult to identify your different states. After a while, you will find it a little easier. To help you identify your self-states, a number of different self-states are listed below. Some of these may apply to you, while others will not. Circle the states below that describe you. Change the descriptions, as needed, by adding or deleting words, so that each state accurately describes the way that you think and feel about yourself. Please use the space below the list for adding self-states that are not listed. When you list your self-states, remember to list states only—that is, experiences that last for a period of time, rather than fleeting feelings or thoughts. During treatment you may want to refer to this list and add further self-states that you have begun to recognize.

Out of control.
Frozen, paralyzed, shut down, blank.
Very special, different from everyone else, brilliant.
Filled with rage.
Terrified, frightened.
Loser, a mess.
Jealous.
Filled with envy—everyone else has things except me.
Angry and resentful, hostile, hate everyone.
Extremely critical of myself, hate myself, contemptuous of myself.
Hurt and humiliated.
Abandoned and rejected by others.
Sulky and resentful; hurt, but won't let anyone know about it.
Safe and secure.
Very protective of myself.
Want to protect everyone.
Frantic and very busy.
Driven to do things.
Give in to everyone, submissive, neglect myself.
Stressed out and unable to cope.
Neglected and ignored.

All powerful, able to do anything.
In charge of things and in control of my life.
Desperately clingy, need to be looked after and taken care of.
Very critical of everyone.
Confused, perplexed, don't know what I think or feel.
Want to hurt myself.
Violent, want to hurt someone.
Vulnerable, easily hurt.
Contemptuous of everyone.
Feel that everyone and everything is against me.
Suspicious, do not trust people, on guard.
Capable, smart, able to do things.
Hate myself.
On top of the world, great.
Not noticeable, invisible, not noticed by anyone.
Dissatisfied, discontented, nothing is going right, whining.
Want to escape, run away, start again, want to get away.
Flirty, seductive, provocative.
Normal.

Now that you have listed the self-states that are important to you, read over the list again to make sure that the words you have used to describe each state really fit your experience. Do not be afraid to change the words or add new items. The above list is provided only to help you to identify your own self-states. When you are satisfied that you have identified the different states that you experience, identify the self-state that you think is the most important for understanding your problems and the one that you would like to change the most. Rank this state number 1, using the space at the end of the description. Then do the same for the second most important, and so on. If two or more states are equally important, give them the same number.

The next pages should be used to describe each state in detail. This information will help you and your therapist understand what triggers each state, the thoughts and feelings that characterize each state, and the way in which you behave in each state.

NAME OR BRIEF DESCRIPTION OF THE STATE

Description of the State

Provide a detailed description of yourself when you are in this state. What sort of person are you? What words do you use to describe yourself? What sorts of things do you say to yourself in this state? What are your major thoughts and concerns?

Feelings

What feelings do you have when you are in this state? How do you feel about yourself?

Behavior

What do you do when you are in this state? How do you tend to react? How do you behave toward other people?

Things That Trigger the State

What kinds of things cause you to get into this state? Often the trigger is a chain of events, thoughts, and feelings. Try to identify the things that seem important.

My Judgments of Other People When I Am in This State

How does this state affect the way that you see other people? Does it affect your impressions of others? What judgments do you make about other people?

Other People's Reactions

How do other people tend to treat you in this state? Does it affect the way that they behave toward you?

References

Abraham, K. (1921). Contributions to the theory of anal character. In *Selected papers on psychoanalysis*. London: Hogarth Press.

Abraham, K. (1925). Character-formation on the genital level of the libido. In *Selected papers on psychoanalysis*. London: Hogarth Press.

Adler G., & Buie, D. (1979a). Aloneness and borderline pathology: The possible relevance of child development issues. *International Journal of Psycho-Analysis, 60,* 83–96.

Adler, G., & Buie, D. (1979b). The psychotherapeutic approach to aloneness in borderline patients. In J. LeBiot (Ed.), *Advances in psychotherapy of the borderline patient* (pp. 433–448). New York: Jason Aronson.

Akhtar, S. (1992). *Hidden structures: Severe personality disorders and their treatment.* Northvale, NJ: Jason Aronson.

Akiskal, H. S. (1991). Cyclothymic, hyperthymic, and depressive temperaments as subaffective variants of mood disorders. In A. Tasman & M. B. Riba (Eds.), *Review of psychiatry* (Vol. 11, pp. 43–62). Washington, DC: American Psychiatric Press.

Akiskal, H. S. (1994). The temperamental borders of affective disorders. *Acta Psychiatrica Scandinavica, 89*(Suppl. 379), 32–37.

Akiskal, H. S. (1995). Toward a temperament-based approach to depression: Implications for neurobiologic research. In G. L. Gessa, W. Fratta, L. Panni, & G. Serra (Eds.), *Depression and mania: From neurobiology to treatment. Advances in biochemical psychopharmacology* (Vol. 49, pp. 99–112). New York: Raven Press.

Akiskal, H. S., Chen, S. E., Davis, G. C., Puzantian, V. R., Kashgarian, M., & Bolinger, J. M. (1985). Borderline: An adjective in search of a noun. *Journal of Clinical Psychiatry, 46,* 41–48.

Alexander, F., & French, T. (1946). *Psychoanalytic therapy: Principles and application.* New York: Ronald Press.

Allen, J. G., Newsom, G. E., Gabbard, G. O., & Coyne, L. (1984). Scales to assess the therapeutic alliance from a psychoanalytic perspective. *Bulletin of the Menninger Clinic, 48,* 383–400.

Allen, J. G., Tarnoff, G., & Coyne, L. (1985). Therapeutic alliance and long-term hospital treatment outcome. *Comprehensive Psychiatry, 38,* 871–875.

Allport, G. W. (1937). *Personality: A psychological interpretation.* New York: Holt, Rinehart & Winston.

Allport, G. W. (1961). *Pattern and growth in personality.* New York: Holt, Rinehart & Winston.

Alnaes, R., & Torgersen, S. (1988). The relationship between DSM-III symptom disorders (Axis I) and personality disorders (Axis II) in an outpatient population. *Acta Psychiatrica Scandinavica, 78,* 485–492.

American Psychiatric Association. (1994). *Diagnostic and statistical manual of mental disorders* (4th ed.). Washington, DC: Author.

American Psychiatric Association. (2001). Practice guidelines for the treatment of patients with borderline personality disorder. *American Journal of Psychiatry,* 158(Oct. Suppl.).

Andrews, J. D. (1984). Psychotherapy with the hysterical personality: An interpersonal approach. *Psychiatry, 47,* 211–232.

Andrews, J. D. (1990). Interpersonal self-confirmation and challenge in psychotherapy. *Psychotherapy, 27,* 485–504.

Andrews, J. D. (1993). The active self model: A paradigm for psychotherapy integration. In G. Stricker & J. R. Gold (Eds.), *Comprehensive handbook of psychotherapy integration* (pp. 165–183). New York: Plenum Press.

Andrulonis, P. A., Glueck, B. C., Stroebel, S. F., Vogel, N. G., Shapiro, A. L., & Aldridge, D. M. (1981). Organic brain dysfunction and the borderline syndrome. *Psychiatric Clinics of North America, 4,* 47–66.

Argyle, M., Tower, P., & Bryant, B. (1974). Explorations in the treatment of personality disorders and neuroses by social skills training. *British Journal of Medical Psychology, 47,* 63–72.

Aronson, T. A. (1989). A critical review of treatments for borderline personality disorder: Historic trends and future directions. *Journal of Nervous and Mental Disease, 177,* 511–527.

Austin, E. J., & Deary, I. J. (2000). The "four A's": A common framework for normal and abnormal personality? *Personality and Individual Differences, 28,* 977–995.

Azim, H. F., Piper, W. E., Segal, P. M., Nixon, G. W., & Duncan, S. C. (1991). The Quality of Object Relations Scale. *Bulletin of the Menninger Clinic, 55,* 323–343.

Bagge, C. L., & Trull, T. J. (in press). DAPP-BQ: Factor structure and relations for personality disorder symptoms in a nonclinical sample. *Journal of Personality Disorders, 17.*

Bandura, A. (1977). Self-efficacy: Toward a unifying theory of behavioral change. *Psychological Review, 84,* 139–157.

Bandura, A. (1982). Self-efficacy mechanism in human agency. *American Psychologist, 37,* 122–147.

Bandura, A. (1999). Social cognitive theory of personality. In D. Cervone & Y. Shoda (Eds.), *The coherence of personality: Social–cognitive bases of consistency, variability, and organization* (pp. 185–241). New York: Guilford Press.

Barnett, J. (1980). Self and character. *Journal of the American Academy of Psychoanalysis, 8,* 337–352.

Bartholomew, K., Kwong, M. J., & Hart, S. D. (2001). Attachment. In W. J. Livesley (Ed.), *Handbook of personality disorders: Theory, research, and treatment* (pp. 196–230). New York: Guilford Press.

Bartlett, F. C. (1995). *Remembering: A study in experimental and social psychology.* New York: Cambridge University Press. (Original work published 1932)

Basŏglu, M., & Mineka, S. (1992). The role of uncontrollability and unpredictability of stress in the development of post-torture stress symptoms. In M. Basŏglu (Ed.), *Torture and its consequences: Current treatment approaches* (pp. 182–225). Cambridge, UK: Cambridge University Press.

Bateman, A., & Fonagy, P. (1999). Effectiveness of partial hospitalization in the treatment of borderline personality disorder: A randomized controlled trial. *American Journal of Psychiatry, 156*, 1563–1569.

Bateman, A., & Fonagy, P. (2001). Treatment of borderline personality disorder with psychoanalytically oriented partial hospitalization: An 18-month follow-up. *American Journal of Psychiatry, 158*, 36–42.

Bateman, A., & Fonagy, P. (2003). Health service utilization costs for borderline personality disorder patients treated with psychoanalytically oriented partial hospitalization versus general psychiatric care. *American Journal of Psychiatry, 160*, 169–171.

Baum, S. (1997). Living on shifting sands: Grounding and borderline personality organization. *Journal of Contemporary Psychotherapy, 27*, 61–86.

Baumeister, R. F. (1989). The problem of life's meanings. In D. M. Buss & N. Cantor (Eds.), *Personality psychology: Recent trends and emerging directions* (pp. 138–148). New York: Springer-Verlag.

Baumeister, R. F. (1991). *Meanings of life.* New York: Guilford Press.

Baumeister, R. F. (1994). The crystallization of discontent in the process of major life change. In T. F. Heatherton & J. L. Weinberger (Eds.), *Can personality change?* (pp. 281–297). Washington, DC: American Psychological Association.

Beck, A. T., & Emory, G., with Greenberg, R. L. (1985). *Anxiety disorders and phobias: A cognitive perspective.* New York: Basic Books.

Beck, A. T., Freeman, A., & Associates. (1990). *Cognitive therapy of personality disorders.* New York: Guilford Press.

Beck, J. S. (1995). *Cognitive therapy: Basics and beyond.* New York: Guilford Press.

Bellack, L. (1980). On some limitations of dyadic psychotherapy and the role of group modalities. *International Journal of Group Psychotherapy, 30*, 7–21.

Benjamin, L. S. (1988). *Short form of the INTREX users' manual.* Madison, WI: INTREX Interpersonal Institute.

Benjamin, L. S. (1993). *Interpersonal diagnosis and treatment of personality disorders.* New York: Guilford Press.

Benjamin, L. S. (1996). *Interpersonal diagnosis and treatment of personality disorders* (2nd ed.). New York: Guilford Press.

Benjamin, L. S., & Pugh, C. (2001). Using interpersonal theory to select effective treatment interventions. In W. J. Livesley (Ed.), *Handbook of personality disorders: Theory, research, and treatment* (pp. 414–436). New York: Guilford Press.

Berkelowitz, M., & Tarnopolsky, A. (1993). The validity of borderline personality disorder: An updated review of recent research. In P. Tyrer & G. Stein (Eds.), *Personality disorder reviewed* (pp. 90–112). London: Gaskell.

Bernstein, D. P., & Fink, L. (1998). *Childhood trauma questionnaire: A retrospective self-report.* San Antonio, TX: Harcourt Brace.

Bernstein, D. P., Stein, J., & Handelsman, L. (1998). Predicting personality pathology among adult patients with substance use disorders: Effects of childhood maltreatment. *Addictive Behavior: An International Journal, 23*, 855–868.

Bernstein, E. M., & Putnam, F. W. (1986). Development, reliability, and validity of a dissociation scale. *Journal of Nervous and Mental Disease, 174*, 727–734.

Beutler, L. E. (1991). Have all won and must all have prizes? Revisiting Luborsky et al's verdict. *Journal of Consulting and Clinical Psychology, 59*, 226–232.

Beutler, L. E., & Clarkin, J. F. (1990). *Systematic treatment selection: Toward targeted therapeutic interventions.* New York: Brunner/Mazel.

Beutler, L. E., & Davison, E. H. (1995). What standard should we use? In S. C. Hayes, V. M. Follette, R. M. Dawes, & K. E. Grady (Eds.), *Scientific standards of psychological practice* (pp. 11–24). Reno, NV: Context Press.

Beutler, L. E., & Harwood, T. M. (2000). *Prescriptive psychotherapy.* Oxford: Oxford University Press.

Blake, D. B., & Sonnenberg, R. T. (1998). Outcome research on behavioral and cognitive-behavioral treatments for trauma survivors. In V. M. Follette, J. I. Ruzek, & F. R. Abueg (Eds.), *Cognitive-behavioral therapies for trauma* (pp. 15–47). New York: Guilford Press.

Blanck, G., & Blanck, R. (1974). *Egopsychology in theory and practice.* New York: Columbia Press.

Blashfield, R. K., & Herkov, M. J. (1996). Investigating clinical adherence to diagnosis by criteria: A replication of Morey and Ochoa (1989). *Journal of Personality Disorders, 10*, 219–228.

Blatt, S. J., Ford, R. Q., Berman, W. H., Cook, B., Cramer, P., & Robins, C. E. (Eds.). (1994). *Therapeutic change: An object relationship perspective.* New York: Plenum Press.

Bongar, B. M. (1991). *The suicidal patient: Clinical and legal standards of care.* Washington, DC: American Psychological Association.

Borden, E. S. (1979). The generalizability of the psychoanalytic concept of the working alliance. *Psychotherapy Theory, Research and Practice, 16*, 252–260.

Borden, E. S. (1994). Theory and research in the therapeutic working alliance: New directions. In A. Horvath & L. S. Greenberg (Eds.), *The working alliance* (pp. 13–37). New York: Wiley.

Bowlby, J. (1971). *Attachment and loss: Vol. 1.* Harmondsworth, UK: Penguin Books.

Bowlby, J. (1973). The making and breaking of affectional bonds. *British Journal of Psychiatry, 130*, 201–210.

Bowlby, J. (1980). *Attachment and loss: Vol. 3. Loss: Sadness and depression.* London: Hogarth Press.

Bradley, S. J. (1979). The relationship of early maternal separation to borderline personality disorder in children and adolescents. *American Journal of Psychiatry, 136*, 424–426.

Bradley, S. J. (2000). *Affect regulation and the development of psychopathology.* New York: Guilford Press.

Bricker, D., Young, J. E., & Flanagan, C. (1993). Schema-focused cognitive therapy: A comprehensive framework for characterological problems. In K. Kuehlwein & H. Rosen (Eds.), *Cognitive therapies in action: Evolving innovative practice* (pp. 88–125). San Francisco: Jossey-Bass.

Brière, J., & Runtz, M. (1986). Suicidal thoughts and behaviors in former sexual abuse victims. *Canadian Journal of Behavioural Science, 20*, 413–423.

Brière, J., & Ziadi, L. Y. (1989). Suicidal thoughts and behaviors in female psychiatric emergency room patients. *American Journal of Psychiatry, 146*, 1602–1606.

Brody, N. (1994). .5 + or −.5: Continuity and change in personal dispositions. In T. F. Heatherton & J. L. Weinberger (Eds.), *Can personality change?* Washington, DC: American Psychological Association.

Bromley, D. B. (1977). *Personality description in ordinary language.* London: Wiley.

Brown, T. A., & Barlow, D. H. (1992). Comorbidity among anxiety disorders: Implications for treatment and DSM-IV. *Journal of Consulting and Clinical Psychology, 60,* 835–844.

Browne, A., & Finkelhor, D. (1986). Impact of child abuse: A review of the literature. *Psychological Bulletin, 99,* 66–77.

Bruner, J. (1990). *Acts of meaning.* Cambridge, MA: Harvard University Press.

Budman, S. H., Demby, A., Soldz, S., & Merry, J. (1996). Time-limited group psychotherapy for patients with personality disorders: Outcomes and dropouts. *International Journal of Group Psychotherapy, 46,* 357–377.

Bugenthal, J. F. T., & Kleiner, R. (1993). Existential psychotherapies. In G. Stricker & J. R. Gold (Eds.), *Comprehensive handbook of psychotherapy integration* (pp. 101–112). New York: Plenum Press.

Buie, D. H., & Adler, G. (1982). The definitive treatment of the borderline personality. *International Journal of Psychoanalytic Psychotherapy, 9,* 51–87.

Buss, A. H., & Plomin, R. (1975). *A temperament theory of personality development.* New York: Wiley.

Byrne, C. P., Cernovsky, A., Velamoor, V. R., Coretese, L., & Losztyn, S. (1990). A comparison of borderline and schizophrenic patients for childhood life events and parent–child relationships. *Canadian Journal of Psychiatry, 35,* 590–595.

Cadoret, R. J. (1978). Psychopathology in adopted-away offspring of biologic parents with antisocial behavior. *Archives of General Psychiatry, 35,* 176–184.

Cantor, N. (1990). From thought to behavior: "Having" and "doing" in the study of personality and cognition. *American Psychologist, 45,* 735–750.

Carver, C. S., & Scheier, M. F. (1998). *On the self-regulation of behavior.* Cambridge, UK: Cambridge University Press.

Caspi, A., & Bem, D. J. (1990). Personality continuity and change across the life course. In L. A. Pervin (Ed.), *Handbook of personality: Theory and research* (pp. 549–575). New York: Guilford Press.

Caspi, A., Bem, D. J., & Elder, G. H. (1989). Continuities and consequences of interactional styles across the life course. Special issue: Long-term stability and change in personality. *Journal of Personality, 57,* 375–406.

Caspi, A., & Herbener, E. S. (1990). Continuity and change: Assortative marriage and the consistency of personality in adulthood. *Journal of Personality and Social Psychology, 58,* 250–258.

Cervone, D., & Shoda, Y. (1999). Social–cognitive theories and coherence of personality. In D. Cervone & Y. Shoda (Eds.), *The coherence of personality: Social–cognitive bases of consistency, variability, and organization* (pp. 3–33). New York: Guilford Press.

Charney, D. S., Nelson, J. C., & Quinlan, D. M. (1981). Personality traits and disorders in depression. *American Journal of Psychiatry, 138,* 1601–1604.

Chessick, R. (1977). *Intensive psychotherapy of the borderline patient.* New York: Jason Aronson.

Chessick, R. (1979). A practical approach to the psychotherapy of the borderline patient. *American Journal of Psychotherapy, 33,* 531–566.

Chessick, R. (1982). Current issues in intensive psychotherapy. *American Journal of Psychotherapy, 36,* 438–449.

Chopra, H. D., & Beatson, J. A. (1986). Psychotic symptoms in borderline personality disorder. *American Journal of Psychiatry, 143,* 1605–1607.

Clark, L. A. (1993). *Manual for the Schedule for Non-adaptive and Adaptive Personality (SNAP).* Minneapolis: University of Minnesota Press.

Clark, L. A., Livesley, W. J., Schroeder, M. L., & Irish, S. L. (1996). Convergence of two systems for assessing specific traits of personality disorder. *Psychological Assessment, 8,* 294–303.

Clark, L. A., Vittengl, J. R., Kraft, D., & Jerrett, R. (in press). To predict depression treatment outcome from personality scores separate trait from state variance. *Journal of Personality Disorders.*

Clarkin, J. F., Hull, J. W., Cantor, J., & Sanderson, C. (1993). Borderline personality disorder and personality traits: A comparison of SCID-II BPD and NEO-PI. *Psychological Assessment, 5,* 472–476.

Clarkin, J. F., Marziali, E., & Munroe-Blum, H. (1991). Group and family treatments for borderline personality disorder. *Hospital and Community Psychiatry, 42,* 1038–1043.

Clarkin, J. F., Widiger, T. A., Frances, A., Hurt, S. W., & Gilmore, M. (1983). Prototypic typology and the borderline personality disorder. *Journal of Abnormal Psychology, 92,* 263–275.

Clarkin, J. F., Yeomans, F. E., & Kernberg, O. (1999). *Psychotherapy for borderline personality disorder.* New York: Wiley.

Cleckley, H. (1976). *The mask of insanity* (5th ed.). St. Louis, MO: Mosby.

Cloninger, C. R. (1987). A systematic method for clinical description and classification of personality variants. *Archives of General Psychiatry, 44,* 573–588.

Cloninger, C. R. (2000). A practical way to diagnose personality disorder: A proposal. *Journal of Personality Disorders, 14,* 99–108.

Cloninger, C. R., Sigvardsson, S., Bohman, M., & van Knorring, A. L. (1982). Predisposition to petty criminality in Swedish adoptees, II: Cross-fostering analysis of gene–environment interaction. *Archives of General Psychiatry, 39,* 1242–1253.

Cloninger, C. R., Svrakic, D. M., & Przybeck, T. R. (1993). A psychobiological model of temperament and character. *Archives of General Psychiatry, 50,* 975–990.

Coccaro, E. F. (2001). Biological and treatment correlates. In W. J. Livesley (Ed.), *Handbook of personality disorders: Theory, research, and treatment* (pp. 124–135). New York: Guilford Press.

Coccaro, E. F., Kavoussi, R. J., & Hauger, R. L. (1995). Physiological responses to d-fenfluramine and ipsapirone challenge: Correlates with indices of aggression in males with personality disorder. *International Clinical Psychopharmacology, 10,* 177–179.

Coccaro, E. F., & Kavoussi, R. J. (1997). Fluoxetine and impulsive aggressive behavior in personality disordered subjects. *Archives of General Psychiatry, 54,* 1081–1088.

Coccaro, E. F., Siever, L. J., Klar, H. M., Maurer, G., Cochrane, K., Cooper, T. B., Mohs, R. C., & Davis, K. L. (1989). Serotonergic studies in patients with affective and personality disorder: Correlates with suicidal and impulsive aggressive behavior. *Archives of General Psychiatry, 46,* 587–599.

Conley, J. J. (1984a). The hierarchy of consistency: A review and model of longitudinal findings on adult individual differences in intelligence, personality, and self-opinion. *Personality and Individual Differences*, 5, 11–26.

Conley, J. J. (1984b). Longitudinal consistency of adult personality: Self-reported psychological characteristics across 45 years. *Journal of Personality and Social Psychology*, 47, 1325–1333.

Conley, J. J. (1984c). Relation of temporal stability and cross-situational consistency in personality: Comment on the Mischel–Epstein debate. *Psychological Review*, 91, 491–496.

Conley, J. J. (1985). Longitudinal stability of personality traits: A multitrait–multimethod–multioccasion analysis. *Journal of Personality and Social Psychology*, 49, 1266–1282.

Connolly, M. B., Crits-Christoph, P., Shappell, S., Barber, J. P., Luborsky, L., & Shaffer, C. (1999). Relation of transference interpretations to outcome in the early session of brief supportive-expressive psychotherapy. *Psychotherapy Research*, 9, 485–495.

Cornelius, J. R., Soloff, P. H., Perel, J. M., & Ulrich, R. F. (1990). Fluoxetine trial in borderline personality disorder. *Psychopharmacological Bulletin*, 26, 151–154.

Cornelius, J. R., Soloff, P. H., Perel, J. M., & Ulrich, R. F. (1993). Continuation pharmacotherapy of borderline personality disorder with haloperidol and phenelzine. *American Journal of Psychiatry*, 150, 1843–1848.

Costa, P. T., & McCrae, R. R. (1980). Influence of extraversion and neuroticism on subjective well-being: Happy and unhappy people. *Journal of Personality and Social Psychology*, 38, 668–678.

Costa, P. T., & McCrae, R. R. (1990). Personality disorders and the five-factor model of personality. *Journal of Personality Disorders*, 4, 362–371.

Costa, P. T., & McCrae, R. R. (1992). *Revised NEO Personality Inventory (NEO-PI-R) and the NEO Five-Factor Inventory (NEO-FFI) professional manual*. Odessa, FL: Psychological Assessment Resources.

Costa, P. T., & McCrae, R. R. (1994). Can personality change? In T. F. Heatherton & J. L. Weinberger (Eds.), *Can personality change?* (pp. 21–40). Washington, DC: American Psychological Association.

Costa, P. T., & Widiger, T. A. (Eds.). (1994). *Personality disorders and the five-factor model of personality*. Washington, DC: American Psychological Association Books.

Costa, P. T., & Widiger, T. A. (Eds.). (2002). *Personality disorders and the five-factor model of personality* (2nd ed.). Washington, DC: American Psychological Association Books.

Cottraux, J., & Blackburn, I. M. (2001). Cognitive therapy. In W. J. Livesley (Ed.), *Handbook of personality disorders: Theory, research, and treatment* (pp. 377–399). New York: Guilford Press.

Cowdry, R. W., & Gardner, D. L. (1988). Pharmacotherapy of borderline personality disorder: Alprazolam, carbamazapine, trifluoperazine, and tranylcypromine. *Archives of General Psychiatry*, 45, 111–119.

Cowdry, R. W., Pickar, D., & Davis, R. (1985). Symptoms and EEG findings in the borderline syndrome. *International Journal of Psychiatry in Medicine*, 15, 201–211.

Dahl, A. A. (1986). Some aspects of the DSM-III personality disorders illustrated by a consecutive sample of hospitalized patients. *Acta Psychiatrica Scandinavica Supplement*, 328, 61–67.

Dahl, A. A. (1994). Heredity in personality disorders: An overview. *Clinical Genetics*, 46, 138–143.

David, J. D., & Pilkonis, P. A. (1996). The stability of personality disorder diagnoses. *Journal of Personality Disorders*, 10, 1–15.

Davidson, K. M., & Tyrer, P. (1996). Cognitive therapy for antisocial and borderline personality disorders: Single case study series. *British Journal of Clinical Psychology*, 35, 413–429.

Dawson, D. F. (1988). Treatment of the borderline patient: Relationship management. *Canadian Journal of Psychiatry*, 33, 370–374.

Dawson, D. F., & MacMillan, H. L. (1993). *Relationship management of the borderline patient*. New York: Brunner/Mazel.

DeCharms, R. (1968). *Personal causation: The internal affective determinants of behavior*. New York: Academic Press.

Deutsch, H. (1942). Some forms of emotional disturbance and their relationship to schizophrenia. *Psychoanalytic Quarterly*, 11, 301–321.

Dick, P., Cameron, L., Cohen, D., Barlow, M., & Ince, A. (1985). Day and full time psychiatric treatment: A controlled comparison. *British Journal of Psychiatry*, 147, 246–250.

DiClemente, C. C. (1994). If behaviors change, can personality be far behind? In T. F. Heatherton & J. L. Weinberger (Eds.), *Can personality change?* (pp. 175–198). Washington, DC: American Psychological Association.

Dodge, K. A., Pettit, G. S., Bates, J. E., & Valente, E. (1995). Social information-processing patterns partially mediate the effect of early physical abuse on later conduct problems. *Journal of Abnormal Psychology*, 104, 632–643.

Dolan-Sewell, R. T., Krueger, R. F., & Shea, M. T. (2001). Co-occurrence with syndrome disorders. In W. J. Livesley (Ed.), *Handbook of personality disorders: Theory, research, and treatment* (pp. 84–104). New York: Guilford Press.

Downs, N. S., Swerdlow, N. R., & Zisook, S. (1992). The relationship of affective illness and personality disorders in psychiatric outpatients. *Annals of Clinical Psychiatry*, 4, 87–94.

Drake, R. E., & Vaillant, G. E. (1985). A validity study of Axis II of DSM-III. *American Journal of Psychiatry*, 142, 553–558.

Dulit, R. A., Fyer, M. R., Leon, A. C., Brodsky, B. S., & Frances, A. J. (1994). Clinical correlates of self-mutilation in borderline personality disorder. *American Journal of Psychiatry*, 151, 1305–1311.

Dweck, C. S. (1996). Implicit theories as organizers of goals and behavior. In P. M. Gollwitzer & J. A. Bargh (Eds.), *The psychology of action: Linking cognition and motivation to behavior* (pp. 69–90). New York: Guilford Press.

Eells, T. D. (1997). Psychotherapy case formulation: History and current status. In T. D. Eells (Ed.), *Handbook of psychotherapy case formulation* (pp. 1–15). New York: Guilford Press.

Ekselius, L., Lindstrom, E., von Knorring, L., Bodlund, O., & Kullgren, G. (1994). A principal component analysis of the DSM-III-R Axis II personality disorders. *Journal of Personality Disorders*, 8, 140–148.

Emde, R. N. (1989). The infant's relationship to experience: Developmental and affective aspects. In A. J. Sameroff & R. N. Emde (Eds.), *Relationship disturbances in early childhood: A developmental approach* (pp. 35–51). New York: Basic Books.

Epstein, S. (1973). The self-concept revisited, or a theory of a theory. *American Psychologist, 28,* 404–416.

Epstein, S. (1990). Cognitive–experiential self-theory. In L. A. Pervin (Ed.), *Handbook of personality: Theory and research* (pp. 165–192). New York: Guilford Press.

Erikson, E. H. (1950). *Childhood and society.* New York: Norton.

Evans, K., Tyrer, P., Catalan, J., Schmidt, U., Davidson, K., Tata, P., Thornton, S., Barber, J., & Thompson, S. (1999). Manual assisted cognitive-behavioral therapy (MACT): A randomized controlled trial of a brief intervention with bibliotherapy in the treatment of recurrent deliberate self-harm. *Psychological Medicine, 29,* 19–25.

Eysenck, H. J. (1987). The definition of personality disorders and the criteria appropriate to their definition. *Journal of Personality Disorders, 1,* 211–219.

Ezriel, H. (1952). Notes on psychoanalytic group therapy: II. Interpretation. *Research Psychiatry, 15,* 119.

Fabrega, H., Jr., Pilkonis, P., Mezzich, J., Ahn, C. W., & Shea, S. (1990). Explaining diagnostic complexity in an intake setting. *Comprehensive Psychiatry, 31*(1), 5–14.

Fairbairn, W. R. D. (1952). *Psychoanalytic studies of the personality.* London: Tavistock.

Feeny, N. C., Zoeller, L. A., & Foa, E. B. (2002). Treatment outcome for chronic PTSD among female assault victims with borderline personality characteristics: A preliminary examination. *Journal of Personality Disorders, 16*(1), 30–40.

Feiner, A. H. (2000). *Interpersonal psychoanalytic perspectives on relevance, dismissal and self-definition.* London: Jessica Young.

Finkelhor, D., Hotaling, G., Lewis, I. A., & Smith, C. (1990). Sexual abuse in a national survey of adult men and women: Prevalence characteristics and risk factors. *Child Abuse and Neglect, 14,* 19–28.

Fishman, S. T., & Lubetkin, B. S. (1983). Office practice of behavioral therapy. In M. Hersen (Ed.), *Outpatient behavioral therapy* (pp. 21–41). New York: Grune & Stratton.

Foa, E. B., & Jaycox, L. H. (1999). Cognitive-behavioral treatment of posttraumatic stress disorder. In D. Spiegel (Ed.), *Psychotherapeutic frontiers: New principles and practices* (pp. 23–61). Washington, DC: American Psychiatric Association Press.

Foa, E. B., & Rothbaum, B. O. (1998). *Treating the trauma of rape: Cognitive-behavioral therapy for PTSD.* New York: Guilford Press.

Foa, E. B., Steketee, G., & Rothbaum, B. O. (1989). Behavioral/cognitive conceptualization of post-traumatic stress disorder. *Behavior Therapy, 20,* 155–176.

Follette, V. M., Ruzek, J. I., & Abueg, F. R. (1998). A contextual analysis of trauma: Assessment and treatment. In V. M. Follette, J. I. Ruzek, & F. R. Abueg (Eds.), *Cognitive-behavioral therapies for trauma* (pp. 3–14). New York: Guilford Press.

Foreman, S. A., & Marmar, C. R. (1985). Therapist actions that address initially poor therapeutic alliances in psychotherapy. *American Journal of Psychiatry, 142,* 922–926.

Fossati, A., Madeddu, F., & Maffei, C. (1999). Borderline personality disorder and childhood sexual abuse: A meta-analytic study. *Journal of Personality Disorders, 13*(3), 268–80.

Frances, A. J. (1992). Foreword. In L. H. Rockland, *Supportive therapy for borderline patients: A psychodynamic approach* (pp. vii–viii). New York: Guilford Press.

Frances, A. J., Clarkin, J. F., Gilmore, M., Hurt, S. W., & Brown, R. (1984). Reliability of criteria for borderline personality disorder: A comparison of DSM-III and the Diagnostic Interview for Borderline Patients. *American Journal of Psychiatry, 141,* 1080–1084.

Frances, A. J., Clarkin, J. F., & Perry, S. (1984). *Differential therapeutic in psychiatry: The art and science of treatment selection.* New York: Brunner/Mazel.

Frank, A. F. (1992). The therapeutic alliances of borderline patients. In J. F. Clarkin, E. Marziali, & H. Munroe-Blum (Eds.), *Borderline personality disorder: Clinical and empirical perspectives* (pp. 220–247). New York: Guilford Press.

Frank, H., & Paris J. (1981). Family experience in borderline patients. *Archives of General Psychiatry, 38,* 1031–1034.

Freud, S. (1962). *Civilization and its discontents* (J. Strachey, Ed. & Trans.). New York: Norton. (Originally published 1908)

Friedman, R. C., Aronoff, M. S., Clarkin, J. F., Corn, R., & Hurt, S. W. (1983). History of suicidal behavior in depressed borderline inpatients. *American Journal of Psychiatry, 140,* 1023–1026.

Fyer, M. R., Frances, A. J., Sullivan, T., Hurt, S. W., & Clarkin, J. F. (1988). Suicide attempts in patients with borderline personality disorder. *American Journal of Psychiatry, 145,* 737–739.

Gabbard, G. O. (1998). Treatment resistant borderline personality disorder. *Psychiatric Annals, 28,* 651–656.

Gabbard, G. O. (2000). Psychoanalysis. In B. J. Sadock & V. A. Sadock (Eds.), *Comprehensive textbook of psychiatry* (Vol. 1, 7th ed., pp. 431–478). Baltimore: Lippincott Williams and Wilkins.

Gabbard, G. O. (2001). Psychoanalysis and psychoanalytic therapy. In W. J. Livesley (Ed.), *Handbook of personality disorders: Theory, research, and treatment* (pp. 359–376). New York: Guilford Press.

Gabbard, G. O., Horwitz, L., Allen, J. G., Frieswyk, S., Newsom, G., Colson, D. B., & Coyne, L. (1994). Transference interpretation in the psychotherapy of borderline patients: A high-risk, high-gain phenomenon. *Harvard Review of Psychiatry, 2,* 59–69.

Gabbard, G. O., Horwitz, L., Frieswyk, S., Allen, J. G., Colson, D. B., Newsom, G., & Coyne, L. (1988). The effect of therapist interventions on the therapeutic alliance with borderline patients. *Journal of the American Psychoanalytic Association, 36,* 697–727.

Gable, S., & Isabella, R. A. (1992). Maternal contributions to infant regulation of arousal. *Infant Behavior and Development, 15,* 95–107.

Gardner, A. R., & Gardner, A. J. (1975). Self-mutilation, obsessionality, and narcissism. *British Journal of Psychiatry, 127,* 127–132.

Gardner, D. L., & Cowdry, R. W. (1985). Alprazolam induced dyscontrol in borderline personality disorder. *American Journal of Psychiatry, 142,* 98–100.

Gaston, L. (1990). The concept of the alliance and its role in psychotherapy: Theoretical and empirical considerations. *Psychotherapy, 27,* 143–153.

George, A., & Soloff, P. (1986). Schizotypal symptoms in patients with borderline personality disorders. *American Journal of Psychiatry, 143,* 212–215.

Giovacchini, P. (1979). *Treatment of primitive mental states.* New York: Jason Aronson.

Gold, J. R. (1990a). Culture, history, and psychotherapy integration. *Journal of Integrative and Eclectic Psychotherapy, 9,* 41–48.

Gold, J. R. (1990b). The integration of psychoanalytic, interpersonal, and cognitive approaches in the psychotherapy of borderline and narcissistic disorders. *Journal of Integrative and Eclectic Psychotherapy*, 9, 49–68.

Gold, J. R. (1996). *Key concepts in psychotherapy integration*. New York: Plenum Press.

Goldberg, L. R. (1990). An alternative "description of personality": The Big-Five factor structure. *Journal of Personality and Social Psychology*, 59, 1216–1229.

Goldberg, L. R. (1993). The structure of phenotypic personality traits. *American Psychologist*, 48, 26–34.

Goldberg, S. C., Schulz, S. C., Schultz, P. M., Resnick, R. J., Hamer, R. M., & Friedel, R. O. (1986). Borderline and schizotypal personality disorders treated with low-dose thiothixene vs. placebo. *Archives of General Psychiatry*, 43, 680–686.

Goldfried, M. R. (1980). Toward the delineation of therapeutic change principles. *American Psychologist*, 35, 991–999.

Goldfried, M. R. (1982). On the history of therapeutic integration. *Behavior Therapy*, 13, 572–593.

Goldfried, M. R. (1983). A behavior therapist looks at rapprochement. *Journal of Humanistic Psychology*, 23, 97–107.

Goldfried, M. R. (1995). *From cognitive-behavior therapy to psychotherapy integration: An evolving view*. New York: Springer.

Goldfried, M. R., & Davison, G. C. (1976). *Clinical behavior therapy*. New York: Holt, Rinehart and Winston.

Goldsmith, H. H. (1983). Genetic influence on personality from infancy to adulthood. *Child Development*, 54, 331–355.

Goldstein, A. P. (1962). *Therapist–patient expectancies in psychotherapy*. Oxford: Pergamon.

Good, M. I. (1989). Substance-induced dissociative disorders and psychiatric nosology. *Journal of Clinical Psychopharmacology*, 9, 88–93.

Greenberg, M. T., Kusche, C. A., & Speltz, M. (1992). Emotional regulation, self-control, and psychopathology: The role of relationships in early childhood. In D. Cicchetti & S. L. Toth (Eds.), *Rochester Symposium on Developmental Psychopathology: Vol. 2. Internalizing and externalizing expression of dysfunction* (pp. 21–55). Hillsdale, NJ: Erlbaum.

Greenwald, A. G. (1980). The totalitarian ego: Fabrication and revision of personal history. *American Psychologist*, 35, 603–618.

Grilo, G. M., & McGlashan, T. H. (1999). Stablity and course of personality disorders. *Current Opinion in Psychiatry*, 12, 157–162.

Guidano, V. F. (1987). *Complexity of the self: A developmental approach to psychopathology and therapy*. New York: Guilford Press.

Guidano, V. F. (1991a). Affective change events in a cognitive therapy systems approach. In J. D. Safran & L. S. Greenberg (Eds.), *Emotion, psychotherapy, and change* (pp. 50–79). New York: Guilford Press.

Guidano, V. F. (1991b). *The self in process: Toward a post-rationalist cognitive therapy*. New York: Guilford Press.

Guidano, V. F., & Liotti, G. (1983). *Cognitive processes and emotional disorders: A structural approach to psychotherapy*. New York: Guilford Press.

Gunderson, J. G. (1984). *Borderline personality disorder*. Washington, DC: American Psychiatric Association.

Gunderson, J. G. (2001). *Borderline personality disorder: A clinical guide*. Washington, DC: American Psychiatric Association.

Gunderson, J. G., Frank, A. F., Ronningstam, E. F., Wachter, S., Lynch, V. J., & Wolf, P. J. (1989). Early discontinuance of borderline patients from psychotherapy. *Journal of Nervous and Mental Disease, 177,* 38–42.

Gunderson, J. G., & Sabo, A. N. (1993). The phenomenological and conceptual interface between borderline personality disorder and PTSD. *American Journal of Psychiatry, 150*(1), 19–27.

Gunnell, D., & Frankel, S. (1994). Prevention of suicide: aspirations and evidence. *British Medical Journal, 308*(6938), 1227–33.

Guntrip, H. (1968). *Schizoid phenomena, objection relations and the self.* London: Hogarth Press.

Gurman, A. S., & Kniskern, D. P. (1981). Family therapy outcome research. In A. S. Gurman & D. P. Kniskern (Eds.), *Handbook of family therapy* (pp. 742–775). New York: Brunner-Mazel.

Haan, N., Millsap, R., & Hartka, E. (1986). As time goes by: Change and stability in personality over fifty years. *Psychology and Aging, 1,* 220–232.

Hall, C. S., & Lindzey, G. (1957). *Theories of personality.* New York: Wiley.

Hanson, R. A. (1975). Consistency and stability of home environmental measures related to IQ. *Child Development, 46,* 470–480.

Hardy, G. E., Barkham, M., Shapiro, D. A., Stiles, W. B., Rees, A., & Reynolds, S. (1995). Impact of Cluster C personality disorders on outcomes of contrasting brief psychotherapies for depression. *Journal of Consulting and Clinical Psychology, 63,* 997–1004.

Hare, R. D. (1991). *Manual for the Hare Psychopathy Checklist—Revised.* Toronto: Multi-Health Systems.

Harpur, T. J., Hakstian, A. R., & Hare, R. D. (1988). Factor structure of the psychopathy checklist. *Journal of Consulting and Clinical Psychology, 66,* 741–747.

Harter, S. (1993). Causes and consequences of low self-esteem in children and adolescents. In R. Baumeister (Ed.), *Self-esteem: The puzzle of low self-regard* (pp. 87–116). New York: Plenum Press.

Hartley, D. E. (1985). Research on the therapeutic alliance in psychotherapy. In R. Hales & A. Frances (Eds.), *Psychiatric update: American Psychiatric Press annual review of psychiatry* (Vol. 4, pp. 532–549). Washington, DC: American Psychiatric Association Press.

Hatcher, R. L., & Barends, A. W. (1996). Patients' view of the alliance in psychotherapy: Explanatory factor analysis of three alliance measures. *Journal of Consulting and Clinical Psychology, 64,* 1326–1336.

Heatherton, T. F., & Nichols, P. A. (1994a). Conceptual issues in assessing whether personality can change. In T. F. Heatherton & J. L. Weinberger (Eds.), *Can personality change?* (pp. 3–18). Washington, DC: American Psychological Association.

Heatherton, T. F., & Nichols, P. A. (1994b). Personal accounts of successful versus failed attempts at life change. *Personality and Social Psychology Bulletin, 20,* 664–675.

Heatherton, T. F., & Weinberger, J. L. (Eds.). (1994). *Can personality change?* Washington, DC: American Psychological Association.

Heckhausen, J., & Schulz, R. (1995). A life-span theory of control. *Psychological Review, 102,* 284–304.

Hellinga, G. (1999). *Lastige lieden* [Difficult people]. Amsterdam: Boom.

Helson, R., & Moane, G. (1987). Personality change in women from college to mid-life. *Journal of Personality and Social Psychology, 53*, 176–186.

Herman, J. L. (1992). *Trauma and recovery*. New York: Basic Books.

Herman, J. L., Perry, J. C., & van der Kolk, B. A. (1989). Childhood trauma in borderline personality disorder. *American Journal of Psychiatry, 146*, 490–495.

Herman, J. L., & van der Kolk, B. A. (1987). Traumatic antecedents of borderline personality disorder. In B. A. van der Kolk (Ed.), *Psychological trauma* (pp. 111–126). Washington, DC: American Psychiatric Press.

Higgins, E. T. (1987). Self-discrepancy: A theory relating self and affect. *Psychological Review, 94*, 319–340.

Higgins, E. T. (1989). Knowledge accessibility and activation: Subjectivity and suffering from unconscious sources. In J. S. Uleman & J. A. Bargh (Eds.), *Unintended thought: The limits of awareness, intention, and control* (pp. 75–123). New York: Guilford Press.

Higgins, E. T. (1996). Ideals, oughts, and regulatory focus: Affect and motivation from distinct pains and pleasures. In P. M. Gollwitzer & J. A. Bargh (Eds.), *The psychology of action: Linking cognition and motivation to behavior* (pp. 91–114). New York: Guilford Press.

Higgins, E. T., & Tykocinski, O. (1992). Self-discrepancies and biographical memory: Personality and cognition at the level of psychological situation. *Personality and Social Psychology Bulletin, 18*, 527–535.

Hinde, R. A., & Groebel, J. (1991). Introduction. In R. A. Hinde & J. Groebel (Eds.), *Cooperation and prosocial behaviour* (pp. 1–8). Cambridge, UK: Cambridge University Press.

Hirschfeld, R. M., Klerman, G. L., Clayton, P. J., Keller, M. D., McDonald-Scott, P., & Larkin, B. H. (1983). Assessing personality: Effects of the depressive state on trait measurement. *American Journal of Psychiatry, 140*, 695–699.

Hirschfeld, R. M., & Russell, J. M. (1997). Assessment and treatment of suicidal patients. *New England Journal of Medicine, 337*, 910–915.

Hoglend, P. (1993). Personality disorders and long-term outcome after brief dynamic psychotherapy. *Journal of Personality Disorders, 7*, 168–181.

Hoglend, P., Sortie, T., Heyerdahl, O., Sorbye, O., & Amlo, S. (1993). Brief dynamic psychotherapy: Patient suitability, treatment length, and outcome. *Journal of Psychotherapy Practice and Research, 2*, 230–241.

Holt, R. R. (1989). *Freud reappraised: A fresh look at psychoanalytic theory*. New York: Guilford Press.

Horowitz, L. M., Rosenberg, S. E., Baer, B. A., Ureno, G., & Villasenor, V. S. (1988). Inventory of interpersonal problems: Psychometric properties and clinical applications. *Journal of Consulting and Clinical Psychology, 56*, 885–892.

Horowitz, M. J. (1979). *States of mind*. New York: Plenum Press.

Horowitz, M. J. (1988). *Introduction to psychodynamics*. New York: Basic Books.

Horowitz, M. J. (1998). *Cognitive psychodynamics*. New York: Wiley.

Horowitz, M. J., & Marmar, C. (1985). The therapeutic alliance with difficult patients. In R. E. Hales & A. J. Frances (Eds.), *Psychiatric update: American Psychiatric Association annual review* (pp. 573–585). Washington, DC: American Psychiatric Association Press.

Horowitz, M. J., Marmar, C. R., Weiss, D. S., Kaltreider, N. B., & Wilner, N. R.

(1986). Comprehensive analysis of change after brief dynamic psychotherapy. *American Journal of Psychiatry, 143,* 582–589.

Horvath, A. O., & Greenberg, L. S. (Eds.) (1994). *The working alliance.* New York: Wiley.

Horvath, A. O., & Symonds, D. B. (1991). Relation between working alliance and outcome in psychotherapy: A meta-analysis. *Journal of Counseling Psychology, 38,* 139–149.

Horwitz, L. (1974). *Clinical prediction in psychotherapy.* New York: Jason Aronson.

Horwitz, L. (1980). Group psychotherapy for borderline and narcissistic disorders. *Bulletin of the Menninger Clinic, 44,* 181–200.

Horwitz, L., Gabbard, G. O., Allen, J. G., Frieswyk, S. H., Colson, D. B., Newsom, G. E., & Coyne, L. (1996). *Borderline personality disorder: Tailoring the psychotherapy to the patient.* Washington, DC: American Psychiatric Press.

Howard, K. I., Kopta, M., Krause, M., & Orlinsky, D. (1986). The dose–effect relationship in psychotherapy. *American Psychologist, 41,* 149–164.

Howard, K. I., Lueger, R., & Shrank, D. (1992). The psychotherapeutic service delivery system. *Psychotherapy Research, 2,* 164–180.

Huesmann, L. R., Eron, L. D., Lefkowitz, M. M., & Walder, L. O. (1984). Stability of aggression over time and generations. *Developmental Psychology, 20,* 1120–1134.

Hull, J. W., Yeomans, F., Clarkin, J., Li, C., & Goodman, G. (1996). Factors associated with multiple hospitalization of patients with borderline personality disorder. *Psychiatric Services, 47,* 638–641.

Hurt, S. W., Clarkin, J. F., Munroe-Blum, H., & Marziali, E. (1992). Borderline behavioral clusters and different treatment approaches. In J. F. Clarkin, E. Marziali, & H. Munroe-Blum (Eds.), *Borderline personality disorder: Clinical and empirical perspectives* (pp. 199–219). New York: Guilford Press.

James, W. (1981). *The principles of psychology* (Vol. 1). Cambridge, MA: Harvard University Press. (Original work published 1890)

Jang, K. L., Livesley, W. J., & Vernon, P. A. (1996a). The genetic basis of personality at different ages: A cross-sectional twin study. *Personality and Individual Differences, 21,* 229–301.

Jang, K. L., Livesley, W. J., & Vernon, P. A. (1996b). Heritability of the big five personality dimensions and their facets: A twin study. *Journal of Personality, 64,* 577–591.

Jang, K. L., Livesley, W. J., Vernon, P. A., & Jackson, D. N. (1996). Heritability of personality disorder traits: A twin study. *Acta Psychiatrica Scandinavica, 94,* 438–444.

Jang, K. L., Paris, J., Zweig-Frank, H., & Livesley, W. J. (1998). Twin study of dissociative experience. *Journal of Nervous and Mental Disease, 186,* 345–351.

Janoff-Bulman, R. (1992). *Shattered assumptions: Towards a new psychology of trauma.* New York: Free Press.

Jary, M. L., & Stewart, M. A. (1985). Psychiatric disorder in the parents of adopted children with aggressive conduct disorder. *Neuropsychobiology, 13,* 7–11.

Jaycox, L. H., & Foa, E. B. (1996). Obstacles to implementing exposure therapy for PTSD: Case discussions and practical solutions. *Clinical Psychology and Psychotherapy, 3,* 176–184.

Jessor, R. (1983). The stability of change: Psycho-social development from adolescence to young adulthood. In D. Magnusson & V. L. Allen (Eds.), *Human devel-*

opment and interactional perspective (pp. 321–341). San Diego, CA: Academic Press.

John, O. P., & Srivastava, S. (1999). The big five trait taxonomy: History, measurement, and theoretical perspectives. In L. Pervin & O. P. John (Eds.), *Handbook of personality: Theory and research* (2nd ed., pp. 102–138). New York: Guilford Press.

Johnson, J. G., Williams, J. B. W., Goetz, R. R., Rabkin, J. G., Lipsitz, J. D., & Remien, R. H. (1997). Stability and change in personality disorder symptomatology: Findings from a longitudinal study of HIV+ and HIV- men. *Journal of Abnormal Psychology, 106*, 154–158.

Johnson, J. J., Cohen, P., Brown, J., Smailes, E. M., & Bernstein, D. P. (1999). Childhood maltreatment increases risk for personality disorders during early adulthood. *Archives of General Psychiatry, 56*, 600–606.

Joseph, B. (1983). On understanding and not understanding: Some technical issues. *International Journal of Psychoanalysis, 64*, 291–298.

Karasu, T. B. (1986). Specificity versus non-specificity. *American Journal of Psychiatry, 143*, 687–695.

Karterud, S., Vaglum, S., Friis, S., Irion, T., Johns, S., & Vaglum, P. (1992). Day hospital therapeutic community treatment for patients with personality disorders. Am empirical evaluation of the containment function. *Journal of Nervous and Mental Disease, 180*, 238–243.

Kavoussi, R. J., Liu, J., & Coccaro, E. F. (1994). An open trial of sertraline in personality disordered patients with impulsive aggression. *Journal of Clinical Psychiatry, 55*, 137–141.

Kelly, G. A. (1955). *The psychology of personal constructs* (Vol. 1). New York: Norton.

Kelly, T., Soloff, P. H., Cornelius, J. R., George, A., & Lis, J. (1992). Can we study (treat) borderline patients: Attrition from research and open treatment. *Journal of Personality Disorders, 6*, 417–433.

Kemperman, I., Russ, M. J., & Shearin, E. (1997). Self-injurious behavior and mood regulation in borderline patients. *Journal of Personality Disorders, 11*, 146–157.

Kent, S., Fogarty, M., & Yellowlees, P. (1995). Heavy utilization of inpatient and outpatient services in a public mental health service. *Psychiatric Services, 46*, 1254–1257.

Kernberg, O. F. (1975). *Borderline conditions and pathological narcissism.* New York: Jason Aronson.

Kernberg, O. F. (1984). *Severe personality disorders.* New Haven, CT: Yale University Press.

Kernberg, O. F. (2001). The suicidal risk of severe personality disorders: Differential diagnosis and treatment. *Journal of Personality Disorders, 15*, 195–208.

Kiesler, D. J. (1986). The 1982 Interpersonal Circle: An analysis of DSM-III personality disorders. In T. Millon & G. L. Klerman (Eds.), *Contemporary directions in psychopathology: Toward the DSM-IV* (pp. 571–597). New York: Guilford Press.

Kjelsberg, E., Eikeseth, P. H., & Dahl, A. A. (1991). Suicide in borderline patients—predictive factors. *Acta Psychiatrica Scandinavica, 94*, 283–287.

Klohnen, E. C., & Bera, S. (1998). Behavioral and experiential patterns of avoidantly and securely attached women across adulthood. *Journal of Personality and Social Psychology, 74*, 211–223.

Knutson, B., Wolkowitz, O. M., Cole, S. W., Chan, T., Moore, E. A., Johnson, R.

C., Terpstra, J., Turner, R. A., & Reus, V. I. (1998). Selective alteration of personality and social behavior by serotonergic intervention. *American Journal of Psychiatry, 155,* 373–379.

Kohut, H. (1971). *The analysis of the self.* New York: International Universities Press.

Kohut, H. (1975). Introspection, empathy, and psychoanalysis: An examination of the relationship between mode of observation and theory. *Journal of Psychotherapy Practice and Research, 4,* 163–177.

Kohut, H. (1977). *The restoration of the self.* New York: International Universities Press.

Kolden, G., & Howard, K. I. (1992). An empirical test of the generic model of psychotherapy. *Journal of Psychotherapy Practice and Research, 1,* 225–236.

Komatsu, L. K. (1992). Recent views of conceptual structure. *Psychological Bulletin, 42,* 500–526.

Koons, C. R., Robins, C. J., Bishop, G. K., Morse, J. Q., Tweed, J. L., Lynch, T. R., Gonzales, A. M., Butterfield, M. I., & Bastian, L. A. (2001). Efficacy of dialectical behavior therapy with borderline women veterans: A randomized controlled trial. *Behavior Therapy, 32,* 371–390.

Kopte, S. M., Howard, K. I., Lowry, L. J. L., & Beutler, L. E. (1994). Patterns of symptomatic recovery in time limited psychotherapy. *Journal of Consulting and Clinical Psychology, 62,* 1009–1016.

Kretschmer, E. (1925). *Physique and character.* London: Kegan, Paul, Trench, and Trubner.

Kroll, J. (1988). *The challenge of the borderline patient.* New York: Basic Books.

Kroll, J. (1993). *PTSD/borderlines in therapy.* New York: Norton.

Kroll, J. (2000). Use of no-suicide contracts by psychiatrists in Minnesota. *American Journal of Psychiatry, 157,* 1684–1686.

Krystal, J. H., Bennett, A. L., Bremner, D. J., Southwick, S. M., & Charney, D. S. (1995). Toward a cognitive neuroscience of dissociation altered memory function in posttraumatic stress disorder. In M. J. Freeman, D. S. Charney, & A. Y. Deutsch (Eds.), *Neurobiological and clinical consequences of stress: From normal adaptation to posttraumatic stress disorder* (pp. 239–269). Philadelphia: Lippincott-Raven.

Kubany, E. S., & Manke, F. P. (1995). Cognitive therapy for trauma-related guilt: Conceptual bases and treatment outlines. *Cognitive and Behavioral Practice, 2,* 23–61.

Kutcher, S., Papatheodorou, G., Reiter, S., & Gardner, D. (1995). The successful pharmacological treatment of adolescents and young adults with borderline personality disorder: A preliminary open trail of flupenthixol. *Journal of Psychiatry and Neuroscience, 20,* 113–118.

Lambert, M. J. (1986). Some implications of psychotherapy outcome research for eclectic psychotherapy. *International Journal of Eclectic Psychotherapy, 16,* 16–45.

Lambert, M. J. (1992). Psychotherapy outcome research: Implications for integrative and electical therapists. In J. C. Norcross & M. R. Goldfried (Eds.), *Handbook of psychotherapy integration* (pp. 94–129). New York: Basic Books.

Lambert, M. J., & Bergen, A. E. (1994). The effectiveness of psychotherapy. In A. E. Bergin & S. L. Garfield (Eds.), *Handbook of psychotherapy and behavior change* (4th ed., pp. 143–189). New York: Wiley.

Lang, J. A. (1987). Two contrasting frames of reference for understanding borderline patients: Kernberg and Kohut. In J. S. Grotstein, M. Solomon, & J. A. Lang (Eds.), *The borderline patient: Emerging concepts in diagnosis, psychodynamics, and treatment* (Vol. 1, pp. 131–146). Hillsdale, NJ: Analytic Press.

Layden, M. A., Newman, C. F., Freeman, A., & Morse, S. B. (1993). *Cognitive therapy of borderline personality disorder*. Needham Heights, MA: Allyn & Bacon.

Leary, T. (1957). *Interpersonal diagnosis of personality: A functional theory and methodology for personality evaluation*. New York: Ronald Press.

Lenzenweger, M. F. (1999). Stability and change in personality disorder features. *Archives of General Psychiatry, 56*, 1009–1015.

Leone, N. (1982). Response of borderline patients to loxapine and chloropromazine. *Journal of Clinical Psychiatry, 43*, 148–150.

Leszcz, M. (1989). Group therapy. In *Task force on treatment of psychiatric disorders* (Vol. 3, pp. 2667–2677). Washington, DC: American Psychiatric Association.

Lewin, B. R. (1935). *A dynamic theory of personality*. New York: McGraw-Hill.

Lichtenberg, J. D., Lachmann, F. M., & Fosshage, J. L. (1992). *Self and motivational systems: Toward a theory of psychoanalytic technique*. Hillsdale, NJ: Analytic Press.

Lieberman, R. P., & Eckman, T. (1981). Behavior therapy versus insight-oriented therapy for repeated suicide attempters. *Archives of General Psychiatry, 38*, 1126–1130.

Linehan, M. M. (1987). Dialectical behavior therapy: A cognitive behavioral approach to parasuicide. *Journal of Personality Disorders, 1*, 328–333.

Linehan, M. M. (1993). *Cognitive-behavioral treatment of borderline personality disorder*. New York: Guilford Press.

Linehan, M. M., Armstrong, H. E., Suarez, A., Allmon, D., & Heard, H. L. (1991). Cognitive-behavioral treatment of chronically parasuicidal borderline patients. *Archives of General Psychiatry, 48*, 1060–1064.

Linehan, M. M., Heard, H. L., & Armstrong, H. E. (1993). Naturalistic follow-up of a behavioral treatment for chronically parasuicidal borderline patients. *Archives of General Psychiatry, 50*, 971–974.

Linehan, M. M., & Kehrer, C. A. (1993). Borderline personality disorder. In D. H. Baslow (Ed.), *Clinical handbook of psychological disorders: A step-by-step treatment manual* (2nd ed., pp. 396–441). New York: Guilford Press.

Linehan, M. M., Schmidt, H. I., Dimeff, L. A., Craft, J. C., Kanter, J., & Comtois, K. A. (1999). Dialectical behavior therapy for patients with borderline personality disorder and drug-dependence. *American Journal of Addictions, 8*, 279–292.

Linehan, M. M., & Shearin, E. N. (1988). Lethal stress: A social–behavioral model of suicidal behavior. In S. Fisher & J. Reason (Eds.), *Handbook of life stress, cognition, and health* (pp. 265–285). Chichester, UK: Wiley.

Linehan, M. M., Tutek, D. A., Heard, H. L., & Armstrong, H. E. (1994). Interpersonal outcome of cognitive behavioral treatment for chronically suicidal borderline patients. *American Journal of Psychiatry, 151*, 1771–1776.

Links, P. S., Heslegrave, R., & van Reekum, R. (1999). Impulsivity: Core aspect of borderline personality disorder. *Journal of Personality Disorders, 13*, 1–9.

Links, P. S., Steiner M., Boiago, I., & Irwin, D. (1990). Lithium therapy for borderline patients: Preliminary findings. *Journal of Personality Disorders, 4*, 173–181.

Links, P. S., Steiner M., & Huxley, G. (1988). The occurrence of borderline personality dsorder in the families of borderline patients. *Journal of Personality Disorders, 2*, 14–20.

Links, P. S., Steiner M., Offord D. R., & Eppel, A. (1988). Characteristics of border-line personality disorder: A Canadian study. *Canadian Journal of Psychiatry, 33,* 336–340.

Linville, P. W. (1982). Affective consequences of complexity regarding self and others. In M. S. Clarke & S. T. Fiske (Eds.), *Affect and cognition: 17th Annual Carnegie Symposium* (pp. 79–95). Hillsdale, NJ: Erlbaum.

Lipschitz, D. S., Bernstein, D. P., Winegar, R. K., & Southwick, S. M. (1999). Hospitalized adolescents' reports of sexual and physical abuse: A comparison of two self-report measures. *Journal of Traumatic Stress, 12,* 641–654.

Livesley, W. J. (1995). Past achievements and future directions. In W. J. Livesley (Ed.), *The DSM-IV personality disorders* (pp. 497–505). New York: Guilford Press.

Livesley, W. J. (1998). Suggestions for a framework for an empirically based classification of personality disorder. *Canadian Journal of Psychiatry, 43,* 137–147.

Livesley, W. J. (1999). The implications of recent research on the etiology and stability of personality and personality disorder for treatment. In J. Derksen, C. Maffei, & H. Groen (Eds.), *The treatment of personality disorders* (pp. 25–37). New York: Plenum Press.

Livesley, W. J. (2000). A practical approach to the treatment of borderline personality. *Psychiatric Clinics of North America, 23,* 211–232.

Livesley, W. J. (2001a). Conceptual and taxonomic issues. In W. J. Livesley (Ed.), *Handbook of personality disorders: Theory, research, and treatment* (pp. 1–38). New York: Guilford Press.

Livesley, W. J. (2001b). A framework for an integrated approach to treatment. In W. J. Livesley (Ed.), *Handbook of personality disorders: Theory, research, and treatment* (pp. 570–600). New York: Guilford Press.

Livesley, W. J. (2001c). The genetic basis of personality and its implications for psychotherapy. *Revista di Psiquiatria do Rio Grande Do Sol, 22,* 218–226.

Livesley, W. J. (2002). Treating the emotional dysregulation cluster of traits. *Psychiatric Annals, 32,* 601–607.

Livesley, W. J. (2003). Diagnostic dilemmas in the classification of personality disorder. In K. Phillips, M. First, & H. A. Pincus (Eds.), *Diagnostic issues for the DSM-V.* Washington, DC: American Psychiatric Association Press.

Livesley, W. J., & Bromley, D. B. (1973). Person perception in childhood and adolescence. Chichester, UK: Wiley.

Livesley, W. J., & Jackson, D. N. (in press). Manual for the dimensional assessment of personality pathology. Port Huron, MI: Sigma Press.

Livesley, W. J., & Jang, K. L. (2000). Toward an empirically based classification of personality disorder. *Journal of Personality Disorders, 14,* 137–151.

Livesley, W. J., Jang, K. L., Jackson, D. N, & Vernon, P. A. (1993). Genetic and environmental contributions to dimensions of personality disorder. *American Journal of Psychiatry, 150,* 1826–1831.

Livesley, W. J., Jang, K. L., & Vernon, P. A. (1998). The phenotypic and genetic architecture of traits delineating personality disorder. *Archives of General Psychiatry, 55,* 941–948.

Livesley, W. J., Jang, K. L., & Vernon, P. A. (2003). Genetic basis of personality structure. In T. Millon & M. J. Lerner (Vol. Eds.) & I. B. Weiner (Ed.), *Handbook of psychology. Vol. 5: Personality and social psychology* (pp. 59–83). Hoboken, NJ: Wiley.

Livesley, W. J., Schroeder, M. L., Jackson, D. N., & Jang, K. L. (1994). Categorical distinctions in the study of personality disorder: Implications for classification. *Journal of Abnormal Psychology, 103,* 6–17.

Loehlin, J. C., & Nichols, R. C. (1976). *Heredity, environment, and personality: A study of 850 sets of twins.* Austin: University of Texas Press.

Luborsky, L. (1976). Helping alliance in psychotherapy. In J. L. Claghorn (Ed.), *Successful psychotherapy* (pp. 92–116). New York: Brunner/Mazel.

Luborsky, L. (1977). Measuring a pervasive psychic structure in psychotherapy: The core conflictual relationship theme. In N. Freedman & S. Grand (Eds.), *Communicative structures and psychic structures* (pp. 367–395). New York: Plenum Press.

Luborsky, L. (1984). *Principles of psychoanalytic psychotherapy.* New York: Basic Books.

Luborsky, L. (1994). Therapeutic alliances as predictors of psychotherapy outcomes: Factors explaining the predictive success. In A. O. Horvath & L. S. Greenberg (Eds.), *The working alliance* (pp. 38–50). New York: Wiley.

Luborsky, L. (1995). Are common factors across different psychotherapies the main explanation for the dodo bird verdict that "everyone has won so all shall have prizes"? *Clinical Psychology: Science and Practice, 2,* 106–109.

Luborsky, L. (1997a). The convergence of Freud's observations about tranference and the CCRT evidence. In L. Luborsky & P. Crits-Christoph (Eds.), *Understanding transference: The core conflictual relationship theme method* (2nd ed.). Washington, DC: American Psychological Association.

Luborsky, L. (1997b). The core conflictual relationship theme: A basic case formulation method. In T. D. Eells (Ed.), *Handbook of psychotherapy case formulation* (pp. 58–83). New York: Guilford Press.

Luborsky, L., Crits-Christoph, P., Alexander, L., & Margolois, M., & Cohen, M. (1983). Two helping alliance methods for predicting outcomes of psychotherapy: A counting signs vs. a global rating method. *Journal of Nervous and Mental Disease, 171,* 480–492.

Luborksy, L., Crits-Christoph, P., Mintz, J., & Auerbach, A. (1988). *Who will benefit from psychotherapy? Predicting therapeutic conditions.* New York: Basic Books.

Luborsky, L., Diguer, L., Luborsky, E., Singer, B., Dichter, D., & Schmidt, K. A. (1993). The efficacy of dynamic psychotherapies: Is it true that "everyone has won and all must have prizes?" In N. E. Miller, L. Luborsky, J. P. Barber, & J. P. Docherty (Eds.), *Psychodynamic treatment research: A handbook for clinical practice* (pp. 497–516). New York: Basic Books.

Luborsky, L., McLellan, A. T., Woody, G. E., O'Brien, C. P., & Auerbach, A. (1985). Therapist success and its determinants. *Archives of General Psychiatry, 42,* 602–611.

Luborsky, L., Singer, B., & Luborsky, L. (1975). Comparative studies of psychotherapies. *Archives of General Psychiatry, 32,* 995–1008.

Ludolph, P. S., Westen, D., & Misle, B (1990). The borderline diagnosis in adolescents: Symptoms and developmental history. *American Journal of Psychiatry, 147,* 470–476.

Ludwig, A. M. (1983). The psychobiological functions of dissociation. *American Journal of Clinical Hypnosis, 26,* 425–434.

MacFarlane, M. (in press). Family treatment of personality disorders. In *Advances in clinical practice.* New York: Haworth Press.

MacKenzie, K. R. (1994). Using personality measurements in clinical practice. In P. T. Costa, & T. A. Widiger (Eds.), *Personality disorders and the five-factor model of personality* (pp. 237–250). Washington, DC: American Psychological Association Books.

MacKenzie, K. R. (1997). *Time-managed group psychotherapy: Effective clinical applications.* Washington, DC: American Psychiatric Association Press.

MacKenzie, K. R. (2001). Personality assessment in clinical practice. In W. J. Livesley (Ed.), *Handbook of personality disorders: Theory, research, and treatment* (pp. 307–320). New York: Guilford Press.

MacKenzie, K. R. (2002). Using personality measurements in clinical practice. In P. T. Costa & T. A. Widiger (Eds.), *Personality disorders and the five-factor model of personality* (2nd ed., pp. 377–390). Washington, DC: American Psychological Association Books.

McRoberts, C., Burlingame, G. M., & Hoag, M. J. (1998). Comparative efficacy of individual and group psychotherapy: A meta-analytic perspective. *Group Dynamics: Theory, Research, and Practice, 2,* 3–14.

Maddi, S. R. (1968). *Personality theories: A comparative analysis.* New York: Guilford Press.

Malan, D. H. (1979). *Individual psychotherapy and the science of psychodynamics.* London: Butterworths.

Malan, D. H., Balfow, F. H. G., Hood, V. G., & Shooter, A. M. N. (1976). Group psychotherapy: A long term follow-up study. *Archives of General Psychiatry, 33,* 1303–1315.

Mann, A. H., Jenkins, R., Cutting, J. C., & Cowen, P. J. (1981). The development and use of a standardized assessment of abnormal personality. *Psychological Medicine, 11,* 839–847.

Mann, J. (1973). *Time-limited psychotherapy.* Cambridge, MA: Harvard University Press.

Mann, J. J., Waternaux, C., Haas, G. L., & Malone, K. M. (1999). Toward a clinical model of suicidal behavior in psychiatric patients. *American Journal of Psychiatry, 156,* 181–189.

Maris, R. W., Berman, A. L., Maltsberger, J. T., & Yufit, R. I. (Eds.). (1992). *Assessment and prediction of suicide.* New York: Guilford Press.

Markovitz, P. (1995). Pharmacotherapy of impulsivity, aggression, and related disorders. In E. Hollander & D. J. Stein (Eds.), *Impulsivity and aggression* (pp. 263–287). Chichester, UK: Wiley.

Markovitz, P. (2001). Pharmacotherapy. In W. J. Livesley (Ed.), *Handbook of personality disorders: Theory, research, and treatment* (pp. 475–493). New York: Guilford Press.

Markovitz, P., Calabrese, J., Charles, S., & Meltzer, H. (1991). Fluoxentine in the treatment of borderline and schizotypal personality disorders. *American Journal of Psychiatry, 148,* 1064–1067.

Markovitz, P., & Wagner, S. (1995). Venlafaxine in the treatment of borderline personality disorder. *Psychopharmacology Bulletin, 31,* 773–777.

Markus, H., & Norius, P. (1986). Possible selves. *American Psychologist, 41,* 954–969.

Marziali, E. A. (1984). Three viewpoints on the therapeutic alliance: Similarities, differences, and associations with psychotherapy outcome. *Journal of Nervous and Mental Disease, 172,* 417–423.

Marziali, E. A., & Munroe-Blum, H. (1994). *Interpersonal group psychotherapy for borderline personality disorder.* New York: Basic Books.

Marziali, E. A., & Sullivan, J. M. (1980). Methodological issues in the content analysis of brief psychotherapy. *British Journal of Medical Psychology, 53,* 19–27.

Marzillier, J. S., Lambert, C., & Kellett, J. (1976). A controlled evaluation of systematic desensitization and social skills training for socially inadequate psychiatric patients. *Behaviour Research and Therapy, 14,* 225–238.

Masterson, J. (1976). *Psychotherapy of the borderline adult.* New York: Brunner/Mazel.

Mattia, J. I., & Zimmerman, M. (2001). Epidemiology. In W. J. Livesley (Ed.), *Handbook of personality disorders: Theory, research, and treatment* (pp. 107–123). New York: Guilford Press.

McAdams, D. P. (1997). A conceptual history of personality psychology. In R. Hogan, J. Johnson, & S. Briggs (Eds.), *Handbook of personality psychology* (pp. 3–39). San Diego, CA: Academic Press.

McAdams, D. P. (1994). Personality, modernity, and the storied self: A contemporary framework for studying persons. *Psychological Inquiry, 7,* 295–321.

McCallum, M., & Piper, W. E. (1997). The Psychological Mindedness Assessment Procedure. In M. McCallum & W. E. Piper (Eds.), *Psychological mindedness* (pp. 27–58). Mahwah, NJ: Erlbaum.

McCann, I. L., & Pearlman, L. A. (1990). *Psychological trauma and the adult survivor: Theory, therapy, and transformation.* New York: Brunner/Mazel.

McCann, I. L., Sakheim, D. K., & Abrahamson, D. J. (1988). Trauma and victimization: A model of psychological adaptation. *Counseling Psychologist, 16,* 531–594.

McConnaughty, E. A., DiClemente, C. C., Prochaska, J. O., & Velicer, W. F. (1989). Stage of change in psychotherapy: A follow-up report. *Psychotherapy: Theory, Research, and Practice, 26,* 494–503.

McCullough Vaillant, L. (1997). *Changing character.* New York: Basic Books.

McGee, M. D. (1997). Cessation of self-mutilation in a patients with borderline personality disorder treated with naltrexone. *Journal of Clinical Psychiatry, 58,* 32–33.

McGlashan, T. H. (1986). The Chestnut Lodge follow-up study: III. Long-term outcome of borderline personalities. *Archives of General Psychiatry, 43,* 20–30.

McGuffin, P., & Thapar, A. (1992). The genetics of personality disorder. *British Journal of Psychiatry, 160,* 12–23.

McKay, D., Kulchycky, S., & Danyko, S. (2000). Borderline personality disorder and obsessive–compulsive symptoms: A community-based longitudinal investigation. *Journal of Personality Disorders, 14,* 57–63.

McLemore, C. W., & Brokaw, D. W. (1987). Personality disorders as dysfunctional interpersonal behavior. *Journal of Personality Disorders, 1,* 270–285.

Mead, G. H. (1934). *Mind, self, and society.* Chicago: University of Chicago Press.

Meadows, E. A., & Foa, E. B. (1998). Intrusion, arousal, and avoidance: Sexual trauma survivors. In V. M. Follette, J. I. Ruzek, & F. R. Abueg (Eds.), *Cognitive-behavioral therapies for trauma* (pp. 100–123). New York: Guilford Press.

Mednick, S. A., Moffitt, T., Gabrielli, J., & Hutchings, B. (1986). Genetic factors in criminal behavior: A review. In F. Olweus, I. Block, & M. Radke-Yarrow (Eds.,), *Development of antisocial and prosocial behavior* (pp. 33–50). New York: Academic Press.

Mehlum, L., Vaglum, P., & Karterud, S. (1994). The longitudinal pattern of suicidal behavior in borderline personality disorder: A prospective follow-up study. *Acta Psychiatrica Scandinavica*, 90, 124–130.

Meichenbaum, D., & Fong, G. (1993). How individuals control their own minds: A constructive narrative perspective. In D. M. Wagner & J. W. Pennabaker (Eds.), *Handbook of mental control* (pp. 473–489). New York: Prentice-Hall.

Meichenbaum, D., & Turk, D. C. (1987). *Facilitating treatment adherence: A practitioner's guidebook.* New York: Plenum Press.

Meijer, M., Goedhart, A. W., & Treffers, P. D. A. (1998). The persistence of borderline personality disorder in adolescence. *Journal of Personality Disorders*, 12, 13–22.

Meissner, W. W. (1984). *The borderline spectrum: Differential diagnosis and developmental issues.* Northvale, NJ: Jason Aronson.

Meissner, W. W. (1991). *What is effective in psychoanalytic therapy?* Northvale, NJ: Jason Aronson.

Menninger, K. (1958). *Theory of psychoanalytic technique.* New York: Basic Books.

Merikangas, K. R., & Wiessman, M. M. (1986). Epidemiology of DSM-III Axis II personality disorders. In *American Psychiatric Association annual review of psychiatry* (Vol. 5, pp. 258–278). Washington, DC: American Psychiatric Association Press.

Meyer, B., & Carver, C. S. (2000). Negative childhood accounts, sensitivity, and pessimism: A study of avoidant personality disorder features in college students. *Journal of Personality Disorders*, 14, 233–248.

Miles, D. R., & Carey, G. (1997). Genetic and environmental architecture of human aggression. *Journal of Personality and Social Psychology*, 72, 207–217.

Miller, L. J. (1989). Inpatient management of borderline personality disorder. *Journal of Personality Disorders*, 3, 122–134.

Miller, T. R. (1991). The psychotherapeutic utility of the five-factor model of personality: A clinician's experience. *Journal of Personality Assessment*, 57, 415–433.

Miller, W. R. (1985). Motivation for treatment: A review with special emphasis on alcoholism. *Psychological Bulletin*, 98, 84–107.

Miller, W. R., & Baca, L. M. (1983). Two-year follow-up of bibliotherapy and therapist-directed controlled drinking for problem drinkers. *Behavior Therapy*, 14, 441–448.

Miller, W. R., Benefield, R. G., & Tonigan, J. S. (1993). Enhancing motivation for change in problem drinking: A controlled comparison of two therapist styles. *Journal of Consulting and Clinical Psychology*, 61, 455–461.

Miller, W. R., & C'de Baca, J. (2001). *Quantum change: When epiphanies and sudden insights transform ordinary lives.* New York: Guilford Press.

Miller, W. R., & Rollnick, S. (1991). *Motivational interviewing: Preparing people to change addictive behavior.* New York: Guilford Press.

Miller, W. R., Taylor, C. A., & West, J. C. (1980). Focused versus broad-spectrum behavior therapy for problem drinkers. *Journal of Consulting and Clinical Psychology*, 48, 590–601.

Mischel, W. (1999). Personality coherence and dispositions in a cognitive-affective personality system (CAPS) approach. In D. Cervone & Y. Shoda (Eds.), *The coherence of personality: Social–cognitive bases of consistency, variability, and organization* (pp. 37–60). New York: Guilford Press.

Morey, L. C., & Ochoa, E. S. (1989). An investigation of adherence to diagnostic criteria: Clinical diagnosis of the DSM-III personality disorders. *Journal of Personality Disorders, 3*, 180–192.

Mortimer, J. T., Finch, M. D., & Kumka, D. (1982). Persistence and change in development: The multi-dimensional self-concept. In P. T. Baltes & O. G. Brim, Jr. (Eds.), *Lifespan development and behavior* (Vol. 4). San Diego, CA: Academic Press.

Mowrer, O. A. (1960). *Learning theory and behavior.* New York: Wiley.

Mulder, R. T., & Joyce, P. R. (1997). Temperament and the structure of personality disorder symptoms. *Psychological Medicine, 27*, 1315–1325.

Munroe-Blum, H., & Marziali, E. (1995). A controlled trial of short-term group treatment for borderline personality disorder. *Journal of Personality Disorders, 9*, 190–198.

Murphy, G. (1947). *Personality: A bio-social approach to origins and structure.* New York: Holt, Rhinehart and Winston.

Nachmias, M., Gunnar, M., Mangelsdorf, S., Parritz, R. H., & Buss, K. (1996). Behavioral inhibition and stress reactivity: The moderating role of attachment security. *Child Development, 67*, 508–522.

Neimeyer, R. A. (1995). Constructivist psychotherapies: Features, foundations, and future directions. In R. A. Neimeyer & M. J. Mahoney, *Constructivism in psychotherapy* (pp. 11–38). Washington, DC: American Psychological Association.

Neimeyer, R. A., & Mahoney, M. J. (1995). *Constructivism in psychotherapy.* Washington, DC: American Psychological Association.

Newcomb, T. M. (1961). *The acquaintance process.* New York: Holt, Rinehart and Winston.

Newell, A., & Simon, H. A. (1972). *Human problem solving.* Englewood Cliffs, NJ: Prentice-Hall.

Nigg, J. T., & Goldsmith, H. H. (1994). Genetics of personality disorders: Perspectives from personality and psychopathology research. *Psychology Bulletin, 115*, 346–380.

Norcross, J. C., & Goldfried, M. R. (Eds.). (1992). *Handbook of psychotherapy integration.* New York: Basic Books.

Norcross, J. C., & Newman, J. C. (1992). Psychotherapy integration: Setting the context. In J. C. Norcross & M. R. Goldfried (Eds.), *Handbook of psychotherapy integration* (pp. 3–45). New York: Basic Books.

Norden, M. J. (1989). Fluoxetine in borderline personality disorder. *Progress in Neuropsychopharmacology and Biological Psychiatry, 13*, 885–893.

Novaco, R. W., & Chemtob, C. M. (1998). Anger and trauma: Conceptualization, assessment, and treatment. In V. M. Follette, J. I. Ruzek, & F. R. Abueg (Eds.), *Cognitive behavioral therapies for trauma* (pp. 162–190). New York: Guilford Press.

Norden, K. A., Klein, D. N., Donaldson, S. K., & Pepper, C. M. (1995). Reports of the early home environment in DSM-III-R personality disorders. *Journal of Personality Disorders, 9*, 213–223.

Ogata, S. N., Silk, K. R., Goodrich, S., Lohr, N. E., Westen, D., & Hill, E. M. (1990). Childhood sexual and physical abuse in adult patients with borderline personality disorder. *American Journal of Psychiatry, 147*, 1008–1013.

Ogrodniczuk, J. S., Piper, W. E., Joyce, A. S., & McCallum, M. (1999). Transference interpretation is short-term dynamic psychotherapy. *Journal of Nervous and Mental Disease, 187*, 572–579.

Oldham, J., Skodol, A. E., Kellman, H. D., Hyler, S. E., Doige, N., Rosnick, L., &

398 References

Gallagher, P. E. (1995). Comorbidity of Axis I and Axis II disorders. *American Journal of Psychiatry, 152,* 571–578.

O'Leary, K. D., & Wilson, G. T. (1987). *Behavior therapy: Application and outcome* (2nd ed.). Englewood Cliffs, NJ: Prentice-Hall.

Olweus, D. (1979). Stability of aggressive reactions in males: A review. *Psychological Bulletin, 86,* 852–875.

Orlinsky, D. E., Grawe, K., & Parks, B. K. (1994). Process and outcome in psychotherapy—Noch Einmel. In A. E. Begin & S. L. Garfield (Eds.), *Handbook of psychotherapy and behavioral change* (3rd ed., pp. 270–376). New York: Wiley.

Orlinsky, D. E., & Howard, K. I. (1986). Process and outcome in psychotherapy. In A. E. Begin & S. L. Garfield (Eds.), *Handbook of psychotherapy and behavioral change* (3rd ed., pp. 311–381). New York: Wiley.

Orlinsky, D. E., & Howard, K. I. (1987). A generic model of psychotherapy. *Journal of Integrative and Eclectic Psychotherapy, 6,* 6–27.

Padesky, C. A. (1994). Schema change processes in cognitive therapy. *Clinical Psychology and Psychotherapy, 1,* 267–278.

Paris, J. (1994). *Borderline personality disorder: A multidimensional approach.* Washington, DC: American Psychiatric Association Press.

Paris, J. (2001). Psychosocial adversity. In W. J. Livesley (Ed.), *Handbook of personality disorders: Theory, research, and treatment* (pp.231–241). New York: Guilford Press.

Paris, J. (2002). Clinical practice guidelines for borderline personality disorder. *Journal of Personality Disorders, 16*(2), 107–108.

Paris J., Brown, R., & Nowlis, D. (1987). Long-term follow-up of borderline patients in a general hospital. *Comprehensive Psychiatry, 28,* 530–535.

Paris, J., & Frank, H. (1992). Childhood factors in adult self-destructive behavior. *American Journal of Psychiatry, 149*(9), 1280–128.

Paris J., Nowlis, D., & Brown, R. (1988). Developmental factors in the outcome of borderline personality disorder. *Comprehensive Psychiatry, 29,* 147–150.

Paris J., Nowlis, D., & Brown, R. (1989). Predictors of suicide in borderline personality disorder. *Canadian Journal of Psychiatry, 34,* 8–9.

Paris, J., & Zweig-Frank, H. (1992). A critical review of childhood sexual abuse in the aetiology of borderline personality disorder. *Canadian Journal of Psychiatry, 37,* 125–128.

Paris, J., Zweig-Frank, H., & Guzder, J. (1994a). Psychological risk factors for borderline personality disorder in female patients. *Comprehensive Psychiatry, 35,* 301–305.

Paris, J., Zweig-Frank, H., & Guzder, J. (1994b). Risk factors for borderline personality in male outpatients. *Journal of Nervous and Mental Disease, 182,* 375–380.

Parker, J. D. A., & Bagby, R. M. (1997). Impulsivity in adults: A critical review of measurement approaches. In C. D. Webster & M. A. Jackson (Eds.), *Impulsivity: Theory, assessment, and treatment* (pp. 142–157). New York: Guilford Press.

Patterson, G. R., & Forgatch, M. S. (1985). Therapist behavior as a determinant of client non-compliance: A paradox for the behavior modifier. *Journal of Consulting and Clinical Psychology, 53,* 846–851.

Perris, C. (1994). Cognitive therapy in the treatment of patients with borderline personality disorders. *Acta Psychiatrica Scandinavica, 89,* 69–72.

Perry, J. C. (1993). Longitudinal studies of personality disorders. *Journal of Personality Disorders, 7,* 63–85.

Perry, J. C., Banon, E., & Ianni, F. (1999). Effectiveness of psychotherapy for personality disorders. *American Journal of Psychiatry, 156*, 1312–1321.

Perry, J. C., & Herman, J. L. (1993). Trauma and defense in the etiology of borderline personality disorder. In J. Paris (Ed.), *Borderline personality disorder, etiology and treatment*. Washington, DC: American Psychiatric Association Press.

Perry, S., Cooper, A. R., & Michels, R. (1987). The psychodynamic formulation: Its purpose, structure, and clinical application. *American Journal of Psychiatry, 144*, 543–550.

Pervin, L. A. (1992). Transversing the individual–environment landscape: A personal odyssey. In W. B. Walsh, K. H. Craik, & R. H. Price (Eds.), *Person–environment psychology: Models and perspectives* (pp. 71–87). Hillsdale, NJ: Erlbaum.

Petrocelli, J. V., Glaser, B. A., Calhoun, G. B., & Campbell, L. F. (2001). Early maladaptive schemas of personality disorder subtypes. *Journal of Personality Disorders, 15*, 546–559.

Pfeiffer, E. (1974). Borderline states. *Diseases of the Nervous System, 35*, 212–219.

Piaget, J. (1926). *Language and thought of the child*. New York: Harcourt, Brace.

Piaget, J. (1952). *The origins of intelligence in children*. New York: International Universities Press.

Pianta, R. C., Sroufe, L. A., & Egeland, B. (1989). Continuity and discontinuity in maternal sensitivity at 6, 24, and 42 months in a high-risk sample. *Child Development, 60*, 481–487.

Pilkonis, P. A., Imber, S. D., Lewis, P., & Rubinsky, P. (1984). A comparative outcome study of individual, group, and conjoint psychotherapy. *Archives of General Psychiatry, 41*, 431–437.

Pincus, A. L., & Wiggins, J. S. (1990). Interpersonal problems and conceptions of personality disorders. *Journal of Personality Disorders, 4*, 342–352.

Piper, W. E. (1993). The use of transference interpretations. *American Journal of Psychotherapy, 47*, 477–478.

Piper, W. E., Azim, H. F. A., Joyce, A. S., McCallum, M., Nixon, G. W. H., & Segal, P. S. (1991). Quality of object relations versus interpersonal functioning as predictors of therapeutic alliance and psychotherapy outcome. *Journal of Nervous and Mental Disease, 179*, 432–438.

Piper, W. E., Debbane, E. G., Bienvenu, J. P., & Garant, J. (1984). A comparative study of four forms of psychotherapy. *Journal of Consulting and Clinical Psychology, 52*, 268–279.

Piper, W. E., & Joyce, A. S. (1996). A consideration of the factors influencing the utilization of time-limited, short-term group psychotherapy. *International Journal of Group Psychotherapy, 46*, 311–328.

Piper, W. E., & Joyce, A. S. (2001). Psychosocial treatment outcome. In W. J. Livesley (Ed.), *Handbook of personality disorders: Theory, research, and treatment* (pp. 323–343). New York: Guilford Press.

Piper, W. E., Marrache, M., & Koenig, A. (1986). Relationships between early and final reports of treatment outcome in long-term group psychotherapy. *Group, 10*, 85–93.

Piper, W. E., McCallum, M., & Azim, H. F. A. (1992). *Adaptation to loss through short-term group psychotherapy*. New York: Guilford Press.

Piper, W. E., Rosie, J. S., Azim, H. F. A., & Joyce, A. S. (1993). A randomized trial of psychiatric day treatment for patients with affective and personality disorders. *Hospital and Community Psychiatry, 44*, 757–763.

Piper, W. E., Rosie, J. S., Joyce, A. S., & Azim, H. F. A. (1996). *Time-limited day treatment for personality disorders: Integration of research and practice in a group program.* Washington, DC: American Psychological Association.

Plomin, R., Chipeur, H. M., & Loehlin, J. C. (1990). Behavior genetics and personality. In L. A. Pervin (Ed.), *Handbook of personality: Theory and research* (pp. 225–243). New York: Guilford Press.

Plutchik, R. (1980). A general psychoevolutionary theory of emotion. In R. Plutchik & H. Kellerman (Eds.), *Emotion, psychopathology, and psychotherapy* (pp. 3–33). New York: Academic Press.

Pollock, V. E., Briere, J., Schneider, L., Knop, J., Mednick, S. A., & Goodwin, D. W. (1990). Childhood antecedents of antisocial behavior: Parental alcoholism and physical abusiveness. *American Journal of Psychiatry, 147*(10), 1290–1293.

Pope, H. G., Jr., Jonas, M. J., & Hudson, J. I. (1983). The validity of DSM-III borderline personality disorders: A phenomenologic, family history, treatment response, and long-term follow-up study. *Archives of General Psychiatry, 40,* 23–30.

Pope, H. G., Jr., Jonas, J. M., Hudson, J. L., Cohen, B. M., & Tohen, M. (1985). An empirical study of psychosis in borderline personality disorder. *American Journal of Psychiatry, 142,* 1285–1290.

Pretzler, J. L., & Beck, A. T. (1996). A cognitive theory of personality disorders. In J. F. Clarkin & M. F. Lenzenweger (Eds.), *Major theories of personality disorder* (pp. 36–105). New York: Guilford Press.

Prochaska, J. O. (1984). *Systems of psychotherapy: A transtheoretical analysis* (2nd ed.). Holmewood, IL: Dorsey Press.

Prochaska, J. O., & DiClemente, C. C. (1986). Toward a comprehensive model of change. In W. R. Miller & N. Heather (Eds.), *Treating addictive behaviors: Processes of change* (pp. 3–27). New York: Plenum Press.

Prochaska, J. O., & DiClemente, C. C. (1992). The transtheoretical approach. In J. C. Norcross & M. R. Goldfried (Eds.), *Handbook of psychotherapy integration* (pp. 300–334). New York: Basic Books.

Prochaska, J. O., DiClemente, C. C., & Norcross, J. C. (1992). In search of how people change. *American Psychologist, 47,* 1102–1114.

Prochaska, J. O., Norcross, J. C., & DiClemente, C. C. (1994). *Changing for good: The revolutionary program that explains the six stages of change and teaches you how to free yourself from bad habits.* New York: William Morrow.

Pukrop, R., Steinbring, I., Gentil, I., Schulte, K., & Klosterkötter, J. (2002, May). *Differential description of personality disorders by the Dimensional Assessment of Personality Pathology questionnaire.* Paper presented at the annual meeting of the Association of European Psychiatry, Stockholm.

Putnam, F. W. (1991). Dissociative phenomena. In A. Tasman & S. M. Goldfinger (Eds.), *American Psychiatric Press review of psychiatry* (Vol. 10, pp. 145–160). Washington, DC: American Psychiatric Press.

Putnam, F. W. (1997). *Dissociation in children and adolescents: A developmental perspective.* New York: Guilford Press.

Raue, P. J., & Goldfried, M. R. (1994). The therapeutic alliance in cognitive-behavioral therapy. In A. O. Horvath & L. S. Greenberg (Eds.), *The working alliance: Theory, research, and practice* (pp. 131–152). New York: Wiley.

Reeve, J., Inck, T. A., & Safran, J. (1993). Toward an integration of cognitive, inter-personal, and experiential approaches to therapy. In G. Stricker & J. R. Gold (Eds.), *Comprehensive handbook of psychotherapy integration* (pp. 113–123). New York: Plenum Press.

Reich, J. H., & Green, A. I. (1991). Effect of personality disorders on outcome of treatment. *Journal of Nervous and Mental Disease, 179,* 74–82.

Reich, J. H., & Vasile, R. G. (1993). Effect of personality disorders on the treatment outcome of Axis I conditions: An update. *Journal of Nervous and Mental Disease, 181,* 475–484.

Reich, W. (1949). *Character analysis* (3rd ed.). New York: Farrar, Straus & Giroux.

Rifkin, A., Levitan, S. J., Glaewski, J., & Klein, D. F. (1972). Emotionally unstable character disorder—a follow-up study. Description of patients and outcome. *Biological Psychiatry, 4,* 65–79.

Rifkin, A., Quitkin, F., Carrillo, C., Blumberg, A. G., & Klein, D. F. (1972). Lithium carbonate in emotionally unstable character disorder. *Archives of General Psychiatry, 27,* 519–523.

Roberts, G. C., Block, J. H., & Block, J. (1984). Continuity and change in parents' child-rearing practices. *Child Development, 55,* 586–597.

Robins, C. J., Ivanoff, A. M., & Linehan, M. M. (2001). Dialectical behavior therapy. In W. J. Livesley (Ed.), *Handbook of personality disorders: Theory, research, and treatment* (pp. 437–459). New York: Guilford Press.

Robins, L. N. (1966). *Deviant children grown up.* Baltimore: Williams and Wilkins.

Rockland, L. H. (1992). *Supportive therapy for borderline patients: A psychodynamic approach.* New York: Guilford Press.

Rogers, C. R. (1951). *Client centered therapy.* Boston: Houghton Mifflin.

Romans, S. E., Martin, J. L., Anderson, J. C., Herbsion, G. P., & Mullen, P. E. (1995). Sexual abuse in childhood and deliberate self harm. *American Journal of Psychiatry, 152,* 1336–1342.

Rosen, L. W., & Thomas, M. A. (1984). Treatment technique for chronic wrist cutters. *Journal of Behavior Therapy and Experimental Psychiatry, 15,* 33–36.

Ross, M. (1989). Relation of implicit theories to the construction of personal histories. *Psychological Review, 96,* 341–357.

Rotter, J. B. (1966). Generalized expectancies for internal versus external control of reinforcement. *Psychological Monographs, 80*(1), 1–28.

Rowe, D. C., Rodgers, J. L., & Meseck-Bushey, S. (1992). Sibling delinquency and the family environment: Shared and unshared influences. *Child Development, 63,* 59–67.

Ruiz-Sancho, A. M., Smith, G. W., & Gunderson, J. G. (2001). Psychoeducational approaches. In W. J. Livesley (Ed.), *Handbook of personality disorders: Theory, research, and treatment* (pp. 460–474). New York: Guilford Press.

Rumelhart, D. E. (1980). On evaluating story grammars. *Cognitive Science, 4,* 313–316.

Rutter, M. (1987). Temperament, personality, and personality disorder. *British Journal of Psychiatry, 150,* 443–458.

Rutter, M., & Maughan, B. (1997). Psychosocial adversities in childhood and adult psychopathology. *Journal of Personality Disorders, 11,* 4–18.

Ryan, R. M., Deci, E. L., & Grolnick, W. S. (1995). Autonomy, relatedness, and the self: Their relation to development and psychopathology. In D. Cicchetti & D. J. Cohen (Eds.), *Developmental psychopathology: Vol. I. Theory and methods* (pp. 618–655). New York: Wiley.

Ryle, A. (1990). *Cognitive analytic therapy: Active participation in change.* Chichester, UK: Wiley.

Ryle, A. (1997). *Cognitive analytic therapy and borderline personality disorder: The model and the method.* Chichester, UK: Wiley.

Ryle, A. (2001). Cognitive analytic therapy. In W. J. Livesley (Ed.), *Handbook of personality disorders: Theory, research, and treatment* (pp. 400–413). New York: Guilford Press.

Sabo, A. N. (1997). Etiological significance of associations between childhood trauma and borderline personality disorder: conceptual and clinical implications. *Journal of Personality Disorders, 11*(1), 50–70.

Safran, J. D., Crocker, P., McMain, S., & Murray, P. (1990). Therapeutic alliance rupture as a therapy event for empirical investigation. *Psychotherapy, 27,* 154–165.

Safran, J. D., & Muran, J. C. (2000). *Negotiating the therapeutic alliance.* New York: Guilford Press.

Safran, J. D., Muran, J. C., & Samstag, L. N. (1994). Resolving therapeutic alliance ruptures: A task analytic investigation. In A. O. Horvath & L. S. Greenberg (Eds.), *The working alliance: Theory, research, and practice* (pp. 225–255). New York: Wiley.

Safran, J. D., & Segal, Z. V. (1990). *Interpersonal process in cognitive therapy.* Northvale, NJ: Jason Aronson.

Salzman, C., Wolfson, A. N., Schatzberg, A., Looper, J., Henke, R., Albanese, M., Schwartz, J., & Miyawaki, E. (1995). Effects of fluoxetine on anger in symptomatic volunteers with borderline personality disorder. *Journal of Clinical Psychopharmacology, 15,* 23–29.

Sanderson, C., & Clarkin, J. F. (1994). Use of the NEO-PI-R personality dimensions in differential treatment planning. In P. T. Costa & T. A. Widiger (Eds.), *Personality disorders and the five-factor model of personality* (pp. 219–235). Washington, DC: American Psychological Association.

Sanderson, C., & Clarkin, J. F. (2002). Further use of the NEO-PI-R personality dimensions in differential treatment planning. In P. T. Costa & T. A. Widiger (Eds.), *Personality disorders and the five-factor model of personality* (2nd ed., pp. 351–375). Washington, DC: American Psychological Association.

Schacht, T. E., Binder, J. L., & Strupp, H. H. (1984). The dynamic focus. In H. H. Strupp & J. L. Binder (Eds.), *Psychotherapy in a new key: A guide to time-limited dynamic psychotherapy* (pp. 65–109). New York: Basic Books.

Schmideberg, M. (1947). The treatment of psychopathic and borderline patients. *American Journal of Psychotherapy, 1,* 45–71.

Schmidt, N. B., Joiner, T. E., Young, J. E., & Telch, M. J. (1995). The schema questionnaire: Investigation of psychometric properties and the hierarchical structure of measure of maladaptive schemas. *Cognitive Therapy and Research, 19,* 295–321.

Schoeneman, T. J., & Curry, S. (1990). Attributions for successful and unsuccessful health behavior change. *Basic and Applied Social Psychology, 11,* 421–431.

Schore, A. N. (1994). *Affect regulation and the origin of the self: The neurobiology of emotional development.* Hillsdale, NJ: Erlbaum.

Schroeder, M. L., Wormsworth, J. A., & Livesley, W. J. (1992). Dimensions of personality disorder and their relationships to the big five dimensions of personality. *Personality Assessment: A Journal of Consulting and Clinical Psychology*, 180, 609–618.

Schulz, S. C., Camlin, K. L., Berry, S. A., & Jesberger, J. A. (1999). Olanzapine safety and efficacy in patients with borderline personality disorder and comorbid dysthymia. *Biological Psychiatry*, 46, 1429–1435.

Segal, Z. (1988). Appraisal of the self schema construct in models of depression. *Psychological Bulletin*, 103, 147–162.

Serban, G., & Siegel, S. (1984). Responses of borderline and schizotypal patients to small doses of thiothixene and haloperidol. *American Journal of Psychiatry*, 141, 1455–1458.

Shapiro, D. (1965). *Neurotic styles*. New York: Basic Books.

Shapiro, D. (1981). *Autonomy and rigid character*. New York: Basic Books.

Shapiro, D. (1989). *Psychotherapy of neurotic character*. New York: Basic Books.

Shea, M. T. (1995). Interrelationships among categories of personality disorders. In W. J. Livesley (Ed.), *The DSM-IV personality disorders* (pp. 397–406). New York: Guilford Press.

Shea, M. T., Widiger, T. A., & Klein, M. H. (1992). Comorbidity of personality disorders and depression: Implications for treatment. *Journal of Consulting and Clinical Psychology*, 60, 857–868.

Sheard, M. H. (1975). Lithium in the treatment of aggression. *Journal of Mental and Nervous Disease*, 160, 108–118.

Sheard, M. H., Marini, J. L., Bridges, C. I., & Wagner, E. (1976). The effect of lithium on impulsive aggressive behavior in man. *American Journal of Psychiatry*, 133, 1409–1413.

Shearer, S. L., Peter, C. P., Quaytman, M. S., & Wadman, B. E. (1988). Intent and lethality of suicide attempts among female borderline patients. *American Journal of Psychiatry*, 145, 1424–1427.

Sheldon, K. M., & Elliot, A. J. (1999). Goal striving, need satisfaction, and longitudinal well-being: The self-concordance model. *Journal of Personality and Social Psychology*, 76, 482–497.

Sheldon, K. M., Ryan, R. M., Rawsthorne, L. J., & Ilardi, B. (1997). Trait self and true self: Cross-role variation in the big-five personality traits and its relations with psychological authenticity and subjective well-being. *Journal of Personality and Social Psychology*, 73, 138—139.

Siegel, D. J. (1999). *The developing mind: Toward a neurobiology of interpersonal experience*. New York: Guilford Press.

Siever, J., & Davies, K. L. (1991). A psychobiologic perspective on the personality disorders. *American Journal of Psychiatry*, 148, 1647–1658.

Sifneos, P. E. (1979). *Short-term dynamic psychotherapy: Evaluation and technique*. New York: Plenum Medical Books.

Silk, K. R., Lohr, N. E., Westen, D., & Goodrich, S. (1989). Psychosis in borderline patients with depression. *Journal of Personality Disorders*, 3, 92–100.

Singer, J. L., & Salovey, P. (1991). Organized knowledge structures and personality: Person schemas, self-schemas, prologues, and scripts. In M. J. Horowitz (Ed.), *Schemas and maladaptive interpersonal patterns* (pp. 33–79). Chicago: University of Chicago Press.

Singer, J. L., Sincott, J. B., & Kollinen, J. (1989). Countertransference and cognition: The psychotherapist's distortions as consequences of normal information processing. *Psychotherapy, 26,* 344–355.

Skinner, E. A. (1996). A guide to constructs of control. *Journal of Personality and Social Psychology, 71,* 549–570.

Skodol, A. E., Buckley, P., & Charles, E. (1983). Is there a characteristic pattern to the treatment history of clinic outpatients with borderline personality? *Journal of Nervous and Mental Disease, 171,* 405–410.

Soloff, P. H. (1994). Is there any drug treatment of choice for the borderline patient? *Acta Psychiatrica Scandinavica, 89*(379, Suppl.), 50–55.

Soloff, P. H. (1998). Algorithms for pharmacological treatment of personality dimensions: Symptom specific treatments for cognitive–perceptual, affective, and impulsive-behavioral dysregulation. *Bulletin of the Menninger Clinic, 62,* 195–214.

Soloff, P. H. (2000). Psychopharmacology of borderline personality disorder. *Psychiatric Clinics of North America, 23,* 169–190.

Soloff, P. H., Cornelius, J. R., George, A., Nathan, S., Perel, J. M., & Ulrich, R. F. (1993). Efficacy of phenelzine and haloperidol in borderline personality disorder. *Archives of General Psychiatry, 50,* 377–385.

Soloff, P. H, George, A., Nathan, R. S., Schultz, D. M., Ulrich, R. F., & Perel, J. M. (1986). Progress in pharmacotherapy of borderline disorders: A double-blind study of amitriptyline, haloperidol, and placebo. *Archives of General Psychiatry, 43,* 691–697.

Soloff, P. H., Lis, J. A., Kelly, T., Cornelius, J., & Ulrich, R. (1994). Self-mutilation and suicidal behavior in borderline personality disorder. *Journal of Personality Disorders, 8,* 257–267.

Soloff, P. H., Lynch, K. G., & Kelly, T. M. (2002). Childhood sexual abuse as a risk factor for suicidal behavior in borderline personality disorder. *Journal of Personality Disorders, 16,* 201–214.

Soloff, P. H., Lynch, K. G., Kelly, T. M., Malone, K. M., & Mann, J. J. (2000). Characteristics of suicide attempts of patients with major depressive episode and borderline personality disorder: A comparative study. *American Journal of Psychiatry, 157,* 601–608.

Soloff, P. H., & Millward, J. W. (1983). Developmental histories of borderline patients. *Comprehensive Psychiatry, 24*(6), 574–88.

Sonne, J. L., & Janoff, D. S. (1979). The effect of treatment attributions on the maintenance of weight reduction: A replication and extension. *Cognitive Therapy and Research, 3,* 389–397.

Sonne, S., Rubey, R., Brady, K., Malcolm, R., & Morris, T. (1996). Naltrexone in the treatment of self-injurious thoughts and behaviors. *Journal of Nervous and Mental Disease, 184,* 192–195.

Sperry, L. (1999). *Cognitive behavior therapy for the DSM-IV personality disorders.* Philadelphia: Brunner/Mazel.

Sroufe, L. A. (1989a). Pathways to adaptation and maladaptation: Psychopathology as developmental deviation. In D. Cicchetti & S. L. Toth (Eds.), *Rochester Symposium on Developmental Psychopathology: Vol. 1. The emergence of a discipline* (pp. 13–40). Hillsdale, NJ: Erlbaum.

Sroufe, L. A. (1989b). Relationships, self, and individual adaptation. In A. J.

Sameroff & R. N. Emde (Eds.), *Relationship disturbances in early childhood: A developmental approach* (pp. 70–94). New York: Basic Books.

Sroufe, L. A. (1991). Considering normal and abnormal together: The essence of developmental psychopathology. *Development and Psychopathology, 2,* 335–347.

Stanford, E. J., Goetz, R. R., & Bloom, J. D. (1994). The No Harm Contract in the emergency assessment of suicidal risk. *Journal of Clinical Psychiatry, 55,* 344–348.

Steiner, J. (1994). Patient-centered and analyst-centered interpretations: Some implications of containment and countertransference. *Psychoanalytic Quarterly, 14,* 406–422.

Stone, M. H. (1989). The course of borderline personality disorder. In A. Tasman, R. E. Hales, & A. J. Frances (Eds.), *American Psychiatric Association review of psychiatry* (Vol. 8, pp. 103–122). Washington, DC: American Psychiatric Association Press.

Stone, M. H. (1990). *The fate of borderline patients: Successful outcome and psychiatric practice.* New York: Guilford Press.

Stone, M. H. (1993). Long-term outcome in personality disorders. *British Journal of Psychiatry, 162,* 299–353.

Stone, M. H. (2001). Natural history and long-term outcome. In W. J. Livesley (Ed), *Handbook of personality disorders* (pp. 259–273). New York: Guilford Press.

Strachey, R. (1934). The nature of the therapeutic action in psychoanalysis. *International Journal of Psycho-Analysis, 15,* 127–159.

Strupp, H. H. (1993). The Vanderbilt psychotherapy studies: Synopsis. *Journal of Consulting and Clinical Psychology, 61,* 431–433.

Strupp, H. H., & Binder, J. (1984). *Psychotherapy in a new way: A guide to time-limited dynamic psychotherapy.* New York: Basic Books.

Strupp, H. H., Fox, R. E., & Lessler, K. (1969). *Patients view their psychotherapy.* Baltimore: Johns Hopkins Press.

Suess, G. J., Grossman, K. E., & Sroufe, L. A. (1992). Effects of infant attachment to mother and father on quality of adaptation in preschool: From dyadic to individual organization of the self. *International Journal of Behavioral Development, 15,* 43–65.

Sullivan, H. S. (1947). *Basic conceptions of modern psychiatry.* Washington, DC: William Alanson White Psychiatric Foundation.

Suyemoto, K. L. (1998). The functions of self-mutilation. *Clinical Psychology Review, 18,* 531–554.

Swann, W. B., Jr. (1983). Self-verification: Bringing social reality into harmony with the self. In J. Suls & A. G. Greenwald (Eds.), *Psychological perspectives on the self* (Vol. 2, pp. 33–66). Hillsdale, NJ: Erlbaum.

Swann, W. B., Jr. (1987). Identity negotiation: Where two roads meet. *Journal of Personality and Social Psychology, 53,* 1038–1051.

Swann, W. B., Jr. (1990). To be adored or to be known? The interplay of self-enhancement and self-verification. In E. T. Higgins & R. M. Sacromentino (Eds.), *Handbook of motivation and cognition. Vol. 2: Motivation & cognition* (pp. 408–448). New York: Guilford Press.

Swann, W. B., Jr., & Pelham, B. W. (2002). The truth about illusions: Authenticity and positivity in social relationships. In C. R. Snyder & S. J. Lopez (Eds.), *Handbook of positive psychology* (pp. 366–381). London: Oxford University Press.

Swann, W. B., Jr., Wenzlaff, R. M., Krull, D. S., & Pelham, B. W. (1992). Allure of negative feedback: Self-verification strivings among depressed persons. *Journal of Abnormal Psychology, 101,* 293–306.

Swenson, C. (1989). Kernberg and Linehan: Two approaches to the borderline patient. *Journal of Personality Disorders, 3,* 26–35.

Swenson, C. (1992). Supportive element of inpatient treatment with borderline patients. In L. H. Rockland, *Supportive therapy for borderline patients: A psychodynamic approach* (pp. 269–283). New York: Guilford Press.

Taylor, S. E. (1983). Adjustment to threatening events: A theory of cognitive adaptation. *American Psychologist, 38,* 1161–1173.

Teasdale, J. D., Segal, Z., & Williams, J. M. G. (1995). How does cognitive therapy prevent depressive relapse and why should attentional control (mindfulness) training help? *Behaviour Research and Therapy, 33,* 25–39.

Thapar, A., & McGuffin, P. (1993). Is personality disorder inherited? An overview of the evidence. *Journal of Psychopathology and Behavioral Assessment, 15,* 325–345.

Thompson, S. C., & Spacaman, S. (1991). Perceptions of control in vulnerable populations. *Journal of Social Issues, 47,* 1–21.

Tickle, J. J., Heatherton, T. F., & Wittenberg, L. G. (2001). Can personality change? In W. J. Livesley (Ed.), *Handbook of personality disorders: Theory, research, and treatment* (pp. 242–258). New York: Guilford Press.

Torgersen S., & Alnaes R. (1992). Differential perception of parental bonding in schizotypal and borderline personality disorder. *Comprehensive Psychiatry, 33,* 34–38.

Torgersen S., Kringlen, E., & Cramer, V. (2001). The prevalence of personality disorders in a community sample. *Archives of General Psychiatry, 58,* 590–596.

Torgersen, S., Lygren, S., Oien, P. A., Skre, I., Onstad, S., Edvardsen, J., Tambs, K., & Kringlen, E. (2000). A twin study of personality disorders. *Comprehensive Psychiatry, 41*(6), 416–25.

Toulmin, S. (1978). Self-knowledge and knowledge of the "self." In T. Mischel (Ed.), *The self: Psychological and philosophical issues* (pp. 291–317). Oxford, UK: Oxford University Press.

Trull, T. J., Sher, K. J., Mink-Brown, C., Durbin, J., & Burr, R. (2000). Borderline personality disorder and substance abuse disorders: A review and integration. *Clinical Psychology Review, 20,* 235–253.

Tupin, J. P., Smith, D. B., Clanon, T. L., Kim, L. I., Nugent, A., & Groupe, A. (1973). The long-term use of lithium in aggressive prisoners. *Comprehensive Psychiatry, 14,* 311–317.

Turkheimer, E. (1998). Heritability and biological explanation. *Psychological Review, 105,* 782–791.

Tyrer, P., Gunderson, J., Lyons, M., & Tohen, M. (1997). Extent of comorbidity between mental state and personality disorders. *Journal of Personality Disorders, 11,* 242–259.

Vaglum, P., Friis, S., Irion, T., Johns, S., Karterud, S., Larsen, S., & Vaglum, S. (1990). Treatment response of severe and nonsevere personality disorders in a therapeutic community day unit. *Journal of Personality Disorders, 4,* 161–172.

Vaillant, G. E. (1992). The beginning of wisdom is never calling a patient a borderline. *Journal of Psychotherapy Practice and Research, 1,* 117–134.

van Reekum, R., Links, P. S., & Boiago, I. (1993). Constitutional factors in borderline personality disorder: Genetics, brain dysfunction, and biological markers. In

J. Paris (Ed.), *Borderline personality disorder* (pp. 13–38). Washington, DC: American Psychiatric Association Press.

Vernon, P. E. (1964). *Personality assessment: A critical survey.* London: Methuen.

Wachtel, P. L. (1977). *Psychoanalysis and behavior therapy.* New York: Basic Books.

Wachtel, P. L. (1991). From eclecticism to synthesis: Toward a more seamless psychotherapeutic integration. *Journal of Psychotherapy Integration, 1,* 43–54.

Wagner, A. W., & Linehan, M. M. (1998). Dissociative behavior. In V. M. Follette, J. I. Ruzek, & F. R. Abueg (Eds.), *Cognitive-behavioral therapies for trauma* (pp. 191–225). New York: Guilford Press.

Waldinger, R. J. (1987). Intensive psychodynamic therapy with borderline patients: An overview. *American Journal of Psychiatry, 144,* 267–274.

Waldinger, R. J., & Gunderson, J. G. (1984). Completed psychotherapies with borderline patients. *American Journal of Psychotherapy, 38,* 190–202.

Waldinger, R. T., & Gunderson, J. G. (1989). *Effective psychotherapy with borderline patients.* Washington, DC: American Psychiatric Association.

Wallerstein, R. S. (1986). How does self psychology differ in practice? In A. Goldberg (Ed.), *Progress in self psychology* (Vol. 2, pp. 63–83). New York: Guilford Press.

Wallerstein, R. S. (1988). One psychoanalysis or many? *International Journal of Psycho-Analysis, 66,* 391–404.

Weiner, B. (1985). An attributional theory of achievement motivation and emotion. *Psychological Review, 92,* 548–573.

Weiss, J. (1993). *How psychotherapy works: Process and technique.* New York: Guilford Press.

Wender, P. H. (1995). *Attention deficit hyperactivity disorder in adults.* New York: Oxford University Press.

Westen, D. (1990). Psychoanalytic approaches to personality. In L. A. Pervin (Ed.), *Handbook of personality* (pp. 21–55). New York: Guilford Press.

Westen, D., & Arkowitz-Westen, L. (1998). Limitations of Axis II in diagnosing personality pathology in clinical practice. *American Journal of Psychiatry, 155,* 1767–1771.

Westen D., Ludolph P., Misle B., Ruffins S., & Block J. (1990). Physical and sexual abuse in adolescent girls with borderline personality disorder. *American Journal of Orthopsychiatry, 60,* 55–66.

Westerman, M. A., Foote, J. P., & Winston, A. (1995). Change in coordination across phases of psychotherapy and outcome: Two mechanisms for the role played by patients' contribution to the alliance. *Journal of Consulting and Clinical Psychology, 63,* 672–675.

Wicklund, R. A. (1975). Objective self-awareness. In L. Berkowitz (Ed.), *Advances in experimental social psychology* (Vol. 8, pp. 233–275). New York: Academic Press.

Wicklund, R. A., & Duval, S. (1971). Opinion change and performance facilitation as a result of objective self-awareness. *Journal of Experimental Social Psychology, 7,* 319–342.

Widiger, T. A. (1993). The DSM-III-R categorical personality disorder diagnoses: A critique and alternative. *Psychological Inquiry, 4,* 75–90.

Widiger, T. A., Frances, A. J., Harris, M., Jacobsberg, L., Fyer, M., & Manning, D. (1991). Comorbidity among Axis II disorders. In J. Oldham (Ed.), *Personality disorders: New perspectives on diagnostic validity* (pp. 163–194). Washington, DC: American Psychiatric Association Press.

Widiger, T. A., & Kelso, K. (1983). Psychodiagnosis of Axis II. *Clinical Psychology Review*, 3, 491–510.

Wiggins, J. S. (Ed.). (1996). *The five-factor model of personality: Theoretical perspectives*. New York: Guilford Press.

Wild, J. (1965). Authentic existence: A new approach to "value theory." In J. M. Edie (Ed.), *An invitation to phenomenology: Studies in the philosophy of experience* (pp. 59–78). Chicago: Quadrangle Books.

Willi, J. (1999). *Ecological psychotherapy*. Seattle, WA: Hogrefe & Huber.

Williams, C. (1998). A classic case of borderline personality disorder. *Psychiatrtic Services*, 49, 173–174.

Williams, W., Weiss, T. W., & Edens, A., Johnson, M., & Thornby, J. I. (1998). Hospital utilization and personality characteristics of veterans with psychiatric problems. *Hospital and Community Psychiatry*, 49, 370–375.

Winnicott, D. W. (1960). Ego distortion in terms of true and false self. In *The maturational processes and the facilitating environment* (pp. 158–165). New York: International Universities Press.

Winnicott, D. W. (1965). *The maturational processes and the facilitating environment*. Oxford, UK: International Universities Press.

Winston, A., & Muran, J. C. (1996). Common factors in the time-limited psychotherapies. In L. J. Dickstein, M. B. Riba, & J. M. Oldham (Eds.), *American Psychiatric Association review of psychiatry* (Vol. 15). Washington, DC: American Psychiatric Association Press.

Winston, A., Pinsker, H., & McCullough, L. (1986). Supportive psychotherapy: A review. *Hospital and Community Psychiatry*, 36, 1105–1114.

Wolff, S., & Chick, J. (1980). Schizoid personality in childhood: A controlled followup study. *Psychological Medicine*, 10, 85–100.

Wolpe, J. (1958). *Psychotherapy by reciprocal inhibition*. Stanford, CA: Stanford University Press.

Wong, J. (1980). Combined group and individual treatment of borderline and narcissistic patients: Heterogeneous versus homogeneous groups. *International Journal of Group Psychotherapy*, 30, 389–404.

Yalom, I. D. (1975). *The principles and practice of group psychotherapy*. New York: Basic Books.

Yeomans, F. E., Hull, J. W., & Clarkin, J. C. (1994). Compulsive exhibitionism successfully treated with fluvoxamine: A controlled case study. *Journal of Clinical Psychiatry*, 55, 86–88.

Young, J. E. (1990). *Cognitive therapy for personality disorders: A schema-focused approach*. Sarasota, FL: Professional Resource Exchange.

Young, J. E. (1994). *Cognitive therapy for personality disorders: A schema-focused approach* (rev. ed.). Sarasota, FL: Professional Resource Exchange.

Young, J. E., & Lindemann, M. D. (1992). An interpretative schema-focused model for personality disorders. *Journal of Cognitive Psychotherapy*, 6, 11–23.

Zanarini, M. C. (1993). Borderline personality disorder as an impulse spectrum disorder. In J. Paris (Ed.), *Borderline personality disorder: Etiology and treatment* (pp. 67–86). Washington, DC: American Psychiatric Association Press.

Zanarini, M. C. (2000). Childhood experiences associated with the development of borderline personality disorder. *Psychiatric Clinics of North America*, 23, 89–101.

Zanarini, M. C., & Frankenburg, F. R. (2001). Olanzapine treatment of female borderline personality disorder patients: A double-blind, placebo-controlled pilot study. *Journal of Clinical Psychiatry, 62,* 849–854.

Zanarini, M. C., Gunderson, J. G., & Frankenburg, F. R. (1990). Cognitive features of borderline personality disorder. *American Journal of Psychiatry, 147,* 57–63.

Zanarini, M. C., Gunderson, J. G., & Marino, M. F. (1989). Childhood experiences of borderline patients. *Comprehensive Psychiatry, 30,* 18–25

Zelli, A., & Dodge, K. A. (1999). Personality development from the bottom up. In D. Cervone & Y. Shoda (Eds.), *The coherence of personality: Social–cognitive bases of consistency, variability, and organization* (pp. 94–126). New York: Guilford Press.

Zetzel, E. (1971). A developmental approach to the borderline patient. *American Journal of Psychiatry, 127,* 867–871.

Zimmerman, M. (1994). Diagnosing personality disorders: A review of issues and research methods. *Archives of General Psychiatry, 51,* 225–245.

Zisook, S., Goff, A., Sledge, P., & Schuchter, S. R. (1994). Reported suicidal behavior and current suicidal ideation in a psychiatric outpatient clinic. *Annals of Clinical Psychiatry, 6,* 27–31.

Zuckerman, M. (1971). Dimensions of sensation seeking. *Journal of Consulting and Clinical Psychology, 36,* 45–52.

Zuckerman, M. (1990). Broad or narrow affect scores for the Multiple Affect Adjective Check List? Comment on Hunsley's "Dimensionality of the Multiple Affect Adjective Check List—Revised." *Journal of Psychopathology and Behavioral Assessment, 12,* 93–97.

Zuckerman, M. (1991). *Psychobiology of personality.* Cambridge, UK: University of Cambridge Press.

Zuckerman, M. (1994a). *Behavioral expressions and biosocial bases of sensation seeking.* Cambridge, UK: Cambridge University Press.

Zuckerman, M. (1994b). Impulsive sensation seeking: The biological foundations of a basic dimension of personality. In J. E. Bates & T.D. Wachs (Eds.), *Temperament: Individual differences at the interface of biology and behavior.* Washington, DC: American Psychological Association.

Zweig-Frank, H., Paris, J., & Guzder, J. (1994). Psychological risk factors for dissociation and self-mutilation in female patients with borderline personality disorder. *Canadian Journal of Psychiatry, 39,* 259–264.

Zwerling, I., & Wilder, J. (1964). An evaluation of the applicability of the day hospital in the treatment of acutely disturbed patients. *Israel Annals of Psychiatry, 2,* 162–185.

Index